Second Edition

Pathophysiology of Blood

ALLAN J. ERSLEV, M.D.

Cardeza Research Professor of Medicine, Jefferson Medical
College of Thomas Jefferson University; Attending Physician,
Thomas Jefferson University Hospital, Philadelphia

THOMAS G. GABUZDA, M.D.

Professor of Medicine, Jefferson Medical College of Thomas Jefferson
University; Chief, Department of Hematology, Lankenau Hospital,
Philadelphia

W. B. SAUNDERS COMPANY / Philadelphia / London / Toronto

W. B. Saunders Company: West Washington Square
Philadelphia, PA 19105

1 St. Anne's Road
Eastbourne, East Sussex BN21 3UN, England

1 Goldthorne Avenue
Toronto, Ontario M8Z 5T9, Canada

Cover: Fenestrated basement membrane of venous sinus in rat bone marrow. Micrograph courtesy of Pierre F. Leblond (Nouv. Rev. Franç. d'Hémat., *13*:771, 1973).

Pathophysiology of Blood   ISBN 0-7216-3403-6

Last digit is the print number: 9   8   7   6   5   4   3   2

PREFACE

The first edition of *Pathophysiology of Blood* was published in 1975 to meet a need for a small, readable, and profusely illustrated paperback on the normal and abnormal physiology of blood cells and their supporting plasma components. Now, four years later, the explosive addition of new information has necessitated the publication of a second edition. All the chapters have been updated and to a great extent rewritten. New illustrations have been added, and we have attempted to present a current review of hematologic physiology and the mechanisms of disease. The text was prepared as one chapter for the sixth edition of the textbook *Pathologic Physiology: Mechanisms of Disease,* published by W. B. Saunders Company, and we are indebted to the editors, Dr. William A. Sodeman, Jr., and Dr. William A. Sodeman, Sr., for permitting us to publish these chapters as a separate monograph.

In the second edition of *Pathologic Physiology,* the corresponding chapters were written by Dr. William B. Castle and Dr. James H. Jandl, investigators renowned for their role in transforming hematology from a static morphologic art to a dynamic metabolic science. We have striven to live up to the standards of scholarship and lucid prose set by these investigators. This monograph is aimed at preparing students for courses in hematology and oncology, house staff for board examinations, and internists for postgraduate programs or recertification. However, it is also hoped that the monograph will be read generally as an enjoyable exposure to hematology and as a help in modern therapy, which is based increasingly on an understanding of disease processes at a molecular level.

As in the first edition, we would like to thank our medical artist, Andrew S. Likens, for his excellent illustrations and photomicrographs. In order to maintain a uniform style, all graphs have been redrawn and all legends on the ordinate have been turned for a more readable horizontal presentation. Our secretaries, Rosemarie Silvano, Doris Riso, and Rosemary McGlynn, have provided valiant support; our associates at the Cardeza Foundation, helpful criticisms; and our wives, patient endurance. For all of this we are most grateful.

ALLAN J. ERSLEV, M.D.
THOMAS G. GABUZDA, M.D.

CONTENTS

Introduction

Hematology is traditionally defined as the study of the formed elements of blood. The combined mass of these elements constitutes an organ of considerable size and complexity. On the average, it measures 30 ml. per kg. body weight or about the same as the liver. The inclusion of active bone marrow, spleen, lymph nodes, and mononuclear macrophage tissue further adds to the size of the hematologic system and to the importance of hematology. Hematology also has close ties with the fluid phase of blood and with the function and kinetics of other organ systems and it has been increasingly difficult to establish its pathophysiologic limits. The erythrocytes need the cooperation of the heart, lungs, vessels and kidneys in order to bring oxygen to the tissues; the granulocytes need a host of supporting plasma factors for their phagocytic mission; the lymphocytes produce and react with immunoglobulins; and the thrombocytes cannot be functionally separated from the coagulation factors. With this in mind, an attempt will be made here to correlate structure, function, and kinetics of the formed elements of blood with those of other organ systems and with over-all human pathophysiology. This correlation and its documentation must of necessity be of an introductory nature, but it is hoped that it will stimulate the reader to seek more information from the monographs and key references listed.

Bone Marrow

With the exception of lymphocytes, blood cell formation in the normal adult is the exclusive prerogative of bone marrow. Even lymphocytes, however, both T and B cells, are bone marrow derived, and multipotential stem cells in the bone marrow cavities are probably directly or indirectly responsible for all blood cell formation. Other areas can support hematopoiesis, but the bones appear to provide an optimal environment for differentiation and multiplication of blood cells. Before bone cavities form during the fifth fetal month, blood cell formation takes place first in the yolk sac and then in the liver and spleen (Fig. 1–1). During the brief yolk-sac phase the erythrocytes produced are nucleated and contain an embryonic hemoglobin but the subsequent crops of fetal erythrocytes produced by the liver, spleen, and bone marrow are non-nucleated and contain

fetal hemoglobin with $\alpha_2\gamma_2$ polypeptide chains. Although the spleen in the human fetus plays only a brief role in hematopoiesis between the third and the seventh months, the splenic microcirculation appears to be well suited for blood cell formation, and the spleen serves as the principal back-up organ for the bone marrow. At time of birth the splenic and hepatic phases have ceased, the slow transformation from fetal to adult hemoglobin production is under way, and all bone cavities are actively involved in blood cell formation.

For the first few years of life there is a precarious balance between the need for blood cells of a rapidly growing infant and the available bone marrow space, and reactivation of hepatic and splenic hematopoiesis takes place whenever there is an increased demand for blood cell forma-

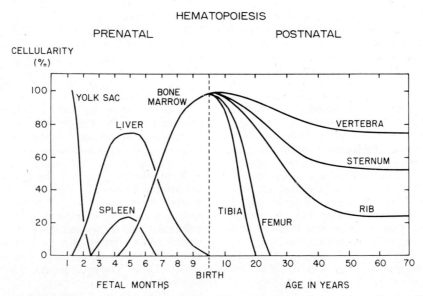

Figure 1–1 Expansion and regression of hematopoietic tissue during fetal and adult life.

tion. At about the age of 4 the growth of bone cavities has outstripped the growth of the circulating blood cell mass, and fatty reserve bone marrow becomes noticeable. Fatty replacement occurs first in the diaphysis of the peripheral long bones, then slowly creeps centripetally until at the age of about 18 hematopoietically active bone marrow is found only in the vertebrae, ribs, sternum, skull, and proximal epiphyses of the long bones. This obviously must mean that the available bone marrow space has continued to grow faster than the circulating blood cell mass, since the ratio between progenitor cells in the marrow and mature cells in the circulation is the same at all ages. In support of this assumption are measurements by Hudson which indicate that the volume of bone marrow cavities increases from about 1.5 per cent of body weight at birth to about 4.5 per cent of body weight in the adult, while the blood volume actually decreases from about 8 per cent of body weight at birth to about 7 per cent of body weight in the adult. During adult life the expansion of bone cavities continues, owing to bone resorption, and there is a gradual increase in the amount of fatty tissue present in all bone marrow areas. Because of the abundant bone marrow space, compensatory reactivation of extramedullary sites rarely takes place in later life, even during periods of accelerated hematopoietic activity. When present, extramedullary hematopoiesis often indicates inappropriate rather than compensatory blood formation.

Measurements of blood flow and hematopoietic activity have shown a close relationship between cellular production and blood supply, and some interesting experiments by Huggins suggest that this relationship goes in both directions and that induced vascularization is followed by increased hematopoietic activity. Huggins and co-workers implanted the tip of a rat's tail into the abdominal cavity or enclosed it in a heating chamber and found after some weeks that the inactive fatty marrow had become red and hematopoietically active. The conclusion from these experiments was initially that the low peripheral temperature in the long bones impairs blood cell formation and is responsible for the centripetal regression of active marrow in the adult. However, fatty marrow appears in the fingers even before birth and active marrow is found in peripheral epiphyses when more proximal diaphyses are completely inactive. It seems more likely that temperature is merely one of many variables which control vascularization and that it is the vascular density of the bone marrow which determines hematopoietic activity. Recent studies by Crosby suggest that this vascular density is inherently lower in the peripheral areas of the body rendering them particularly vulnerable to decreased temperature.

Structurally, the bone marrow is highly organized with a spokelike pattern of venous sinuses and cords of hematopoietic tissue (Fig. 1–2). The cords are percolated by arterial blood draining into the central venous sinuses through a fenestrated basement membrane (Fig. 1–3) partly covered on the inside by endothelial cells and on the outside by reticular cells. Projections from the reticular cells subdivide the cords and provide support for hematopoietic cells (Fig. 1–4). They also control available hematopoietic space by gaining or losing lipid globules. Within the cords, the megakaryocytes lie close to the outside of the sinus wall and appear to reel off strings of cytoplasmic platelets directly into the sinus. The erythroblasts also lie close to the venous sinuses in distinctive clusters or islands. Each island consists of a central macrophage, or nurse cell, with maturing and dividing erythroblasts nestled in cytoplasmic pockets (Fig. 1–5). When mature enough for independent existence, the erythroblasts squeeze through the sinus apertures usually losing their pyknotic and non-deformable nuclei (Fig. 1–6). The maturing and dividing granulocytic precursors are situated deep in the hematopoietic cords and do not move toward the sinus wall until they reach a motile metamyelocytic stage.

The nervous supply to the bone marrow is quite extensive, as everyone having experienced a bone marrow aspiration can attest. Some of the nerves are in close contact with the hematopoietic islands and may sense pressure changes caused by cellular proliferation. If such signals are transmitted to the nerves attached to the vessel walls, an autoregulatory system may well exist, adjusting the blood flow to permit undisturbed proliferation and maturation before the cells are released into the circulation.

The fatty tissue which in the adult fills about 50 per cent of the bone cavities probably serves merely as a space-occupying material. Attempts have been made to assign primary regulatory functions to it, but the evidence presented so far has been unimpressive.

As described in the section on the spleen, the bone marrow is one of the major lymphomacrophage organs and is involved in antigen processing, cellular and humoral immunity, and the recognition and removal of senescent cells. Its main mission is, however, the production of differentiated blood cells (Fig. 1–7). These cells are derived from pools of self-perpetuating stem cells — a multi- or pluripotential pool capable of differentiation in several directions and unipotential pools committed to erythropoiesis, granulopoiesis, or thrombopoiesis (Boggs and Chervenick, 1970). The multipotential stem cells are believed to provide a dormant bone marrow reserve. They are not destroyed by tritiated thymi-

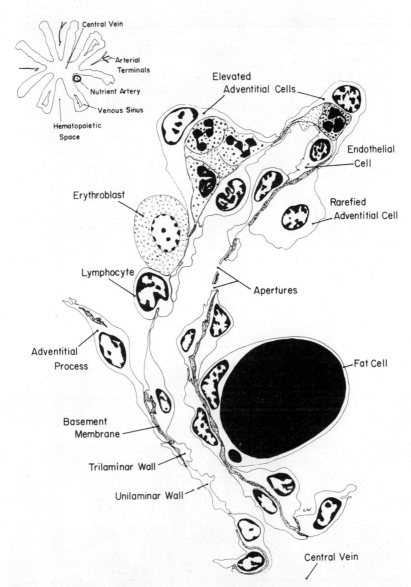

Figure 1–2 Sketch in upper left depicts cross section of bone marrow with spokelike sinusoids draining into a central longitudinal vein. Larger sketch depicts sinusoidal basement membrane covered on the outside by adventitial reticular cells guarding the tenestrations in the basement membrane and providing structural support for hematopoietic cells. (From Weiss, L.: In Gordon, A. S. (Ed.): Regulation of Hematopoiesis. Vol. 1. New York, Appleton-Century-Crofts, 1970.)

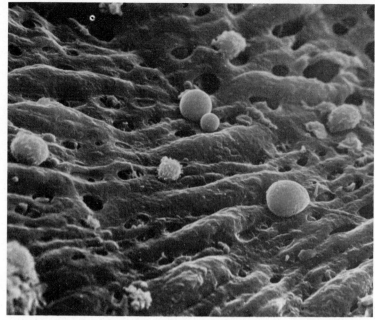

Figure 1–3 Fenestrated basement membrane of venous sinus in rat bone marrow (Courtesy of LeBlond, P.-F., Nouv. Rev. Franc. d'Hemat., *13*:771, 1973).

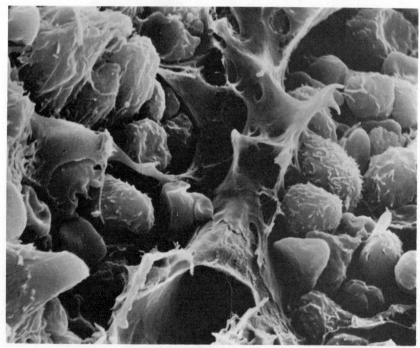

Figure 1–4 A venous sinus crossing the field with luminal endothelium exposed to the right but otherwise covered by adventitial reticular cells. The cytoplasm of these cells extends far into the hematopoietic compartment and provides structure and support for hematopoietic cells. (Courtesy of Weiss L.: Anat. Rev., *186*:161, 1976.)

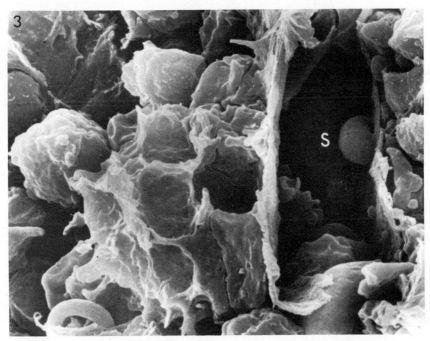

Figure 1–5 An erythropoietic island lying on the wall of a sinusoid (s) in rat bone marrow. The erythroblasts, nestled in the pockets of the island, were removed during the preparation of this scanning electron microscopic picture. (Courtesy of Weiss, L. Anat. Rev., *186*:161, 1976.)

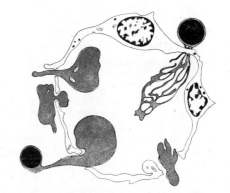

Figure 1–6 Nucleated and non-nucleated red blood cells squeezing through basement pores into a venous sinusoid. The nucleus is incapable of the necessary deformation and is snared off. (Courtesy of Bessis M. Life Cycle of the Erythrocyte. Sandoz Pharm., 1966.)

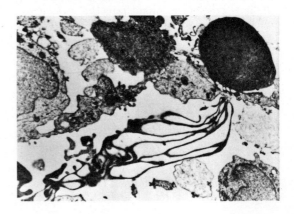

HEMATOPOIESIS

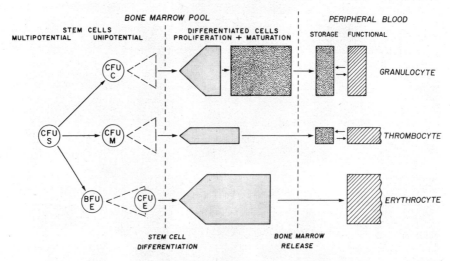

Figure 1–7 A dynamic model of hematopoietic activity.

dine when given in doses which will cause radiation-induced "suicide" of all cells using thymidine in the synthesis of DNA, unless they first have become activated by bone marrow depletion or injury. Such activation into a regenerative and differentiating cell cycle was first described by Till and McCulloch in their classic observations of the spleens of irradiated mice in which surviving or transplanted marrow attempts to replenish the hematopoietic tissues. Initially, the few available stem cells enter into intense proliferative activity and produce minute clonal colonies of undifferentiated stem cells. After the fifth day, specific differentiation takes place and discrete bone marrow colonies can be observed macroscopically on the surface of the spleen and microscopically in the parenchyma of the spleen and the bone marrow (Fig. 1–8). Since chromosomal studies have shown conclusively that each colony is derived from a single stem cell, it is possible to quantitate the number of multipotential stem cells [CFU — S (colony forming units — spleen)] present initially. In the mouse, it has been estimated that there are about 1 to 3 multipotential stem cells per 1000 nucleated bone marrow cells, or about 1 per 100 nucleated red blood cells.

In the human, CFU — S have been isolated by Barr and Wang-Peng in the lymphocyte fraction when peripheral blood cells were separated by velocity sedimentation. In this fraction they could be separated from B and T lymphocytes by their failure to form rosettes with sheep red cells, but otherwise they were found to be morphologically identical with small lymphocytes.

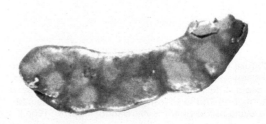

Figure 1–8 Each white raised plaque on the surface of the lower mouse spleen contains a colony of bone marrow cells. These colonies were found 7 days after total body radiation immediately followed by a transfusion of bone marrow cells obtained from an isogeneic donor. Each colony is derived from a single sequestered multipotential stem cell. The upper spleen is a normal control.

Studies on the distribution and composition of bone marrow colonies in the spleen have provided valuable information about the interrelationship between parenchymal structure and cellular differentiation. Each colony is made up of a mixture of hematopoietic cellular elements, usually with one cell type dominating. Although the specific differentiation probably is determined by humoral stimuli, it has been demonstrated by Trentin that the immediate cellular environment or HIM (hematopoietic inductive microenvironment) modifies the effectiveness of the stimuli. Colonies derived from stem cells lodged on the surface of the spleen are primarily erythroid, while colonies from cells lodged in the center of the spleen or in the bone marrow are primarily granulocytic and megakaryocytic. This effect of the microenvironment on cellular differentiation is undoubtedly of major importance for normal hematopoiesis but it is not known whether it is caused by a modification of the activities of stem cells or of differentiated cells.

The unipotential stem cells have been shown, by the use of "suicide" techniques, to be in active cell cycle and capable of self-renewal for a considerable period of time. However, they need the stimulus of a humoral "poietin" in order to undergo blast transformation and further differentiation. Erythropoietin is known to be the specific "poietin" for stem cells committed to erythropoiesis but there is also mounting evidence for the existence of a leukopoietin and a thrombopoietin responsible for the differentiation of stem cells committed to granulocytopoiesis and thrombopoiesis.

In the presence of even small amounts of erythropoietin, bone marrow suspensions plated on fibrin clots or on methyl cellulose plates will form tiny erythroid colonies consisting of from 8 to 64 hemoglobin-containing erythroblasts (Fig.

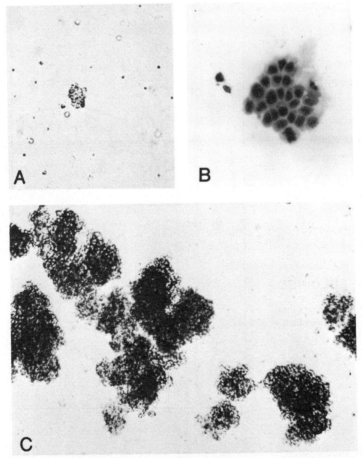

Figure 1–9 The appearance of a single CFU-E (*A*) and a single BFU-E (*C*) grown on a methyl cellulose medium (× 120) (courtesy of Gregory C. J. and Eaves A. C.: Blood, *49*:855, 1977) and of a single CFU-E (*B*) × 1,000.

1–9). The responsible cell has been identified by Clarke and Housman as a small mononuclear "lymphocyte." It has been designated as a CFU-E (colony forming unit-erythroid) and it is probably identical with the unipotential, erythropoietin-responsive stem cell. In addition to these early occurring CFU-E, a second kind of colony begins to appear after eight to ten days of culture if the medium contains large amounts of erythropoietin. These colonies grow to macroscopic size and may contain thousands of erythroblasts. Because of their irregular outline with many CFU-E subcolonies they are called "bursts," and the responsible cell is called a "burst forming unit-erythroid" or BFU-E. BFU-E have been demonstrated both in peripheral blood and bone marrow while CFU-E have been found only in the bone marrow (Fig. 1–10).

Apparently, erythropoietin promotes both stem cell proliferation and blast transformation. Whether this dual effect is accomplished by a single effect of erythropoietin on stem cells or by multiple sequential actions (or multiple erythropoietin species) is not known. A current hypothesis envisions BFU-E as early descendants of CFU-S (Fig. 1–7). They contain a few erythropoietin receptors enabling them to respond to large concentrations of erythropoietin with proliferation and maturation. According to Gregory and Eaves, the progeny will contain an increasing number of erythropoietin receptors until at a certain point of maturation the stem cells acquire the properties of CFU-E and undergo blast transformation to hemoglobin-producing erythroblasts. A problem with this hypothesis is that erythropoietin-responsive stem cells appear to be in

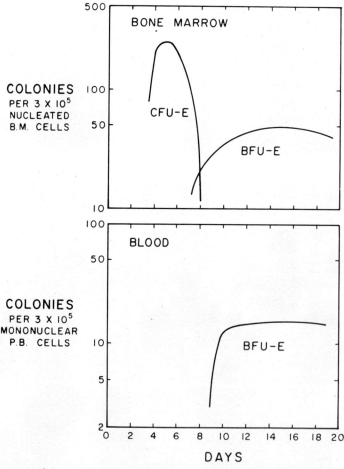

Figure 1–10 The sequential appearance and disappearance of erythroid colonies in bone marrow and peripheral blood suspensions plated on a methyl cellulose medium. (Slightly modified from Ogawa M. et al., Blood, *50*:1081, 1977.)

REFERENCES

Baikie, A. G., Court Brown, W. M., Buckton, K. E., Harnden, D. G., Jacobs, P. A., and Tough, I. M.: A possible specific chromosome abnormality in human chronic myeloid leukaemia. Nature (London), *188*:1165, 1960.

Barr, R. D., and Whang-Peng, J.: Hemopoietic stem cells in human peripheral blood. Science, *190*:284, 1975.

Boggs, D. R., and Chervenick, P. A.: Hemopoietic stem cells. *In* Greenwalt, T. J., and Jamieson, G. A. (Eds.): Formation and Destruction of Blood Cells. J. B. Lippincott Co., Philadelphia, 1970, p. 240.

Clarke, B. J., and Houseman, D.: Characterization of an erythroid cell of high proliferative capacity in normal human peripheral blood. Proc. Nat. Acad. Sci. USA, *74*:1105, 1977.

Craddock, C. G., Longmire, R., and McMillan, R.: Lymphocytes and the immune response. N. Engl. J. Med., *285*:324, 1972.

Crosby, W. H.: Experience with Injured and Implanted Bone Marrow: Relation of Function to Structure. *In* Stohlman, F. Jr. (ed.): Hematopoietic Cellular Proliferation. Grune & Stratton, New York, 1970, p. 87.

Ebbe, S.: Thrombopoietin. Blood, *44*:605, 1974.

Erslev, A. J.: Feedback circuits in the control of stem cell differentiation. Am. J. Pathol., *65*:629, 1971.

Finch, C. A.: Pathophysiologic aspects of sickle cell anemia. Am. J. Med., *53*:1, 1972.

Finch, C. A., Harker, L. A., and Cook, J. D.: Kinetics of the formed elements of human blood. Blood, *50*:699, 1977.

Gregersen, M. I., and Rawson, R. A.: Blood volume. Physiol. Rev., *39*:307, 1959.

Gregory, C. J., and Eaves, A. C.: Human marrow cells capable of erythropoietic differentiation in vitro. Definition of three erythroid colony responses. Blood *49*:855, 1977.

Hudson, G.: Bone marrow volume in the human foetus and newborn. Br. J. Haematol., *11*:446, 1965.

Huggins, L., and Blockson, B. H.: Changes in outlying bone marrow accompanying a local increase of temperature within physiologic limits. J. Exp. Med., *64*:253, 1956.

Killmann, S. A., Cronkite, E. P., Fliedner, T. M., and Bond, V. P.: Mitotic indices of human bone marrow cells. III. Duration of some phases of erythrocyte and granulocytic proliferation computed from mitotic indices. Blood, *24*:267, 1964.

Kretchmar, A. L.: Erythropoietin: Hypothesis of action tested by analog computer. Science, *152*:367, 1966.

Nakeff, A., and Daniels-McQueen, S.: In vitro colony assay for a new class of megakaryocyte precursor: Colony-forming unit megakaryocyte (CFU-M). Proc. Soc. Exp. Biol. Med., *151*:587, 1976.

Ogawa, M., Grush, O. C., O'Dell, R. F., Hara, H., and MacEachern, M. D.: Circulating erythropoietic precursors assessed in culture: Characterization in normal men and patients with hemoglobinopathies. Blood, *50*:1081, 1977.

Reissmann, K. R., and Udupa, R. B.: Effect of erythropoietin on proliferation of erythropoietin-responsive cells. Cell Tissue Kinet., *5*:481, 1972.

Robinson, W. A., and Mangalik, A.: The kinetics and regulation of granulopoiesis. Seminars Hematol., *12*:7, 1975.

Till, J. E., and McCulloch, E. A.: A direct measurement of the radiation sensitivity of normal mouse bone marrow cells. Radiat. Res., *14*:213, 1961.

Trentin, J. J.: Determination of bone marrow stem cell differentiation by stromal hemopoietic inductive microenvironment (HIM). Am. J. Pathol., *65*:621, 1971.

Weiss, L.: The hemopoietic microenvironment of the bone marrow: An ultrastructural study of the stroma in rats. Anat. Rev., *186*:161, 1976.

Weiss, L.: The histology of the bone marrow. *In* Gordon, A. S. (Ed.): Regulation of Hematopoiesis. Appleton-Century-Crofts, New York, 1970, p. 79.

Weiss, L., and Chen, L. T.: The organization of hematopoietic cords and vascular sinuses in bone marrow. Blood Cells, *1*:617, 1975.

Wu, A. M., Till, J. E. Siminovitch, L., and McCulloch, E. A.: A cytological study of the capacity for differentiation of normal hemopoietic colony-forming cells. J. Cell. Physiol., *69*:177, 1967.

2

Spleen

STRUCTURE

The máture normal spleen — no longer involved in hematopoiesis — is the largest of the lymphoid organs. Yet it is also a unique filtration bed for the circulating blood well equipped with macrophages to remove undesired particles from the circulation. The parenchyma or "pulp" is partitioned by fibrous trabeculae, through which run the arteries, veins, and lymphatics. Arterioles run out from the trabeculae into the white pulp, branch at right angles into the marginal zone, and then terminate in the red pulp (Fig. 2–1). The venous drainage system originates in the sinus system of the red pulp. The blood then flows out through the trabecular veins and on into the portal system. The efferent lymphatic drainage runs into the thoracic duct.

In the white pulp, a sleeve of T lymphocytes — the "periarterial lymphatic sheath" — is wrapped around the central artery (Fig. 2–2). Nodular accumulations of lymphocytes, often at the sites of the right angled vascular branches, form follicles along the course of the central arteriole. These contain germinal centers rich in B lymphocytes surrounded by mantle zones of T lymphocytes and macrophages. The cellular structure is held together by a network of fibrillar reticular cells.

The marginal zone is an ill-defined boundary between the white and red pulp. Into its interstices, also held together by fibrillar reticular cells, empty many arteriolar branches filling the spongy network with blood cells. Under provocative stimuli, macrophages readily migrate into this area.

Blood from the marginal zone as well as from central arterial terminals drains into the red pulp, either directly into venous sinuses and on out through the efferent veins, or into the cords that lie between the sinuses (Fig. 2–3). The blood cells that enter the cords must pass through the fenestrated wall separating the cords from the sinuses before gaining access to the venous drainage system. They are thus delayed to varying degrees in their transit. The fenestrations in the wall separating the cords and sinuses are about 3 μ in diameter, so small that erythrocytes must be squeezed through with effort. They pass through because their pliability and deformability is normally very great (Fig. 2–4). The sinus side of the wall is lined by reticular endothelial cells lying upon the fenestrated basement membrane. The cordal side of the wall is made up of the adventitial network of reticular cells and macrophages surrounding and separating the sinuses.

Blood flow through the spleen, thus, is both fast and slow. Rapid transit is achieved by the fraction that bypasses the cords and enters directly into the sinuses. The slow transit fraction is temporarily detained in the cords. Normally, this detention is not very great; the time required for complete mixing of blood within the spleen as measured with tagged erythrocytes is only about 2 minutes. When the spleen enlarges, however, the detention time of the "slow flow" fraction may increase to as long as an hour, with potentially deleterious effects on the survival time of erythrocytes, particularly if they do not have their customary flexibility and become more easily entrapped in the splenic cords.

Plasma skimming is another important aspect of the splenic circulation. Laminar flow in the central arteries directs leukocyte-rich plasma

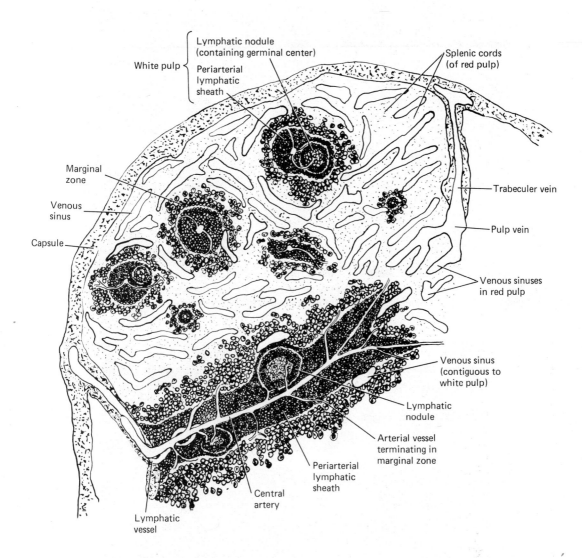

Figure 2-1 The structure of the spleen. The white pulp consists of the periarterial lymphatic sheath and lymphatic nodules with germinal centers. The red pulp contains the splenic cords and sinuses. The marginal zone is interposed between white and red pulp. The central artery sends branches out into the marginal zone and then terminates in the red pulp. Blood from the splenic cords passes through a fenestrated wall into the sinuses and is then collected into the splenic veins. (From Weiss, L., and Tavassoli, M.: Sem. in Hematol., 7, 372, 1970, Reprinted from Histology, by L. Weiss, and R. O. Greep, Copyright © 1977, McGraw-Hill Book Company.

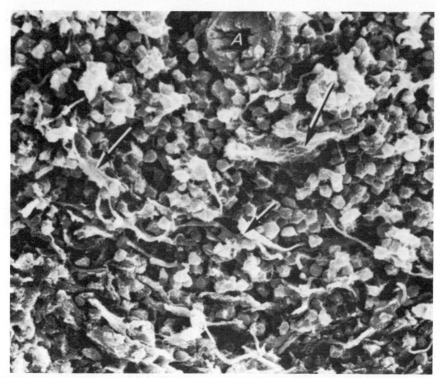

Figure 2–2 Scanning electron micrograph of the splenic white pulp in the region of the periarterial lymphatic sheath. A sea of lymphocytes is held together by reticular cells and their associated fibrils (shown by arrows). The central arteriole (A) is shown in cross section near the upper margin. (From Weiss, L. Blood *43*:665, 1974.)

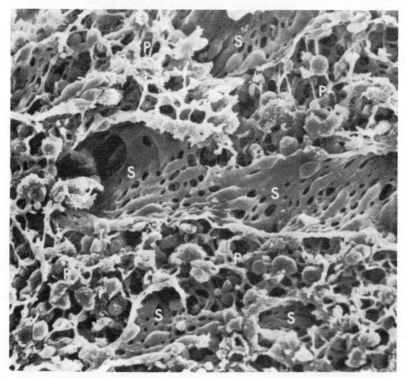

Figure 2–3 Scanning electron micrograph of the splenic red pulp, showing the fenestrated sinuses (S) and the spongy cords (P) that lie between the sinuses and consist of hematogenous cells enmeshed in an adventitial reticular network. (From Miyoshi, M., and Fujita, T. Arch. Histol. Japan *33*:225–246, 1971.)

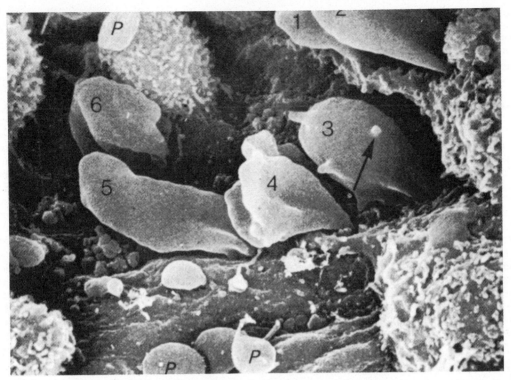

Figure 2–4 Scanning electron micrograph demonstrating erythrocytes (numbered 1 through 6) squeezing through the fenestrated wall in transit from the splenic cord to the sinus. The view shows the endothelial lining of the sinus wall, to which platelets (P) adhere, along with "hairy" white cells, probably macrophages. (From Weiss, L. Blood *43*:665, 1974.)

into the perpendicular branches feeding the germinal follicles and the marginal zone. This leaves behind more viscous high hematocrit blood in the central artery to flow on into hemoconcentrated red pulp.

FUNCTION

The circulating blood passes through no more discriminating a filter than that of the spongy red pulp of the spleen. While the liver, by virtue of its larger blood flow, performs the lion's share of phagocytic clearance of unwanted particles from the circulation, the spleen is more discriminating and is able to pick out for destruction more subtly altered cells. Warm antibody coated erythrocytes and the sensitized platelets of autoimmune thrombocytopenic purpura are examples of such altered cells usually missed by the hepatic macrophages past which they circulate too rapidly to be trapped, but selected for destruction in the spleen.

Erythrocytes undergo a certain degree of re-structuring as they percolate through the splenic cords. Reticulocytes endure preferential splenic delay in transit, possibly because their transferrin coating makes them more "sticky" than mature erythrocytes. Intracytoplasmic inclusions left over after extrusion of the newly formed erythrocyte into the marrow sinusoid are plucked by splenic macrophages from the cell interior, usually without detriment to the integrity of the self sealing red cell membrane. These inclusions include iron granules, hemoglobin precipitates, fragments of DNA, or even the entire erythroid cell nucleus. They are not numerous unless bone marrow function is hyperactive or abnormal, such as in Cooley's anemia or sickle cell anemia. In these conditions, the asplenic state is characterized by large numbers of circulating normoblasts and inclusion-containing erythrocytes. Loss of membrane surface along with membrane cholesterol accompanies the cellular grooming during splenic transit.

In man, the spleen is an important reservoir of platelets, as reported by Aster. About 30 per cent of the body's platelets are sequestered there in slow transit and in dynamic equilibrium with the circulating pool. The splenic platelets are immediately moved into the circulation after stress or injection of epinephrine. The transitory platelet increase is accompanied by a parallel increase in Factor VIII level. Neither response is seen in the splenectomized individual. There is .no significant storage pool of red or white cells in the human spleen, although in some animals, such as the dog, horse, or sheep, muscular contraction of the splenic capsule abruptly increases the peripheral hematocrit by means of "autotransfusion" of a reservoir of splenic blood.

The spleen is a dispensible organ in the adult, but young children may suffer sudden overwhelming infection in its absence, as reported by Erickson and co-workers in 1968. Children with Cooley's anemia or other severe systemic disorders are the most susceptible. There are even occasional reports of sudden fatal sepsis in splenectomized adults. The first immunologic response to antigen introduced directly into the circulation appears to take place in the spleen after phagocytosis by splenic macrophages. Possibly this function of the spleen is more vital in the early years. of life. Likhite has reported that removal of the

spleen is in fact followed by a significant drop in plasma concentration of IgM.

PATHOPHYSIOLOGY

ASPLENIA

The asplenic state is usually the result of surgical removal, performed either in the hematologically normal individual who has suffered traumatic rupture or for such hematologic indications as hereditary spherocytosis, idiopathic thrombocytopenic purpura, or staging operation for Hodgkin's disease. In sickle cell anemia repeated splenic infarctions lead to "autosplenectomy" during childhood. Atrophy of the spleen occurs in association with malabsorption syndromes (Wardrop and associates, 1975). Although true congenital asplenia is a rare condition, "functional asplenia" is found in normal neonates, especially the premature. Chronic hemolysis may also cause functional asplenia, presumably because erythrophagocytosis blocks the splenic macrophages.

The removal of the spleen is followed by a rise

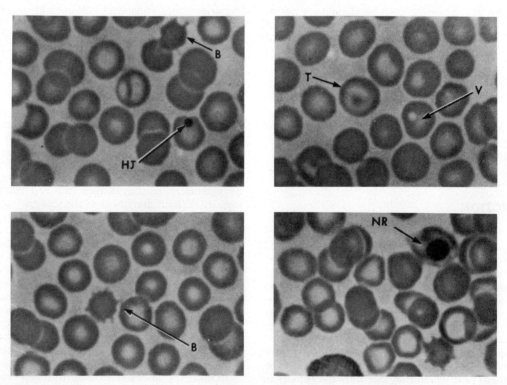

Figure 2–5 Morphologic signs in the peripheral blood of asplenia. HJ–Howell-Jolly body (fragment of DNA); T-target cell; V–vacuole; B–"burr" cell; NR–nucleated red cell. (From Holroyde, C. P. *In* Custer, R. P.: An Atlas of the Blood and Bone Marrow. Philadelphia, W. B. Saunders Co., 1974, p. 125.)

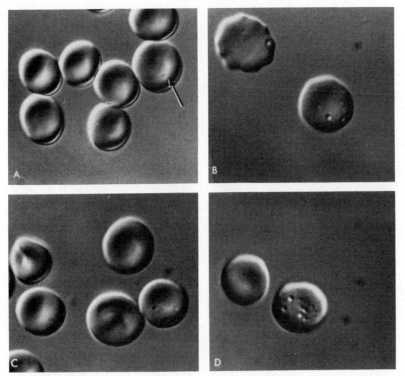

Figure 2–6   Interference contrast microscopy of erythrocytes. A. Normal adult with intact spleen. Only 1-2% of the cells have vacuoles; B. Normal adult after splenectomy performed because of ruptured spleen. About 50% of the cells contain vacuoles; C. Full term infant, and D. premature infant demonstrate an increased proportion of vacuole-containing cells, the latter to a more striking degree. (From Holroyde, C. P. *In* Custer, R. P.: An Atlas of the Blood and Bone Marrow. Philadelphia, W. B. Saunders Co., 1974, p. 134.)

in platelet and granulocyte counts, often reaching peaks after about ten days of more than one million and 30,000 per mm³, respectively. The elevated counts gradually return to normal values in most cases. Late postsplenectomy effects include an absolute lymphocytosis, monocytosis, and the presence of occasional immature cells in the peripheral blood. Interaction between the spleen and bone marrow has been postulated to explain these changes, but experimental proof for this hypothesis has never come forth.

The asplenic state can usually be suspected by the presence of red cell inclusions, especially Howell–Jolly bodies, which otherwise are removed by the normal spleen (Fig. 2–5). In pathologic states these may be very numerous. Significant numbers of target cells and spiculated erythrocytes, or "burr" cells, are also present, along with a parallel increase in erythrocyte membrane surface, membrane cholesterol content, and osmotic resistance. Reticulocytes may be slightly increased and a few giant platelets are seen in the circulation. Special microscopic techniques demonstrate erythrocyte vacuoles which give the cell surface a pitted appearance (Fig. 2–6).

SPLENOMEGALY

Occasionally splenic enlargement is caused by a disorder intrinsic to the spleen, such as a cyst, but more often it occurs as a feature of a systemic disease process (Table 2–1). A reactive response of the lymphoid white pulp is seen in infections, especially viral, while neoplastic proliferation is responsible for the splenomegaly of the lymphoproliferative disorders. The splenic pool of macrophages hypertrophies when subjected to a chronic work load. This may be caused by bacterial infections, such as subacute bacterial endocarditis or miliary tuberculosis, or from the state of chronic hemolysis itself. Hypertrophy of the splenic pool of lipid-laden macrophages is responsible for the splenomegaly of the lipidoses.

The spleen may return to shades of its past

TABLE 2-1   CLASSIFICATION OF SPLENOMEGALY

Lymphatic Disorders
   Reactions to infections, especially viral (e.g., infectious mononucleosis)
   Reactions to connective tissue disorders (e.g., disseminated lupus erythematosus)
   Lymphoproliferative disorders (e.g., lymphatic leukemia, lymphoma)

Macrophage Disorders
   Reactions to infections (e.g., subacute bacterial endocarditis, miliary tuberculosis, tropical splenomegaly)
   "Work hypertrophy" secondary to chronic hemolytic anemia
   Lipidoses (e.g., Gaucher's disease)
   Proliferative disorders (e.g., histiocytic medullary reticulosis, Letterer-Siwe disease)

Infiltrative Disorders
   Myeloproliferative disorders
   Extramedullary hematopoiesis secondary to chronic hemolytic anemia (e.g., Cooley's anemia)
   Amyloidosis

Increased Splenic Vein Pressure (Congestive Splenomegaly)
   Splenic or portal vein thrombosis
   Liver cirrhosis

Miscellaneous
   Sarcoidosis
   Congenital cyst ("true", epithelial lined, "primary")
   Post traumatic cyst (not lined, "secondary")
   Rare tumors, primary and metastatic
   Non-tropical idiopathic splenomegaly

developmental history and become swollen with hematopoietic myeloid tissue. Severe chronic hemolytic anemia is one stimulus for extramedullary hematopoiesis, especially in Cooley's anemia. Splenic infiltration with hematogenous elements also occurs as a common feature of the myeloproliferative syndromes. In temperate zones, some of the largest spleens occur in patients with myelofibrosis and myeloid metaplasia.

Vascular congestion — "congestive splenomegaly" — is seen most often as a consequence of portal hypertension secondary to hepatic cirrhosis, but obstructions of the portal or splenic vein are other etiologic considerations. Marked splenomegaly in patients living in tropical regions — "tropical splenomegaly" — apparently is caused by chronic malarial infestation or other infections endemic to the region. "Non-tropical idiopathic splenomegaly" was so designated by Dacie and associates because of the non-diagnostic histology of the spleen after its removal in patients without evidence of other coexisting disease. A significant proportion of such patients subsequently develop lymphoma.

ACCESSORY SPLEENS

Small accessory spleens are found in the splenic hilum, the mesentery, the region of the tail of the pancreas or elsewhere in about 10 per cent of normal individuals. They may enlarge after splenectomy and cause relapse of the hematologic condition for which the operation was originally done. This is, however, an unusual occurrence. "Splenosis" follows the seeding of multiple small implants of spleen tissue in the peritoneal cavity as a result of rupture of the splenic capsule. The spleen cells colonize and develop into nodules of spleen tissue studded on serosal surfaces.

THE SPLEEN AS A TRAP

"Hypersplenism" is a term honored by both time and usage, but in the light of present concepts of the interactions of the hematogenous cells with the spleen, it lacks pathophysiologic precision. It is characterized by (1) reduction in erythrocytes, platelets, granulocytes, or any combination of these cellular elements of the peripheral blood; (2) splenomegaly; (3) a cellular marrow implying adequate marrow compensation in response to the cytopenia; and (4) correction of the cytopenia by splenectomy. Strictly speaking the term should thus not be used until successful response to splenectomy has been documented.

The splenic blood volume, normally about 50 ml., may increase to such a degree in splenomegalic states that it contains as much as 25 per cent of the total blood volume, and up to 90 per cent or more of the total pool of platelets. However, the platelets, if otherwise untainted, withstand this altered distribution quite nicely. They easily escape from the splenic cords into the sinuses, where they are found temporarily adhering to the vascular wall, happily bathed by flowing blood with excellent preservation of their viability. Granulocytes, if otherwise normal, also seem to endure sequestration in the enlarged spleen without suffering undue damage. Red cells, dependent upon glycolysis for energy, are susceptible to deterioration during repeated passages through the splenic cords. The depressed glucose concentration in the splenic red pulp, as low as a third the level in the blood, and the inhibitory action of the low pH, the result of lactic acid accumulation, severely limit glycolysis. Hemoconcentration and low Po_2 add insult to injury — especially in sickle cell disorders. The larger the spleen the greater the likelihood of clinically significant sequestration phenomena, but precise correlation with the degree of splenomegaly is not always possible. Differences in the extent of cell entrapment in the splenic cords among patients with comparable degrees of splenomegaly may be explained by differences in the partition of splenic blood flow into rapid and slow transit streams.

The rigid inelastic cells of sickle hemoglobinopathy, homozygous Hemoglobin C disease, or the Heinz body hemolytic anemias are more easily trapped and damaged in the spleen than normal erythrocytes. The erythrocyte in hereditary spherocytosis, by virtue of its high glycolytic requirement, is exquisitely sensitive to erythrostasis, and the stress of repeated passages through the splenic environment produces fragmentation at the membrane surface with sphering and ultimately entrapment and lysis. The state of chronic hemolysis provokes work hypertrophy of the spleen which in turn may adversely reciprocate and worsen the hemolysis. In Cooley's anemia, the spleen may enlarge so massively that transfused erythrocytes do not survive sufficiently long to enable the patient to maintain adequate hemoglobin levels. Splenectomy then becomes mandatory. If the massive splenomegaly in the patient with myelofibrosis and myeloid metaplasia is responsible for intolerable transfusion requirements or for bleeding due to severe thrombocytopenia, splenectomy may be beneficial even in the face of marrow failure.

THE SPLEEN AND AUTOANTIBODIES

Erythrocytes or platelets coated with 7S antibody are selectively taken up and destroyed in the spleen. In autoimmune hemolytic anemia and thrombocytopenic purpura, the antibody is of endogenous origin. During splenic transit the antibodies on the cell surfaces cause adhesion to macrophages, the instruments of cell damage and destruction. The notion that an autoantibody is responsible for granulocyte destruction in the spleen in patients with splenic neutropenia or Felty's syndrome is still inferential. When cells are more grossly affected with autoantibody and such phenomena as agglutination or complement mediated membrane damage occur in the circulation, cell destruction in extrasplenic sites predominates.

The observation that some patients achieve permanent remission after splenectomy with eventual disappearance of the autoantibody has led to the hypothesis that in these instances the spleen is the major or even the sole site of its synthesis. If this is true, the concentration of the autoantibody would be much higher in the splenic plasma, possibly leading to instantaneous cell destruction, with little or no evidence of the presence of antibody coated cells in the circulation. Indeed, the concentration of antibody in the

plasma may be so much less in the general circulation than in the spleen that its detection would be difficult. Such phenomena would explain instances in which laboratory detection of such autoimmune states has been elusive. The recent experiments of Karpatkin and associates, corroborated by those of McMillan and coworkers, have provided direct evidence that spleen cells prepared from the excised spleens of patients with autoimmune idiopathic thrombocytopenic purpura do indeed synthesize an anti-platelet antibody, leading to platelet destruction by the splenic macrophages.

THE SPLEEN, INTRAVASCULAR VOLUME, AND PORTAL HYPERTENSION

In patients with massive splenomegaly (Table 2–2), the blood flow through the organ increases from its normal value of 5 per cent to as much as 50 per cent of the cardiac output. The large volume of blood draining out through the splenic vein distends the portal vascular tree with two important consequences, "dilutional" anemia and portal hypertension.

Although anemia in the presence of massive splenomegaly may be primarily related to pooling of a quarter or more of the red cell mass along with varying degrees of hemolysis, measurement of the total red cell mass may reveal that it is actually normal or even increased with an even greater expansion of total plasma volume and blood volume, i.e., there is a dilutional anemia. The mechanism of these changes in intravascular volume has been described by Hess and coworkers. The portal vascular bed is expanded at the expense of the remainder of the intravascular space, including the renal circulation. Stimulation of the renin-angiotensin-aldosterone system retains salt and water. Reduced colloid osmotic pressure then stimulates albumin synthesis. Normal albumin concentrations are restored and the total albumin pool is expanded.

Massive splenomegaly is also associated with high cardiac output, hypermetabolism, and a

TABLE 2–2   SOME CAUSES OF CHRONIC MASSIVE SPLENOMEGALY

Myelofibrosis with myeloid metaplasia
Chronic granulocytic leukemia
"Hairy cell" leukemia
Chronic lymphocytic leukemia
Lymphosarcoma
Cooley's anemia
Gaucher's disease
Kala-azar
Malaria

wide pulse pressure. Decreased peripheral vascular resistance, necessary to meet the needs of heat dispersion, also compromises the renal circulation and stimulates renin secretion to expand intravascular volume.

If the spleen is surgically removed, the expanded blood volume only gradually returns to normal over a matter of several months. The reason for this slow reversal probably is the long time necessary for normal catabolic processes to dispose of the excess in the total body albumin pool.

Portal hypertension secondary to massive splenomegaly may be complicated by esophageal and gastric varices and risks of upper gastrointestinal hemorrhage. Varices may also form secondary to splenic vein thrombosis because of the increased blood flow from splenic accessory veins into the venous system of the greater curvature of the stomach and lower esophagus. When the spleen is the cause of serious portal hypertension, its removal may be the cure. However, outflow obstruction due to hepatic cirrhosis is by far the commonest cause of portal hypertension, for which splenectomy is almost never helpful except perhaps when bleeding occurs in association with unusually severe thrombocytopenia.

REFERENCES

Aster, R. H.: Pooling of platelets in the spleen. Role in the pathogenesis of "hypersplenic" thrombocytopenia. J. Clin. Invest. 45:645, 1966.

Dacie, J. V., Brain, M. C., Harrison, C. V., Lewis, S. M., and Worlledge, S. M.: Non-tropical idiopathic splenomegaly ("primary hypersplenism"); a review of ten cases and their relationship to malignant lymphomas. Br. J. Haematol. 17:317, 1969.

Erickson, W. D., Burgert, E. O., Sr., and Lynn, H. B.: The hazard of infection following splenectomy in children. Am. J. Dis. Child. 116:1, 1968.

Fujita, T. Application of scanning electron microscopy to hematological studies. Acta Haematol. Jap. 35:453, Aug. 1972.

Hess, C. E., Ayers, C. R., Sandusky, W. R., Carpenter, M. A., Wetzel, R. A., and Mohler, D. N. Mechanism of dilutional anemia in massive splenomegaly. Blood, 47, 629, 1976.

Holroyde, C. P. Asplenia. In Custer, R. P.: An Atlas of the Blood and Bone Marrow. Philadelphia, London, Toronto, W. B. Saunders Co., 1974, p. 123.

Karpatkin, S., Strick, N., and Siskin, G. W.: Detection of splenic antiplatelet antibody synthesis in idiopathic autoimmune thrombocytopenic purpura (ATP). Br. J. Haematol. 23:167, 1972.

Kevy, S. V., Tefft, M., Vawter, G. F., and Rosen, F. S.: Hereditary splenic hypoplasia. Pediatrics 42:752, 1968.

Likhite, V. V. Immunologic impairment and susceptibility to infection after splenectomy. J.A.M.A., 236, 1376, 1976.

McMillan, R., Longmire, R. L., Tavassoli, M., Armstrong, S., and Yelenosky, R.: In vitro platelet phagocytosis by splenic leukocytes in idiopathic thrombocytopenic purpura. N. Engl. J. Med. 290:249, 1974.

Wardrop, C. A. J., Lee, F. D., Dyet, J. F., Dagg, J. H., Singh, H., and Moffat, A.: Immunological abnormalities in splenic atrophy. Lancet, 2, 4, 1975.

Weed, R. I., and Weiss, L.: The relationship of red cell fragmentation occurring within cell to cell destruction. Trans. Assoc. Am. Physicians, 79:426, 1966.

Weiss, L.: A scanning electron microscopic study of the spleen. Blood. 43:665, 1974.

Weiss, L., and Tavassoli, M.: Anatomical hazards to the passage of erythrocytes through the spleen. Seminars Hematol. 7:372, 1970.

3

Erythrocytes

STRUCTURE

The ultrastructure of the erythroid cells has by now been so closely correlated with metabolic activities that structure and function cannot be separated and will be dealt with together in this section. However, the morphology of blood cells stained with the Romanovsky dyes deserves some separate remarks, since stained blood and bone marrow smears are cornerstones in the clinical management of patients with hematologic disorders.

The earliest nucleated red blood cell, the proerythroblast is a large cell with a diameter of about 20 to 25 μ and a nucleus occupying about three fourths of the cell (Fig. 1–11). The nuclear chromatin, stained dark violet with the usual Wright or Giemsa stain, is finely dispersed, and the nucleus with its one or several nucleoli is clearly separated from the deep-blue cytoplasm by a distinct membrane. The nucleus is usually perfectly round and the cytoplasm devoid of granules. The subsequent proliferation and maturation through the stages of basophilic, polychromatophilic, and orthochromatic erythroblasts are characterized by a stepwise reduction in cellular and nuclear size, by a condensation of the nuclear chromatin into well-defined chunks, and by a dilution of the blue staining cytoplasmic ribosomes with newly synthesized hemoglobin. At the orthochromatic stage, the nucleus has become condensed into a small pyknotic mass and is extruded. Hemoglobin synthesis continues for a few more days until the nucleus-dependent synthetic machinery is exhausted. During this period precipitation and condensation of the remaining basophilic ribosomes with oxidant dyes such as brilliant cresyl blue and methylene blue will result in the characteristic appearance of the reticulocyte on a blood smear. The final transformation of reticulocytes to mature cells is associated with a considerable loss in volume due to cytoplasmic dehydration and loss of cellular membrane.

The mature erythrocyte is a biconcave disk with an average diameter of about 8 μ and a central pallor occupying the middle third of the cell. Owing to a relative excess of surface over volume, the cell is soft and pliable, accounting for the ease with which it can pass through tissue capillaries and splenic fenestrations with diameters considerably less than its own. Its membrane has a remarkable self-healing capacity, and red cell injury may cause the production of viable fragments rather than intravascular hemoglobin leakage. As the cell grows older it becomes slightly more dense, but it maintains its normal pliable biconcave appearance until enzymatic failure leads to rigidity, macrophage trapping, and destruction.

FUNCTION

ERYTHROBLASTS

Erythroblastic function is exclusively inner-directed. Each proerythroblast is programmed to undergo three to four mitotic divisions and to synthesize hemoglobin until its eight to 16 daughter cells contain about 300 million hemoglobin molecules each. This program has general and special metabolic requirements. The general requirements are common to all actively proliferating cells and include the building blocks and coenzymes needed for cellular construction. The special requirements are those needed for the synthesis of hemoglobin molecules and of enzymes designed to protect the integrity and function of these molecules. The various synthetic functions and their influence on red cell production have been reviewed by Marks and Rifkind and by Nienhuis and Benz and will be described later.

ERYTHROCYTES

The red blood cells are usually considered to be functionally quite unsophisticated, since their only obligations appear to be the transport and protection of the oxygen-carrying pigment, hemoglobin. Nevertheless, the survival of cells containing neither nuclei nor mitochrondria for about 4 months in a high oxygen and sodium environment demands the presence of efficient metabolic defenses and long-lived enzymes. The cargo of enzymes provided during the nucleated phase of development has to provide sufficient energy to maintain hemoglobin iron in its active ferrous state; to power the cation pump needed to maintain intracellular sodium and potassium concentrations despite the presence of unfavorable concentration gradients; to keep the sulfhydryl groups of globins, enzymes, and membranes in an active reduced state; and to preserve the integrity of the membrane. The metabolic pathways responsible for maintaining structure and function of the red cells will be described in the section dealing with the pathophysiology of red cell survival.

As mentioned earlier, the raison d'être for the existence of erythroid tissue and circulating red blood cells is the synthesis, transport, and protection of hemoglobin molecules. The importance of these molecules for oxygen transport has been known since 1862, when Hoppe-Seyler first isolated hemoglobin and demonstrated its affinity for oxygen. However, the molecular structure making a reversible oxygen binding possible has been clarified only recently.

The hemoglobin molecule is a tetramer consisting of two α and two β polypeptide chains, each with an attached heme group. The sequential mapping of the 141 amino acids of the α chain and 146 amino acids of the β chain has been of great importance for our identification of abnormal hemoglobins with specific amino acid substitutions. However, normal function of the hemoglobin molecules and the functional impact of such amino acid substitutions was not comprehended until the spatial positioning of the chains and of the individual amino acids had been established. Recent studies initiated by the classic x-ray crystallographic observations by Perutz and co-workers have shown that each of the four chains coils into eight helices (Fig. 3–1), forming an eggshaped molecule with a central cavity (Fig. 3–2). The polar, hydrophilic amino acid residues cover the surfaces while hydrophobic residues line four superficial pockets, each containing a heme group with its iron positioned between two histidine radicals. The proximal histidine is firmly bound to the ferrous atom while the distal histidine provides a protective and reversible link for deoxygenated iron. In our sequential nomenclature these histidine radicals are far apart (histidine 58 and 87 for α chains and histidine 63 and 92 for β chains) (Fig. 3–1), but spatially they are close together in the wells of the heme pockets.

The uptake and delivery of oxygen by the hemoglobin molecules are associated with considerable spatial rearrangement of the hemoglobin molecule, and as Perutz has pointed out, the well-known oxygen dissociation curve can best be explained on the basis of such rearrangement (Fig. 3–3). The oxygen affinity of deoxygenated hemoglobin is low, and it takes a relatively large increase in oxygen tension to attach an oxygen molecule to the first heme group. However, the oxygenation of this heme group causes a wide-

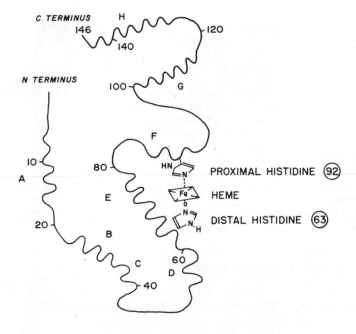

Figure 3–1   Diagram of the β polypeptide chain of hemoglobin with its eight helices (A to H) and the histidine enclosed heme group. (Adapted from Giblett, E. R.: Genetic Markers in Human Blood. Oxford, Blackwell Scientific Publications, 1969, p. 349.)

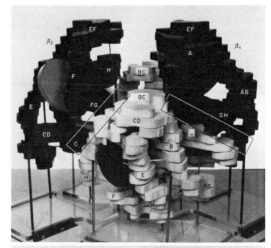

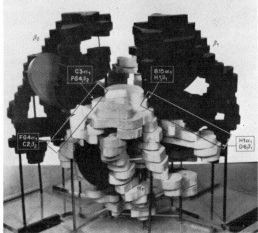

Figure 3–2 Model of the hemoglobin molecule depicting the α-β contact areas and the sliding motions which occur in the transformation from a deoxygenated form with a large central cavity (*top*) to an oxygenated form with a small cavity (*bottom*). (From Muirhead, H., et al.: J. Molec. Biol., 13:646, 1965.)

spread molecular displacement, presumably initiated by changes in the distal histidine radical which formerly was linked to the ferrous atom (Fig. 3–2). A sliding motion in the α-β contact area reduces the size of the central cavity and makes the other heme pockets more available, so that two more oxygen molecules can be attached with only slight additional increases in the oxygen tension. Further molecular rearrangement is finally responsible for the fact that the last heme group has a low oxygen affinity and demands a considerable oxygen pressure to be oxygenated.

The sequential changes in oxygen affinity are reflected in the sigmoid shape of the oxygen dissociation curve and are responsible for the ease with which hemoglobin can be loaded with oxygen in the lungs and unloaded in the tissues. Hemoglobin variants with amino acid substitution in a heme pocket or in the α-β contact area

often have altered oxygen dissociation curves. If these substitutions cause a shift to the left in the curve, the oxygen affinity is increased, the tissues become hypoxic, and a compensatory polycythemia ensues (Fig. 3–3). If the substitution causes a shift to the right, the oxygen affinity is decreased and the tissues can be provided with adequate amounts of oxygen at low hemoglobin concentrations. Obviously, if the amino acid substitutions involve the proximal or distal histidine in the heme pockets, much more severe changes will occur, with loss of the oxygen-carrying capacity of the heme pockets involved. The oxygen dissociation curve for hemoglobins made up by like chains such as β^4 in hemoglobin H or γ^4 in hemoglobin Bart's are not sigmoid but are shifted far to the left, making these hemoglobin variants useless as oxygen carriers.

It has been known for many years that the shape of the oxygen dissociation curve is dependent on the pH (Fig. 3–3). This so-called Bohr effect is responsible for the fact that the curve is shifted to the right in the acid microenvironment of hypoxic tissues, causing an enhanced capacity to release oxygen where it is most needed. The reason for this favorable shift in the oxygen affinity of hemoglobin is related to the oxygen-dependent acidity of the hemoglobin molecule. Oxyhemoglobin is a stronger acid than deoxyhemoglobin, and an acid environment will consequently facilitate deoxygenation.

In addition to the Bohr effect, the oxygen dissociation curve is also responsive to the intracellular concentration of certain organic phosphates. This recent discovery has explained the fact that

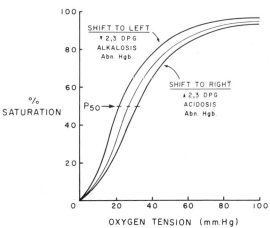

Figure 3–3 Oxygen dissociation curve of normal human blood showing that a shift to the right with an increase in P_{50} (the oxygen tension at which 50% of hemoglobin is deoxygenated) is found under conditions of acidosis or increased 2,3 DPG or with certain abnormal hemoglobins, whereas a shift to the left with a decrease in P_{50} is found under conditions of alkalosis or decreased 2,3 DPG or with other abnormal hemoglobins.

oxygen affinity can be adapted to compensate for a decreased oxygen supply, such as at high altitudes, or an impaired oxygen supply system, such as in anemia. In both these conditions there is an alkalosis, respiratory hyperventilation alkalosis at high altitude and intracellular alkalosis due to accumulation of the more alkaline reduced hemoglobin in anemia. Since alkalosis stimulates glycolysis, there is an increase in the intracellular concentration of 2,3-diphosphoglycerate (2,3-DPG). Furthermore, the binding of increased quantities of 2,3 DPG to deoxyhemoglobin depletes the unbound pool and thus also stimulates the increased synthesis of the low molecular weight phosphate. This phosphate fits into the expanded central cavity of deoxygenated hemoglobin and impedes the transformation of deoxyhemoglobin with a low oxygen affinity to oxyhemoglobin with a high oxygen affinity. The result is that the oxygen dissociation curve shifts to the right, permitting more oxygen to be released at a given tissue tension of oxygen. The opposite of such a facilitated oxygen unloading occurs in conditions in which the 2,3-DPG concentration is decreased, such as in stored bank blood. Here the shift of the curve is to the left, and the tissues may become hypoxic despite a normal oxygen carrying capacity of the perfusing blood.

The respiratory function of hemoglobin also includes support for carbon dioxide transport from the tissues to the lungs. Carbon dioxide will diffuse into the red cells and catalyzed by carbonic anhydrase becomes transformed into carbonic acid. The hydrogen ions of carbonic acid will be buffered by the relatively alkaline deoxyhemoglobin and the bicarbonate ion diffuses back into plasma. In the pulmonary capillary the same process in reverse will liberate carbon dioxide for

pulmonary elimination. In addition to this so-called Bohr effect on carbon dioxide transport, the amino groups of globin form reversible carbamino groups with carbon dioxide and are responsible for about 10 per cent of carbon dioxide transport and excretion.

KINETICS

SELF-RENEWAL AND DIFFERENTIATION

The earliest recognizable erythroid cell is the proerythroblast. However, since it is synthesizing and accumulating hemoglobin from the time of its appearance, it cannot renew itself merely through mitotic division but must be replenished from an earlier undifferentiated stem cell (Fig. 3–4). The existence of such a precursor cell is supported by the fact that nonerythroid cells in an erythropoietically inactive mouse spleen are capable of being transformed into proerythroblasts (Fig. 3–5). The morphologic identity of this precursor cell has not as yet been firmly established, but it probably is a mononuclear lymphoid cell called BFU — E or CFU — E in accord with its cultural characteristics. As described in the bone marrow section, it is replenished from an earlier multipotential stem cell pool (CFU — S) but it is in active cell cycle and capable of some degree of self-renewal. It is solely committed to the erythroid series, and it is generally accepted that the hormone erythropoietin will induce proliferation, activate its potential as a hemoglobin synthesizing cell and transform it into a proerythroblast.

The mechanism by which erythropoietin in-

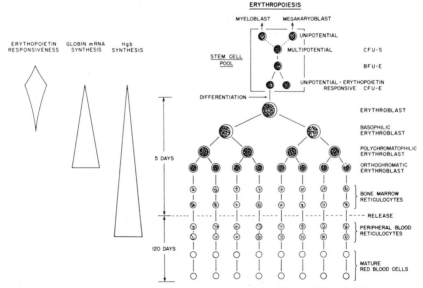

Figure 3–4   A pictorial model of the stem cell compartment and its differentiation by the action of erythropoietin to proliferating, maturing and hemoglobin producing erythroid cells.

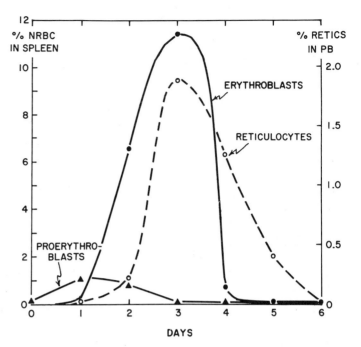

Figure 3–5 Erythropoietic effect of a single injection of erythropoietin at day 0 on a mouse spleen rendered erythropoietically inactive by prior hypertransfusion. (Redrawn from Filmanowicz, E., and Gurney, C. W.: J. Lab. Clin. Med., 57:65–72, 1961.)

duces proliferation and blast transformation is still obscure as noted in a 1978 report by Nienhuis and co-workers. It may directly cause a derepression of the production of a messenger RNA coded for a key enzyme in the synthesis of hemoglobin such as ALA synthetase. It is also possible that it acts indirectly on DNA transcription by activating a membrane adenyl cyclase, which in turn increases the production of cyclic AMP, a common second messenger for hormonal action. In either case, the activated cell appears to differentiate and proliferate according to a preformed program with only little additional stimulation by erythropoietin (Fig. 3–5).

MULTIPLICATION AND MATURATION

Following erythropoietin-induced blast transformation of the unipotential erythropoietin-sensitive stem cells, the emerging proerythroblasts immediately begin an integrated and controlled process of protoporphyrin production, globin-chain synthesis, iron uptake, and hemoglobin assembly. In the mitochondria the newly formed ALA synthetase initiates synthesis of protoporphyrin by condensing activated glycine and succinic acid to ALA. The final step in this synthetic chain occurs again in the mitochondria and consists of the formation of heme from protoporphyrin and iron. Simultaneously, alpha and beta globin chains are produced in ribosomes strung together by m RNA. The synthesis of heme and globins is closely coordinated and it appears that heme plays an essential role in this coordination. It not only exerts an end-product control on ALA synthetase activity but also a control on the transcription or processing of alpha and beta m RNA. The synthesis of other red cell proteins, such as membrane receptors, antigens and glycolytic enzymes, are also closely integrated with the formation of heme and globins.

Iron necessary for the transformation of protoporphyrin to heme is provided from iron-charged transferrin which becomes attached to specific receptors on the immature red cell membrane. The iron passes through the membrane while the iron-free transferrin possibly after a brief sojourn inside the cell is released and reused for shuttling iron from the macrophage system to erythroid cells. The intracellular iron is transported to the mitochondria for heme production or temporarily deposited as ferritin complexes in the cytoplasm. The fate of these so-called siderotic granules is not known. They may provide storage iron for further heme production, or they may be extruded and returned to the circulating iron pool.

Although transferrin-mediated delivery presumably provides adequate amounts of iron to the maturing cell, a second supply exists with iron provided by macrophages through direct cell-to-cell delivery. Since such an intercellular transport system also could facilitate removal or pitting of intracellular iron by the macrophages, the exact role played by these cells in cellular maturation is not clear. Nevertheless, it is known that erythroid development occurs in close physical proximity with macrophages (Fig. 3–6). This

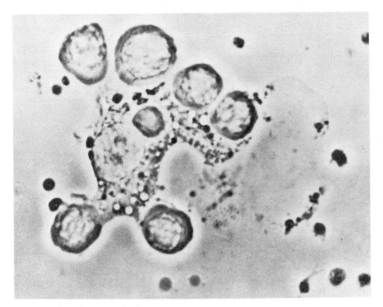

Figure 3–6 Phase contrast picture of a macrophage (nurse-cell) "servicing" attached erythroblasts. (From Lessin, L. S., and Bessis, M.: *In* Williams et al. (Eds.): Hematology. New York, McGraw-Hill Book Co., 1977, p. 105, by permission of Sandoz Ltd., Basel, Switzerland.)

proximity is not always apparent from observing regular bone marrow smears, since the cells are torn apart from each other and from the thin, wide-flung cytoplasmic veil of the macrophages. However, biopsy sections and in-vitro bone marrow cultures often show the presence of characteristic erythropoietic islands, each consisting of a macrophage and nucleated red cells at the same stage of maturation. As the cells mature and proliferate, the islands increase in size until they break up and release their finished cellular products.

Concurrently with the cytoplasmic maturation, the cell will undergo three to four mitotic divisions, causing a stepwise reduction in volume. Since all nucleated red cells are diploid, the reduction in nuclear size must be caused by a progressive condensation of nuclear protein, a condensation which eventually results in the appearance of a dense pyknotic nucleus incapable of further DNA synthesis. Occasionally in normal bone marrow and frequently in bone marrow from patients with accelerated red cell production the last division may be incomplete, with the production of a cloverleaf nucleus or satellite nuclear pieces, so-called Howell-Jolly bodies. In most non-mammalian species, the condensed nucleus is carried as an inert inclusion by the mature circulating red blood cells. In mammals, however, it is extruded by a process of intracellular demarcation and extracellular pressure. The cell is pitted either when it forces its way into the circulation through narrow endothelial openings in the bone marrow sinusoids or when it passes a similar sievelike hazard in the spleen. The extruded nucleus is surrounded by a thin layer of hemoglobin, and in patients with accelerated red cell formation the breakdown of this

hemoglobin may contribute significantly to the concentration of circulating bilirubin.

After the nucleus has been extruded, hemoglobin synthesis continues but at a gradually diminishing rate for another three to four days. The cells lose membrane receptors for transferrin-iron, the mitochondria diminish in number, and the polyribosomes disaggregate. When the ribosomes finally disappear, the cells no longer show the characteristic staining qualities of a reticulocyte and they have become mature red blood cells. The cells also diminish in size, and the stickiness which characterizes immature red cells is lost. This stickiness may be caused by a coating of transferrin, and the diminishing number of iron receptors could be responsible in part for the loss of cellular cohesion and adhesion and could promote the release of cells into the circulating blood.

According to nuclear size and degree of cytoplasmic maturation, the developing bone marrow cell goes through five stages designated respectively as proerythroblasts, basophilic erythroblasts, polychromatic erythroblasts, orthochromatic erythroblasts, and bone marrow reticulocytes. Since each of the first three stages appears to be separated from the next by a mitotic division, it is possible to estimate their duration or generation time by enumerating mitotic figures. The fraction of cells in mitosis (mitotic index) depends on the duration of the mitosis (about 30 to 60 minutes) and on the generation time:

$$\text{Mitotic Index} = \frac{\text{Number of cells in mitosis}}{\text{Total number of cells}}$$

$$= \frac{\text{Mitotic time}}{\text{Generation time}}$$

The mitotic index has been measured to be about 2.5 per cent for proerythroblasts, 5 per cent for basophilic erythroblasts, and 6 per cent for polychromatic erythroblasts, and the generation times are calculated to be 30 hours, 15 hours, and 13 hours, respectively. Unfortunately, when generation times are measured by other techniques, the results have been somewhat different. The most popular alternate method has been based on using tritiated thymidine to label cells during their synthetic phase (lasting about six hours) and employing radioautography to measure fraction of cells labeled, the so-called labeling index.

$$\text{Labeling Index} = \frac{\text{Number of cells in synthetic phase}}{\text{Total number of cells}}$$

$$= \frac{\text{Synthetic time}}{\text{Generation time}}$$

The generation times calculated from such studies by Skårberg are 11 hours for proerythroblasts, 16 hours for basophilic erythroblasts and 26 hours for polychromatic erythroblasts. In the absence of more consistent data, it seems permissible to use as a practical approximation 24 hours for each maturation phase. Since the orthochromatic erythroblasts and the bone marrow reticulocytes do not synthesize DNA or undergo mitotic divisions, the time spent in each of these stages is estimated from the turnover of appropriately labeled cells and is about 24 hours and 48 hours, respectively. Using a model based on these values (Fig. 3–4) one can estimate that the number of erythropoietic cells in the bone marrow is about 3 per cent of the circulating red cells, or, if the red cell mass is 30 ml. per kg. body weight and the mean red cell volume is $90\mu^3$, about 10×10^9 cells per kg body weight. More accurate methods for enumeration of erythropoietic bone marrow cells have disclosed somewhat higher values (Table 3–1), but a basic numerical agreement exists supporting the validity of the model presented in Figure 3–4.

TABLE 3–1   ERYTHROID POOLS

Cell Types	Number of Cells in 10^9 per kg. Body Weight
Proerythroblast	0.10
Basophilic erythroblast	0.48
Polychromatophilic erythroblast	1.47
Orthochromatic erythroblast	2.95
Marrow reticulocytes	8.20
Blood reticulocytes	3.10
Mature red blood cells	307.00
Daily production and destruction	3.00

(Adapted from Donohue D. M., et al.: J. Clin. Invest., 37:1571, 1958 and from Finch C. A., et al., Blood, 50: 699, 1977.)

Part of the transformation of nucleated red cells to mature red cells takes place in circulating blood which contains about one third the reticulocyte pool. Under normal conditions, the reticulum persists for about one to two days, but in patients with accelerated red cell production, reticulocytes are released earlier and stay longer in the blood. As has been emphasized by Hillman and Finch, this has to be taken into account when reticulocytes are used to estimate the rate of red cell production. The earlier release of reticulocytes is also reflected by the fact that these so-called "stress reticulocytes" are larger and more immature than normal circulating reticulocytes and that the bone marrow transit time is shortened. It has been suggested by Leblond and coworkers that the early release is caused by a direct action of erythropoietin on the bone marrow release mechanism. However, it could also be due to ecologic crowding of the bone marrow by new erythroid cells derived from an overstimulated stem cell pool.

REGULATION

Maturation and proliferation of nucleated red cells proceed at an integrated speed and rate. Changes in the speed of cellular maturation or in the rate of cellular proliferation could influence the total output of red cells from the bone marrow but cannot be solely responsible for the remarkable range of erythropoietic activity. A shortened maturation time or an early release of cells will only augment the circulating red cell mass slightly, and several extra mitotic divisions are needed in order to provide the bone marrow with its capacity to increase its rate of red cell production five- to tenfold. Since most studies indicate that an accelerated rate of red cell production is associated with a shortened transit time, it seems most unlikely that added mitotic divisions can be squeezed in. Furthermore, direct measurements of cellular generation times have suggested that the maturation and proliferation of immature red cells proceed at fixed rates independent of the overall erythropoietic activity. Consequently, it seems more likely that the rate of red cell production depends on the number of operational erythropoietic units rather than on the activity within each unit. According to this widely accepted erythropoietic quantum theory, the rate of red cell production is controlled primarily, if not exclusively, by the rate at which stem cells differentiate to proerythroblasts and initiate the formation of an erythropoietic unit.

Under normal steady-state conditions the rate of differentiation provides just enough red cells to replace the daily loss of cells. Maintenance of such a homeostatic balance demands the existence of a feedback system responsive to red cell loss and capable of inducing the necessary adjustment in the production of red cells. Occasionally the reticulocyte count displays the oscillatory pattern which characterizes all feedback control systems (Fig. 3–7), but under normal conditions the system is usually too finely tuned to be visibly oscillatory. Under pathologic conditions with increased loss or destruction of red cells the compensatory adjustment in the rate of red cell production becomes evident. The triggering event in the activation of the adjustment must in some way be related to the physical or functional effect of red cell loss, and it has variously been suggested that red cell production is controlled by a device responsive to breakdown products of red cell destruction, to blood viscosity, to red cell volume, or to oxygen transport. Of these possibilities, a responsiveness to oxygen transport is by far the most likely, since oxygen transport is the main function of the red cell mass. Furthermore, numerous studies have shown that a decreased supply of oxygen to the tissues almost invariably is associated with an increased rate of red cell production.

The existence of an erythropoietic feedback system responsive to the tissue tension of oxygen was first suspected by Dennis Jourdanet, a French physician who in the 1860's practiced medicine in the highlands of Mexico. He observed that the dark blood of his surgical patients was thick and flowed slowly, and he suggested that

there was a connection between a low arterial content of oxygen and thick blood. Subsequent studies by the famous Parisian physiologist, Paul Bert, on the physiologic effect of low barometric pressure led to the hypothesis that decreased arterial oxygen tension stimulates red cell production. Supporting evidence came from the fact that many patients with chronic pulmonary disorders or with right-to-left shunts were polycythemic. Since anemia, despite normal arterial oxygen tension, is also associated with increased red cell production, it was concluded that erythropoietic stimulation is caused by tissue hypoxia due to either a decreased oxygen tension or a decreased oxygen content of arterial blood.

Subsequent observations of the effect of an increased supply of oxygen to the tissues showed that the rate of red cell production is suppressed and that the tissue tension of oxygen apparently influences or controls the full range of red cell production. Direct confirmation of this hypothesis has been difficult to achieve because of our ignorance of the exact cellular location of the oxygen sensor. Measurements of the oxygen tension of subcutaneous tissue have disclosed an inverse relationship between oxygen tension and erythropoietic stimulation (Fig. 3–8). However, the oxygen sensor is probably not located in the subcutaneous tissue, and measurements of the oxygen tension in the kidney, a more likely site,

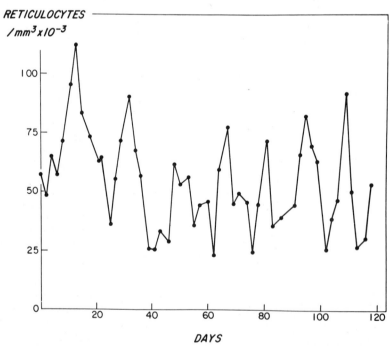

Figure 3–7 Absolute reticulocyte counts of a dog showing regularly spaced oscillations. The period is about 16 days, presumably twice the time from stem cell differentiation to reticulocyte maturation. (Redrawn from Morley, A., and Stohlman, F., Jr.: Science, 165:1025, 1969. Copyright 1969 by the American Association for the Advancement of Science.)

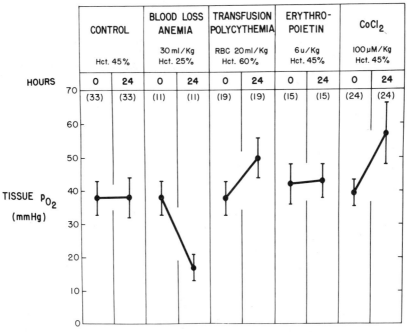

Figure 3–8 Oxygen tension of air pockets introduced subcutaneously in rats. The effects of bleeding, transfusion, erythropoietin, and cobalt on the oxygen tension are given. As expected, bleeding causes hypoxia, transfusion causes hyperoxia and erythropoietin has no immediate effect. Cobalt causes tissue hyperoxia, presumably reflecting reduced oxygen utilization because of inhibited cellular oxidative metabolism.

have not been too informative. This may be related to the fact that the oxygen sensor appears not to be responsive directly to the intercellular tissue tension of oxygen, but rather to a component of intracellular oxidative metabolism. Cobalt chloride administration, for example, causes an accelerated rate of red cell production despite an increase in the tissue tension of oxygen (Fig. 3–8), and the triggering event for the increase in both red cell production and tissue tension of oxygen appears to be impaired intracellular oxidative metabolism and oxygen utilization.

The mechanism which links the oxygen sensor to the bone marrow has recently been clarified and appears to consist of a feedback system mediated in one direction by red cell-bound oxygen and in the opposite direction by erythropoietin, a renal erythropoietic hormone (Fig. 3–9).

The suggestion that tissue hypoxia causes the release of a humoral mediator was given its first solid experimental support in 1950 when Reissmann demonstrated that hypoxia induced in one rat of a parabiotic pair caused increased red cell production in both partners. A few years later an erythropoietic factor was found in the serum of anemic rabbits (Fig. 3–10), and since then this factor, named erythropoietin, has been isolated and partially characterized.

Erythropoietin is a glycoprotein with a molecular weight of about 35,000 and a sialic acid content of about 13 per cent. It is present in both

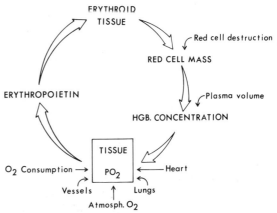

Figure 3–9 The feedback circuit that links red cell production to the tissue tension of oxygen. (From work reviewed by Erslev, A. J.: Medicine, *43*:661, 1964. © 1964. The Williams & Wilkins Company, Baltimore.)

plasma and urine of all mammals tested, and similar substances have been described in birds and fish. It man, it has a biologic half-life of about 4 to 6 hours, but its renal clearance is quite low (about 0.5 ml. per min.). Attempts to characterize and purify erythropoietin and to elucidate its site of production have been impeded by our crude and cumbersome assay technique. Agglutination inhibition tests and radioimmunoassays are being developed, but the only acceptable technique for measurement at present involves bioassay in mice. This assay utilizes mice in which endogenous erythropoietin production is first abolished by transfusion or by hypoxia-induced polycythemia. The technique is unfortunately not sensitive enough to detect erythropoietin in normal serum since its level of sensitivity is 50 mU/ml., and the normal level is about 5 to 20 mU/ml. (Fig. 3–11). Assay of urine, concentrated about 50 times, has shown that there is a linear relationship between the 24 hour erythropoietin excretion and the hemoglobin concentration and has also shown that the daily erythropoietin excretion in normal men is about 2 units and in normal women 3 units (Fig. 3–11).

Following the observations by Jacobson and co-workers that the production of erythropoietin ceases after bilateral nephrectomy, it has generally been accepted that erythropoietin has a renal origin. Support for this hypothesis has come from the observation that erythrocytosis occasionally occurs in patients with compromised renal blood supply or with renal ischemia due to space-occupying lesions. Although hypernephromas specifically have been reported to be a source of inappropriate production of erythropoietin, other tumors, as well as cysts or hydronephroses, have been associated with an increased rate of red cell production, and it seems more likely that erythropoietin is released by the compressed normal kidney tissues rather than by the pathologic lesion. Intrarenal injury due to experimental induction of microinfarcts or as a consequence of tissue rejection after kidney transplantation may also lead to overproduction of erythropoietin and erythrocytosis. However, the usual consequence of renal injury and renal failure is impaired erythropoietin production and anemia.

In order for the normal kidney to adjust erythropoietin production to the oxygen requirements of the body it appears that it, in addition to erythropoietin-producing tissue, also must contain an oxygen-sensitive device. The exact location of these two tissues is still unknown. The cortex appears most unsuited to act as an oxygen sensor since its large supply of blood with a high hematocrit (due to plasma skimming) should make it quite insensitive to small changes in the oxygen-carrying capacity of blood. The medulla, however, is relatively hypoxic owing to the shunting of oxygen between the descending and ascending capillaries at its base, and the apex of the medulla could serve as an oxygen-sensing apparatus. The fact that renal cysts made up of

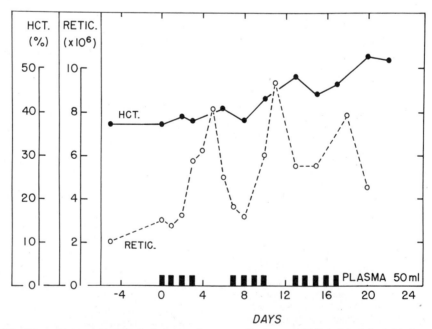

Figure 3–10 The erythropoietic effect of plasma from anemic donor rabbits when infused in large amounts to normal rabbits. (Redrawn from Erslev, A.J.: Blood, 8:349-357, 1953, by permission of Grune & Stratton Inc., New York.)

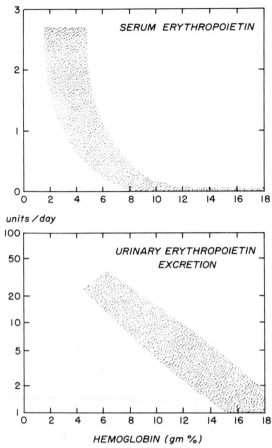

units/ml

SERUM ERYTHROPOIETIN

units/day

URINARY ERYTHROPOIETIN
EXCRETION

HEMOGLOBIN (gm %)

Figure 3–11 The relationship between hemoglobin concentration and the content of erythropoietin in plasma (*upper panel*) and the 24 hour excretion of erythropoietin in urine (*lower panel*).

dilated tubules occasionally contain erythropoietin would also suggest that the site of the erythropoietin-producing tissue may reside in the medulla. On the other hand, studies of the juxtaglomerular apparatus in anemia have suggested that this may be the site of erythropoietin production, a suggestion supported by the fact that fluorescent-tagged antibodies to erythropoietin are attracted to the glomerular tuft. In order to correlate some of these observations, it has been proposed that an oxygen sensor in the medulla controls erythropoietin production in the cortex by means of a short-range releasing hormone, but so far such a hormone has not been demonstrated.

The validity of many of these observations and speculations has recently been questioned because studies of renal extracts have disclosed that kidney tissue is not erythropoietically active. A possible explanation for this surprising finding

has been provided by Gordon and co-workers. They suggest that the kidney does not produce erythropoietin directly but rather produces an enzyme which is capable of transforming a circulating erythropoietin precursor into the active hormone. Considerable experimental support has been marshaled for the existence of such a renal erythropoietic enzyme, and the hypothesis has received wide acceptance because of its close analogy to the renin-angiotensinogen system and to many other cascade-activation schemes. Unfortunately, only trace amounts of erythropoietin can be generated by mixing the renal erythropoietic enzyme with normal plasma. Furthermore, in a 1975 study Erslev has shown that the isolated kidney perfused with a plasma-free amino acid mixture can synthesize erythropoietin almost as well as a kidney perfused with plasma. Consequently it appears that the kidney is the source of erythropoietin and that alternate explanations for the erythropoietic inactivity of renal homogenate must exist. One of these proposed by Erslev and co-workers is that erythropoietin is inactivated by an erythropoietin inhibitor during the processing of the kidney extract. Such an inhibitor has been demonstrated in crude renal homogenate and in its lipid component. This inhibitor is extremely powerful and could completely conceal the presence of many thousands of units of erythropoietin in kidney tissue. Whether or not this lipid inhibitor plays a physiologic role in the storage and release of erythropoietin is not known, but if erythropoietin is present in the kidneys, in an inactive lipid-bound form, practical recovery will have to await methods for inactivating the inhibitor or breaking the erythropoietin-inhibitor bond.

Recent studies of anephric animals and humans have disclosed that extrarenal erythropoietin production occurs. It amounts to a fraction of what is normally produced but the erythropoietic material produced is immunologically similar to renal erythropoietin. The site of production appears to be the liver and/or the mononuclear macrophage system. Since the production here is enhanced by severe anemia and hypoxia, the extrarenal site, like the kidney, must be linked to local or distant oxygen sensors. Extrarenal erythropoietin production has been described in association with various neoplasms, particularly cerebellar hemangiomas and hepatomas, but the relationship between this inappropriate secretion by neoplastic cells and the slight but appropriate secretion found in anephric mammals is completely unknown.

The action of erythropoietin on red cell precursors is better understood, although the exact target cells have not been morphologically identified or isolated. As outlined in Figure 3–4, the target cells are undoubtedly the unipotential stem cells committed to erythroid development. Stimulating effects on other cell types have been described, but at present such effects appear to be related to increased stem cell activity rather than to a direct action of erythropoietin. Changes in granulocyte and thrombocyte counts are frequently observed under conditions of increased erythropoietin release. However, these changes are temporary and may depend on a secondary activation of multipotential cells with either an increased rate of differentiation in all directions or a possible competition by the unipotential stem cell pools for the attention of the multipotent cell compartment. Since an erythropoietin-stimulated bone marrow regularly displays a shortened erythroid transit time with an early release of large immature reticulocytes, a direct effect of erythropoietin on red cell maturation and release has been postulated. However, this effect could also be caused by the rapid growth of the early erythroid cells stressing the physical capacity of bone marrow to provide room for maturing erythroid cells.

Although the capacity of renal hypoxia to generate erythropoietin and in turn to accelerate red cell production explains most clinical and experimental observations on the control of red cell production, the existence of additional regulatory mechanisms has been proposed. The pituitary, hypothalamus, and carotid bodies have all been claimed to be involved in the physiologic regulation of red cell production, but the experimental support for such neuroendocrine control is not convincing. More impressive are reports suggesting that hemolyzed red cells may exert an end product feedback stimulation on red cell production. Because of the high reticulocyte count in hemolytic anemias, it has usually been assumed that these anemias exert a more powerful stimulation on red cell production than similar anemias caused by blood loss. However, the difference in the rate of red cell production between the two kinds of anemia may actually not be as pronounced as suggested by the reticulocyte counts, since hemolysis often causes a selective destruction of old red cells, leaving relatively more reticulocytes in the circulation. Nevertheless, hemolyzed red cells do appear to have some effect on red cell production, mediated either by their iron content or by a "stimulatory" effect on the erythropoietin-producing cells in the kidney or elsewhere.

In summary, it appears that the main, if not only, feedback system regulating red cell production is based on the capacity of the kidneys to sense tissue hypoxia and translate this information into production of erythropoietin. Figure 3–12 shows an updated feedback model which incorporates current concepts of erythropoietin production and action and more recent information about the compensatory adjustments of oxygen transport.

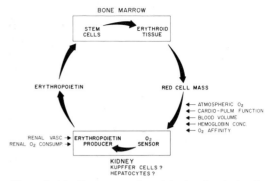

Figure 3–12   Current version of the feedback circuit.

PATHOPHYSIOLOGY

DEFINITION AND CLASSIFICATION OF POLYCYTHEMIAS AND ANEMIAS

The polycythemias and anemias are defined as hematologic disorders with either too many or too few red cells in the circulation. Functionally the polycythemias are better characterized by an increased hematocrit (more than 53 per cent) since their clinical manifestations are not caused by a change in oxygen delivery but rather by hypervolemia and hyperviscosity, both consequences of a high hematocrit. The anemias on the other hand are functionally better characterized by a reduced hemoglobin concentration (less than 12 gm. per cent) since the clinical manifestations depend on the oxygen-carrying capacity of blood.

Based on the size of the red cell mass, both polycythemias and anemias can be classified as either relative, caused by changes in the plasma volume, or absolute, caused by changes in the red cell mass. Strictly speaking, the relative polycythemias or anemias are not primary hematologic disorders. However, from a differential diagnostic point of view they play a considerable role in hematology.

The absolute polycythemias traditionally are subdivided into primary and secondary polycythemias, whereas the absolute anemias can be classified further into anemias caused by decreased red cell production or decreased red cell survival (Table 3–2).

POLYCYTHEMIA

General Effects of Polycythemia

The pathophysiologic manifestations of polycythemia, or more correctly of erythrocytosis, are caused by hyperviscosity and hypervolemia associated with an increase in the red cell mass. Under normal conditions, the red cell mass is maintained carefully at about 30 ml. per kg. body

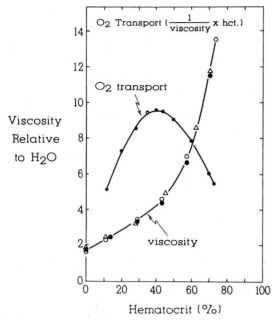

Figure 3–13 Oxygen transport as calculated from blood oxygen carrying capacity (hematocrit) and blood flow (reciprocal of viscosity).

weight, a value which presumably must be considered optimal. The reason for not maintaining a higher red cell mass does not reside in any bone marrow limitation, since a mere doubling of the rate of red cell production would sustain a red cell mass twice normal size. The reason seems to be that an increased red cell mass will be associated with a high viscosity and sluggish flow of circulating blood.

Such sluggish blood flow is responsible in part for the tendency to thrombosis found in patients with polycythemia and would, if not compensated for, result in decreased oxygen flow to the tissues (Fig. 3–13) and obviate any benefits derived from the development of secondary polycythemia. Fortunately, the high hematocrit and high viscosity are associated with an increase in blood volume (Fig. 3–14), and the resulting vasodilatation will enhance the tissue perfusion with blood and oxygen. Using measurement for cardiac output it can be shown directly that oxygen transport at a given hematocrit is greater in hypervolemic than in normovolemic dogs (Fig. 3–15). Furthermore, the optimal value for oxygen transport, which is about 45 per cent for normovolemic animals, is also increased, facilitating the mutual adjustment between hematocrit, red cell mass, and oxygen transport.

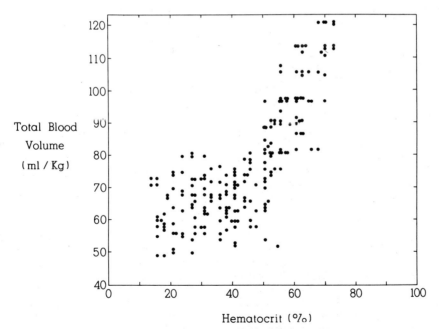

Figure 3–14 Relationship between blood volume and hematocrit. A reduction in hematocrit to about 15 per cent does not cause a significant change in blood volume, but an increase in hematocrit above 50 per cent appears to cause hypervolemia. (Data from Metcalfe, J., et al.: Circ. Res., 25:47, 1969, by permission of The American Heart Association, Inc.)

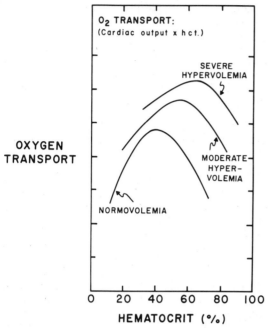

Figure 3–15 Calculated in vivo oxygen transport in normovolemic and hypervolemic conditions. As can be seen, the oxygen transport in hypervolemia is better than that in normovolemic states, even at higher hematocrits. The curves also indicate that the optimal value for oxygen transport is higher at higher blood volumes. (From Murray, J. F., et al.: J. Clin. Invest., 42:1150, 1963, and Thorling, E. B., and Erslev, A.J.: Blood, 31:332, 1968, by permission of Grune & Stratton, Inc., New York.)

The high blood volume in polycythemia is tolerated quite well, though symptoms such as headache, tinnitus, and dizziness and signs such as nose-bleeding and ruddy cyanosis probably are caused by the vascular dilatation needed to accommodate the blood volume. Since the increase in red cell production needed to sustain a polycythemia is quite moderate, clinical or laboratory signs of bone marrow hyperactivity are usually absent. However, a slight increase in uric acid, and lactic dehydrogenase levels may occur, reflecting an increase in the number of red cells destroyed daily.

Relative Polycythemia

A relative erythrocytosis with a hematocrit of more than 53 per cent can be found after severe fluid loss and the hematocrit may serve as a useful gauge of dehydration. A relative erythrocytosis has also been observed in otherwise healthy individuals with no apparent fluid volume deficit. Careful measurements by Brown and co-workers of red cell mass and fluid volume in such patients have suggested that the increase in hematocrit is spurious and merely caused by the combination of a borderline high red cell mass and a borderline low plasma volume. Since many patients with such spurious polycythemia are tense, chain-smoking individuals, the condition has been called "stress polycythemia." However, tobacco by itself produces carbon monoxide hemoglobin leading to a compensatory increase in the red cell mass, and nicotine may have a diuretic, plasma volume lowering effect. Consequently "stress polycythemia," as pointed out by Smith and Landow, probably should be called "tobacco polycythemia" and designated as a secondary rather than a relative polycythemia.

Absolute Polycythemia

Primary. Polycythemia vera is a "myeloproliferative" disorder characterized by an uncontrolled proliferation of erythroid, myeloid, and megakaryocytic bone marrow elements. The proliferation is predominantly erythroid, and the circulating red cell mass is increased during the early part of the disease. The concomitant increase in granulocytes and platelets has led to the assumption that polycythemia vera is caused by an inappropriate activation of multipotential stem cells. However, the unipotential committed stem cells must also be involved in the disease process, since the erythropoietin-sensitive stem cells undergo differentiation despite the fact that the production of erythropoietin is almost completely suppressed.

Recent studies by Adamson, Prchal and co-workers have shown that polycythemia vera is a clonal disorder caused by autonomous overactivity of a single abnormal multipotential stem cell. These authors studied two polycythemic women who were heterozygous for the X-linked A and B glucose-6-phosphate dehydrogenase isoenzymes. As expected, their skin and bone marrow fibroblasts showed a mosaicism of cells with A and B isoenzymes, but all red cells, granulocytes, and platelets contained the same isoenzymes, type A, presumably derived from a single, type A, multipotential stem cell. Bone marrow from these patients cultured in the absence of erythropoietin grew out erythroid colonies, all with the same type A isoenzyme. When erythropoietin was added, the number of type A colonies increased but in addition, colonies with type B isoenzyme appeared. These findings suggest that the autonomous clones of polycythemia vera are responsive to the stimulating effect of erythropoietin and that the bone marrow from patients with polycythemia vera in addition contains a number of normal erythropoietin-dependent clones.

The cause for this autonomous overactivity of the stem cell pool is unknown, but the existence of a viral-induced polycythemia in mice has raised the possibility that the human disorder also is virus-related. However, as is the case for most neoplastic proliferative disorders, firm evidence for a viral etiology is not available.

The increased rate of red cell production causes a steady rise in red cell blood count and hematocrit. The plasma volume remains unchanged or increases slightly, and the erythrocytosis becomes characterized by an increase in both the red cell mass and the blood volume. This process may be quite slow and may be accomplished by a slight but sustained excess of red cell production over red cell destruction. For example, a mere doubling of the rate of red cell production for a period of four months will result in a doubling of the size of the red cell mass. Since the establishment of a clinically recognizable polycythemia may take much longer, it is not surprising that a routine bone marrow examination may not show evidence of much erythroid hyperactivity.

Ferrokinetic studies, measuring total bone marrow activity, are more apt to demonstrate the presence of a slight increase in erythroid bone marrow mass. Such studies also show that the red cell production in patients with polycythemia vera is effective with the release of normal, long-lived red blood cells. Because of the increase in the number of erythroid cells in the bone marrow and circulating blood, a greater than normal amount of iron is "trapped" in the hemoglobin of these cells, and the tissue iron stores may become depleted. This trend is aggravated by the frequent therapeutic use of phlebotomy, by spontaneous nose and gastric bleedings, and by the lack of an "anemic stimulus" to intestinal iron absorbtion, and leads to an iron-deficient erythropoiesis. Fortunately, the production of microcytic and hypochromic cells may be of considerable symptomatic benefit, since the hematocrit and in turn the viscosity will become disproportionately lower than the red cell count.

Most symptoms are related to hypervolemia and hyperviscosity and are alleviated by phlebotomy. They frequently consist merely of nonspecific headaches, dizziness, blurred vision, and a feeling of "fullness in the head." Engorgement of thin-walled vessels may cause nose and gastric bleedings, serving as convenient means for spontaneous bloodletting. However, more serious symptoms may occur if the hyperviscosity causes venous stagnation, thrombosis, and embolization. Such events can cause fatal vascular accidents when they occur in cerebral, coronary, hepatic or intestinal veins.

The characteristic splenomegaly found in polycythemia vera may be caused in part by vascular engorgement but is probably more closely related to the development of extramedullary hematopoiesis, especially extramedullary granulocytopoiesis. The granulocyte count in polycythemia vera is regularly increased, although it rarely exceeds 30,000 cells per cu. mm. The resulting increase in granulocyte turnover is often reflected by an increase in serum and urine muramidase levels and in the concentration of B_{12} and B_{12} binders in serum. The granulocytes are usually mature and normally functioning, but more immature granulocytic elements may be present. The leukocyte alkaline phosphatase is either normal or high, a finding of uncertain functional significance but of use in distinguishing the granulocytosis of polycythemia vera from the granulocytosis of chronic myeloid leukemia. The granulocytes of polycythemia vera reportedly contain an increased amount of histidine decarboxylase, an enzyme involved in the production of histamine from histidine. Excessive histamine may be responsible for the common complaint of itching, especially following warm baths or showers.

The platelet count is regularly increased, but frequently not as much as would be expected from examining bone marrow specimens. These often reveal sheets of megakaryocytes, a finding which may justify bone marrow aspiration as a differential diagnostic test in the polycythemias. The characteristic tendency of patients with polycythemia vera to develop thrombotic complications is frequently related to the increased platelet count. However, morphologic and functional studies of platelets indicate that their adhesiveness is reduced and that despite their increased numbers they may not be responsible for these complications. Actually, studies by Spaet and co-workers on the coagulation process in this disease suggest the presence of impaired hemostasis with poor clot formation rather than hypercoagulability. In evaluating the results from such studies, it is important to realize that the plasma volume is relatively decreased in polycythemic blood and that the amount of available coagulation factors may not be adequate for the establishment of a firm red cell clot.

It is usually not difficult to make a diagnosis of polycythemia vera in patients with full-blown pancytosis and splenomegaly. However, early in the course, polycythemia vera may be more difficult to recognize, and Table 3–3 gives some of the findings of value in the differential diagnosis of various polycythemias. As the disease progresses, patients with polycythemia vera develop specific and characteristic complications not seen in the other polycythemias. The paradoxic occurrence of both thromboses and hemorrhages occurs quite frequently, and cerebral, coronary, mesenteric, or portal thrombosis may cause life-threatening situations in a patient who displays nasal, gastric, or dermal hemorrhages. In a considerable number of patients the disease slowly changes in character, with myelofibrosis and myeloid metaplasia becoming predominant features. These features are the results of excessive fibroblastic activity, an integral part of the general myelo-

TABLE 3-2   CLASSIFICATION OF POLYCYTHEMIAS
AND ANEMIAS

Polycythemias
       Dehydration
       "Stress", "Spurious", "Tobacco"
   Absolute
    Primary
       Polycythemia Vera
    Secondary
      Appropriate
       Altitude
       Cardio-pulmonary disease
       Hemoglobin abnormality
       Cobalt
      Inappropriate
       Renal cyst and tumor
       Various neoplasms

Anemias
   Relative
      Pregnancy
      Macroglobulinemia
   Absolute
    Stem Cell Disorders
     Multipotential
      Aplastic Anemia
     Unipotential
      Anemia of renal disease
      Anemia of chronic disease
      Anemia of endocrine disorders
      Pure red cell aplasia

    Multiplication Disorders
     Vitamin B_{12} deficiency
     Folate deficiency
     Refractory megaloblastic anemias
     Antimetabolite therapy (methotrexate, 6 mercaptopurine)

    Cytoplasmic Maturation Disorders
     Porphyrias
      Hereditary porphyrias
      Acquired porphyrias (lead poisoning)

stimulatory disease process. The reduction in available bone marrow space and the increase in splenic size will lead first to anemia and eventually to pancytopenia.

Acute myelogenous leukemia develops ultimately in about 10 to 15 per cent of patients with polycythemia vera. The occurrence of this dreaded complication has been reviewed by Modan and Lilienfeld and it was believed initially to be related to the therapeutic use of radioactive phosphorus. Recent reports, however, suggest that the use of so-called radiomimetic agents such as busulfan also may be followed by the development of acute myelogenous leukemia. Polycythemia vera was the first "neoplastic" disease with a long enough survival to make possible prolonged follow-up studies after the use of myelosuppressive agents. The more recent successes in the treatment of Hodgkin's disease, breast cancer, chronic lymphatic leukemia, and transplantation rejection have permitted similar prolonged follow-ups after the use of other forms of radiation or radiomimetic drugs, and it has become clear that the development of acute myelogenous leukemia is an appreciable therapeutic hazard. So far the therapeutic results have been well worth the risk, but obviously these agents should be used with reluctance and caution.

Secondary. Secondary polycythemia is a condition characterized by an enhanced, erythropoietin-mediated stimulation of red cell production and an increased red cell mass. In most cases the erythropoietin release is an appropriate response to tissue hypoxia, but in some the

TABLE 3–2 *Continued* CLASSIFICATION OF
POLYCYTHEMIAS AND ANEMIAS

    Iron
        Iron deficiency anemia
        Iron loading anemias
    Globin
        Structural Abnormality
            Hemoglobinopathies (Sickle Cell Anemia)
        Quantitative Abnormality
            Thalassemias

Survival Disorders
   Intrinsic
        Hereditary spherocytosis
        Hereditary elliptocytosis
        Paroxysmal nocturnal hemoglobinuria
        Enzymopathies (G-6-PD, P.K.)
        Hemoglobinopathies
   Extrinsic
    Toxic Factors
        Thermal burn
        Chemical damage
        Infection (malaria)
        Hyperoxia (hyperbaric conditions)
        Oxidative hemolysis due to drugs (sulfonamides)
    Hypersplenism
    Mechanical Factors
        March hemoglobinuria
        Traumatic cardiac hemolysis
        Microangiopathic hemolytic anemia
    Plasma Lipid Abnormality
        Spur cell anemia of cirrhosis
        Hereditary acanthocytosis
    Immune Hemolysis
        Isoimmune
            Transfusion reaction
            Erythroblastosis fetalis
        Autoimmune
            Cold type
            Warm type
   Blood Loss
        Acute blood loss anemia

most cases the erythropoietin release is an appropriate response to tissue hypoxia, but in some the release is inappropriate and the resulting erythrocytosis presumably serves no useful function.

APPROPRIATE SECONDARY POLYCYTHEMIA

High Altitude. The erythrocytosis experienced by high altitude dwellers is probably the most common of the secondary polycythemias and it must be considered an appropriate physiologic adaptation rather than a pathologic disorder. However, sustained physiologic adaptations are usually achieved at a certain biologic cost, and individuals at high altitudes pay for an enhanced oxygen transport by problems related to hypervolemia, hyperviscosity, and hyperventilation.

Most studies of high-altitude polycythemia have been carried out in the small town of Morococha at 15,000 feet in the Peruvian Andes. Only a few precarious settlements exist above this altitude, the highest permanent settlement probably being Aucanguilcha in the Chilean Andes at 17,500 feet. At this level the atmospheric oxygen pressure is not much higher than the mean capillary oxygen pressure at sea level, making it very difficult to provide a downhill gradient for oxygen from air to cells. Above 17,500 feet only short-term sojourns are possible and no one has yet managed to reach the top of the world, Mt Everest, at 29,000 feet without being sustained by supplemental oxygen (Fig. 3–16).

The ability of the inhabitants of the mining town of Morococha to live active, strenuous lives

TABLE 3–3   DIFFERENTIAL DIAGNOSIS
OF POLYCYTHEMIAS

	Relative Polycythemia	Polycythemia Vera	Secondary Polycythemia
Hematocrit	Increased	Increased	Increased
Red blood cell mass	Normal	Increased	Increased
Erythropoietin	Normal	Absent	Increased
White blood count	Normal	Increased	Normal
Platelet count	Normal	Increased	Normal
Bone marrow	Normal	Hyperplastic	Erythroid hyperplasia
Spleen	Normal	Enlarged	Normal
Arterial oxygen saturation	Normal	Normal	Decreased or normal
Serum iron	Normal	Decreased	Normal
Serum B$_{12}$	Normal	Increased	Normal
Leukocyte alkaline phosphatase	Normal	Increased	Normal
Muramidase	Normal	Increased	Normal

at 15,000 feet is directly related to their adaptable oxygen transport system. The tissue requirements for oxygen are the same as or higher than at sea level, but increased pulmonary function, increased oxygen carrying capacity of blood and increased blood volume succeed in reducing the oxygen gradient needed to bring oxygen from the air to the tissues (Fig. 3–17). Such a reduction will ensure that the oxygen molecules in the capillaries are under enough pressure for their subsequent diffusion into the tissues.

Sustained hyperventilation causes a reduction in the oxygen gradient between ambient and alveolar air. Because of the inherent effect of dead space and water vapors, this part of the gradient can only be moderately reduced. However, hyperventilation causes a pulmonary "stretch" with enlargement of the alveolar diffusing area and almost eliminates the alveolar-capillary gradient. The most important reduction occurs in the arterial-venous gradient, permitting unloading of oxygen throughout the length of the capillary at a relatively high pressure. Since the tissue demands for oxygen are not reduced, the maintenance of a shallow gradient demands an increased flow of oxygen-carrying red blood cells through the tissues. Although an increase in cardiac output would accomplish just this, the added workload on a vital organ is unacceptable for chronic adjustments. Of more importance for the maintenance of an increased oxygen flow to the tissues is an increase in the red blood cell count.

Tissue hypoxia will lead to the release of erythropoietin which in turn will increase the rate of red cell production and enhance the oxygen carrying capacity of blood. Furthermore, the increased rate of red cell production will cause an increase in blood volume, with dilatation and opening of vessels, and an increase in tissue perfusion. This dual effect on oxygen flow far outweighs the moderate disadvantages derived from the higher viscosity of circulating blood.

A shift in the oxygen dissociation curve to the right would also reduce the arteriovenous gradient and enhance the unloading of oxygen in the

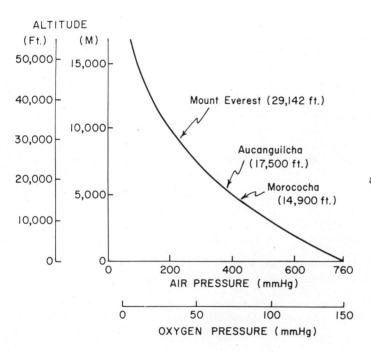

Figure 3–16   The oxygen pressure at altitudes inhabited or visited by man.

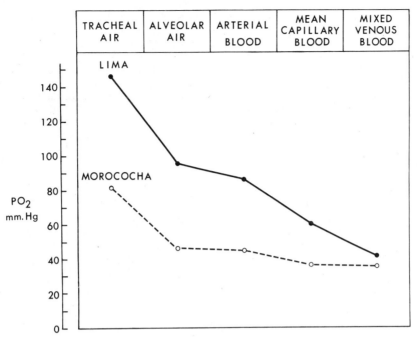

TRACHEAL AIR	ALVEOLAR AIR	ARTERIAL BLOOD	MEAN CAPILLARY BLOOD	MIXED VENOUS BLOOD

Figure 3–17 The oxygen gradient from lungs to tissues at sea level (Lima) or at 15,000 feet (Morococha). (Redrawn from Hurtado, A.: *In* Weihe, W. H. (ed.): Physiological Effects of High Altitude. New York, Pergamon Press, 1964, p.1.)

tissue capillaries (Fig. 3–18). Such a shift is undoubtedly of great importance in the initial adaptation to high altitudes, especially since it will tend to counteract the disadvantageous shift to the left induced by acute hyperventilation alkalosis. However, it is less certain whether it plays a significant role in chronic acclimatization. At that point the blood pH is usually normal and, as emphasized by Finch and Lenfant, an excessive shift to the right might significantly reduce the loading of hemoglobin in the lungs, an important consideration when the ambient oxygen pressure is about one half normal. It is of interest that the animals indigenous to high altitudes such as llamas and vicunas have oxygen dissociation curves positioned far to the left, suggesting that the adjustments of the shape of the curve in sustained acclimatization is aimed at improving the loading of oxygen in the lungs rather than at the unloading in the tissues.

The clinical manifestation of chronic high altitude acclimatization is dominated by ruddy cyanosis and physiologic emphysema. The vascular enlargement can be observed readily in the conjunctiva, mucous membrane, and skin and may contribute to the remarkable capacity of Sherpas to walk barefoot and sleep on ice and snow.

The blood studies reveal a normochromic and normocytic erythrocytosis, with increased red cell mass but only borderline increases in granulocyte or platelet counts. The plasma iron concentration is normal in contradistinction to polycythemia vera, in which it is usually low. This may be due merely to blood loss and to therapeutic phlebotomies in polycythemia vera, but it has been suggested that tissue hypoxia as experienced at high altitudes enhances intestinal iron absorption. Erythropoietin titers in plasma and urine are increased, also in contradistinction to polycythemia vera, in which they are extremely low.

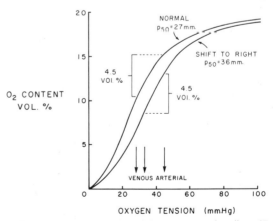

Figure 3–18 At low arterial oxygen tension (i.e., 45 mm.) the delivery of 4.5 vol % of oxygen from normal hemoglobin with a P_{50} of 27 mm. will reduce venous oxygen tension to 28 mm. A shift to the right, however, will permit the delivery of the same volume of oxygen with less reduction in venous oxygen tension (33 mm.).

It is difficult to evaluate the biologic cost of chronic acclimatization to high altitudes, since very few reliable data on the longevity and morbidity of high altitude dwellers exist. However, the compensatory reserves are undoubtedly decreased and the effect of cardiopulmonary disorders must be more serious than at sea level. So-called "chronic mountain sickness" (Monge's disease) is caused by an acquired refractoriness of the respiratory center leading to relative alveolar hypoventilation and excessive tissue hypoxia. Since this in turn will cause an increase in an already expanded red cell mass and higher blood viscosity, cardiovascular decompensation occurs. Therapeutic venesection provides symptomatic relief, but the individuals suffering from Monge's disease usually need to be brought down to sea level for permanent improvement.

Pulmonary Disease. Chronic pulmonary disease associated with cyanosis, clubbing, and arterial oxygen unsaturation is not always accompanied by an increase in hemoglobin concentration (Fig. 3–19). In some cases a concomitant increase in plasma volume may conceal the effect of an increased red cell mass, but in most cases true secondary polycythemia does not occur. The release of erythropoietin appears to be commensurate to the degree of tissue hypoxia, but for unknown reasons there is an unresponsiveness of the stem cells to this hormone or an impairment in the subsequent proliferation of nucleated red cells.

Cardiovascular Disease. Right-to-left shunt in congenital heart disease is characteristically associated with cyanosis, clubbing, and often extreme secondary appropriate polycythemia. Despite high hematocrit, hyperviscosity symptoms are rarely present, probably owing to the simultaneous increase in total blood volume. Whether or not to perform phlebotomy on blue babies prior to surgery is still an unanswered question, but most surgeons feel more comfortable if the hematocrit is brought down below 60 per cent by judicious phlebotomies. It certainly will provide a little more reserve if fluid intake becomes inadequate.

In acquired heart disease with chronic decompensation, erythrokinetic studies by Chodos and co-workers have shown that a mild increase in red cell production and red cell mass is usually present. However, the increased plasma volume prevents an accurate assessment of the size of the red cell mass from hematocrit determinations alone.

Alveolar Hypoventilation. Alveolar hypoventilation, whether related to central or peripheral impairment, causes arterial hypoxemia, cyanosis, and secondary polycythemia. Its two most colorful variants are Monge's chronic mountain sickness (see earlier) and the Pickwickian syndrome. In the latter syndrome, named by Ratto and co-workers, obesity, peripheral hypoventilation, hypercapnia, somnolence and central hypoventilation are involved in a vicious circle lead-

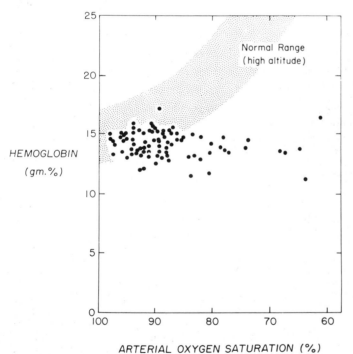

Figure 3–19 Hemoglobin concentrations of patients with various degrees of arterial oxygen desaturation due to chronic pulmonary disease. (Redrawn from Gallo, R.C., et al.: Arch. Intern, Med., *113*:559, 1964. Copyright 1964, American Medical Association.)

ing to the proverbial somnolent cyanosis of Mrs. Wardle's boy, Joe.

Defective Oxygen Transport. Secondary polycythemia is occasionally observed in patients with cyanosis due to acquired or congenital methemoglobinemia. However, the erythropoietic response in these patients is less than would be anticipated in cyanotic patients. Cyanosis may actually be present with as little as 1.5 grams of methemoglobin per 100 ml. in the circulation, an amount which in itself should not result in significant tissue hypoxia. An increase in oxygen affinity is also present in hemoglobin partially combined with carbon monoxide and is probably responsible for the polycythemia observed in heavy smokers.

Familial polycythemias have recently been described in a number of individuals with abnormal hemoglobins. In most of these, the amino acid substitution occurs in the contact area between the alpha and beta chains. Such substitutions interfere with the release of oxygen to the tissues, decrease the P_{50} and result in a compensatory erythrocytosis despite fully oxygenated arterial blood.

Drug-induced Tissue Hypoxia. Although a number of drugs and chemicals can induce histiotoxic anoxia, only cobalt has convincingly been associated with the development of a secondary appropriate polycythemia. Several recent studies have shown that cobalt administration causes the release of erythropoietin, and that this release presumably is related to its inhibitory effect on intracellular oxidative metabolism in the kidneys. Since histiotoxic anoxia is generalized (Fig. 3–8), the use of cobalt in the treatment of refractory anemias is of little benefit to the patient. His oxygen carrying capacity may increase, but merely enough to counteract the effect of the additional tissue hypoxia induced by cobalt.

INAPPROPRIATE SECONDARY POLYCYTHEMIA (TABLE 3–4)

Renal Disorders. A partial obstruction of the renal artery or its tributaries may cause localized renal hypoxia, the stimulus for erythropoietin production. However, an impaired blood supply to the kidneys usually causes structural damage and impaired erythropoietin production, and it is only the rare patient who responds with an increased release of erythropoietin and a secondary polycythemia. It is of potential importance that intrarenal vascular obstruction as observed in transplanted kidneys undergoing rejection will cause the release of erythropoietin. Unfortunately, the current assays are too laborious to permit the erythropoietin titer to be used to detect threatening rejection. However, the appearance of an increased number of nucleated red cells or reticulocytes in the circulating blood may be used as a warning signal.

TABLE 3–4 INAPPROPRIATE SECONDARY POLYCYTHEMIA

Location	Pathologic Condition	Number of Case Reports Until 1972
Kidney		
	Hypernephroma	118
	Other tumors	13
	Hydronephrosis	14
	Cystic disease	35
	Renal artery stenosis	2
	Transplantation rejection	7
	Bartter's syndrome	1
Liver		
	Hepatoma	64
Uterus		
	Leiomyoma	24
Cerebellum		
	Hemangioblastoma	50
Adrenal Gland		
	Pheochromocytoma	5

(Data from Thorling, E. B.: Scand. J. Haemat., Suppl. 17, 1972.)

A more common cause of secondary polycythemia is the presence of space-occupying renal lesions. These lesions can be cysts, either solitary or part of polycystic renal disease, hydronephrosis, or a variety of renal neoplasms. Erythropoietin assays of cyst fluid have disclosed the presence of erythropoietin, and it has been proposed that the tubular lining of cysts is capable of secreting erythropoietin. In regard to the neoplasms, assays of tumor extracts, especially extracts of hypernephromas, for erythropoietin have occasionally been positive. However, the fact that so many histologically different lesions can lead to an excessive production of erythropoietin has raised the suspicion that it is not the tumor cells which are engaged in inappropriate erythropoietin production, but it is the adjoining normal parenchyma which secretes this hormone in response to pressure-induced hypoxia.

Successful removal of renal tumors in patients with polycythemia has in many cases resulted in a normalization of the red blood cell count. Subsequent metastases in the opposite kidney have been associated with a recurrence of the polycythemia. However, the important question of whether or not extrarenal metastases can cause polycythemia has still not been answered.

Extrarenal Disorders. Cerebellar hemangiomas are an infrequent cause of secondary, inappropriate polycythemia. Cyst fluid from the tumor has, in a few cases, been shown to contain erythropoietic stimulatory material indistinguishable from erythropoietin. However, the proximity of the tumor to the respiratory center and to the hypothalamus has also suggested that central hypoventilation plays a role or that a hypothetical hypothalamic-renal connection is involved. In areas such as Hong Kong with a high incidence of hepatocarcinoma, 10 per cent of afflicted patients develop erythrocytosis. The most favored explanation is that the tumor is responsible for inappropriate secretion of erythropoietin, an explanation supported by direct assays of tumor extracts and by the finding that the liver normally produces small amounts of extrarenal erythropoietin. The rare polycythemia observed in patients with large uterine myomas may be caused by mechanical interference with renal blood supply. An inappropriate neoplastic production of erythropoietin by these fibrous, differentiated tumors seems unlikely in view of their histologic character. The occasional association with certain endocrine lesions such as Cushing's syndrome and pheochromocytomas is intriguing but has not been too informative. Steroid hormones appear to stimulate bone marrow activity mildly but the relationship between hypertension and erythropoietin is still quite tenuous. Although androgen-producing lesions have not been associated with polycythemia, androgens have empirically been found to be potent stimulators of erythropoiesis. This was first pointed out by Kennedy and co-workers, who 20 years ago observed the development of plethora and high hematocrits in women treated with androgens for breast cancer. The effect may be mediated via a release of renal erythropoietin, although some data suggest a direct action of androgens on the bone marrow stem cell pool.

ANEMIA

General Effects of Anemia

The pathophysiologic effects of a reduced oxygen carrying capacity of blood are all related to tissue hypoxia and to the compensatory mechanisms mobilized to alleviate this hypoxia. Tissue hypoxia occurs when the pressure head of oxygen in the capillaries is too low to provide distant cells with enough oxygen for their metabolic needs. This may happen despite the presence of several times the needed oxygen in the circulating blood. Using approximate figures for a normal adult, the red cell mass has to provide the tissues with about 250 ml. of oxygen per minute to support life. Since the oxygen-carrying capacity of normal blood is 1.34 ml. per gram hemoglobin or about 20 ml. per 100 ml. of normal blood and the cardiac output is about 5000 ml. per minute, 1000 ml. of oxygen per minute is made available at the tissue level. The extraction of one fourth of this amount will reduce the oxygen tension of 100 mm. Hg in the arterial end of the capillary to 40 mm. Hg in the venous end. This partial extraction will maintain a diffusion pressure throughout the capillaries sufficient to provide all cells within a truncated cone segment with enough oxygen for their metabolism (Fig. 3–20). In anemia, the extraction of the same amount of oxygen would lead to greater hemoglobin desaturation and a lower oxygen tension at the venous end of the capillary. Since this would result in destructive cellular hypoxia or anoxia in the immediate vicinity, compensatory and frequently symptomatic adjustment in the supply of blood and oxygen must be mobilized in order to keep the oxygen gradient almost unchanged (see review by Finch and Lenfant in 1977).

Decreased Oxygen Affinity. One of the earliest and least traumatic adjustments is a shift in the oxygen dissociation curve to the right, permitting the extraction of increased amounts of oxygen without a decrease in oxygen pressure. As mentioned before, the position of the oxygen dissociation curve is in part dependent on the intracellular pH. At an acid pH, as experienced in tissues in which anemic hypoxia has led to anaerobic metabolism and lactic acid accumulation, the curve will be shifted to the right, the so-called Bohr effect (Fig. 3–3). More important, however, is a stimulation of the production of 2,3 diphosphoglycerate. The reason for this stimulation in anemia is not clear, but it has been suggested that the binding of free 2,3-DPG to deoxygenated hemoglobin, present in increased amounts in anemia, will result in a compensatory increase in glycolysis and 2,3-DPG production. Alternately, deoxygenated hemoglobin may cause enough intracellular alkalosis to stimulate glycosis and 2,3-DPG production. The binding of 2,3-DPG to reduced hemoglobin stabilizes the molecule in its low-affinity state and facilitates the unloading of oxygen in the tissues. According to Torrance et al., this change in oxygen affinity plays a substantial role in reducing the arteriovenous oxygen pressure gradient and in minimizing cellular hypoxia (Fig. 3–21).

Increased Tissue Perfusion. Redistribution of blood from tissues with fairly low oxygen requirements and high blood supply such as skin or kidneys to oxygen-dependent tissues such as brain and myocardium provides an early and efficient protection of these vital tissues. The metabolic price for maintaining a high oxygen tension in some selective organs or tissues appears reasonable. Subcutaneous vasoconstriction and oxygen deprivation are tolerated well, since dermal blood supply is geared more toward temperature regulation than toward oxygen delivery. The same is true for the kidney, in which the blood supply is far in excess of the oxygen requirement. The effect on renal excretory function is relatively minor, since

Partial O₂

Extraction

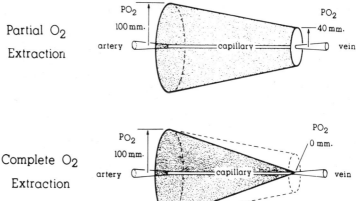

Figure 3–20 A hypothetical model of the tissue cone provided by oxygen when the blood is partially or completely extracted of oxygen.

Complete O₂

Extraction

the decrease in blood supply is offset by the increase in "plasma crit" of the perfusing anemic blood.

Increased Cardiac Output. In mild to moderate anemia, the combined effects of decreased oxygen affinity and selective redistribution of blood maintain oxygen pressure at close to normal levels, and these anemias are usually quite asymptomatic. However, with more severe anemias it becomes necessary to increase cardiac output in order to provide the tissues with enough oxygen. Although the low viscosity of anemic blood and the peripheral vasodilatation reduce the workload on the heart, the metabolic cost and the wear and tear on the moving part of the cardiac pump make an increase in cardiac output an undesirable device for long-term compensation.

The clinical manifestations of severe anemia are to a great extent caused by the compensatory cardiac overactivity. Pallor is due primarily to dermal vasoconstriction and blood redistribution, but tachycardia and symptoms of decreased cardiac reserve are related to cardiac stress. The characteristic shortness of breath of severe anemia may be a sign of incipient cardiopulmonary failure rather than a manifestation of ventilatory compensation to the anemia. Owing to the almost complete saturation of anemic blood with oxygen in the lungs, a pulmonary compensation would actually be of little practical importance.

Increased Red Cell Production. The most appropriate but also the slowest compensatory device in anemia is an increase in the rate of red cell production. Tissue hypoxia will lead to increased erythropoietin production within four to seven hours, but owing to the time lag from stem cell differentiation to the release of reticulocytes from the bone marrow, a compensatory increase in the number of circulating red cells does not begin until four to five days later. Increased erythropoietin titers in serum and urine (Fig. 3–11) causing increased bone marrow activity may be associated with sternal pain or tenderness and

the presence of large immature reticulocytes on the blood smear.

These compensatory mechanisms are all designed to keep the capillary oxygen pressure up and the oxygen delivery adequate for the cellular needs. However, a complete rectification of tissue hypoxia cannot occur until the hemoglobin concentration has been restored to normal. Some degree of tissue hypoxia is needed in order to provide a driving force for the various compensatory devices. The symptomatology of such remaining hypoxia is difficult to separate from that of the compensatory mechanisms, but leg cramps, angina pectoris, and light-headedness appear to be caused directly by tissue hypoxia.

Stem Cell Disorders

Under physiologic conditions, the red cell mass is maintained at an optimal size by appropriate adjustments in the rate of transformation of stem cells to nucleated red blood cells. These adjustments are accomplished by feedback systems, and

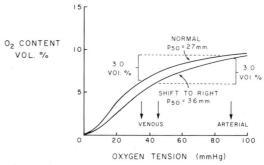

Figure 3–21 This figure depicts the effect on venous oxygen tension when 3.0 vol. % of oxygen is extracted from normal hemoglobin in an anemic individual. A shift to the right will permit this extraction of 3 vol. % with less reduction in venous oxygen tension and therefore an enhanced tissue oxygenation.

a disruption at any point in the circuits of these systems will lead to disordered stem cell function and anemia. A disordered function of the multipotential stem cells such as observed in patients with aplastic anemia is usually believed to be caused by an intrinsic defect of the stem cells themselves. However, very little is known of their regulation, and it is possible that cellular dysfunction is secondary to defective feedback signals from the immediate microenvironment.

The feedback system regulating the unipotential erythropoietin-sensitive stem cells is much better understood, and it is now possible to relate various aregenerative anemias to defects in specific key stations in this circuit. The major distinction between disorders of the multipotential and the unipotential stem cells is that multipotential stem cell disorders are characterized by pancytopenia and unipotential stem cell disorders by erythrocytopenia.

Disorders of Multipotential Stem Cells

APLASTIC ANEMIA.   Aplastic anemia is a bone marrow disorder characterized by a reduction in the number and function of multipotential stem cells. This reduction leads in turn to a decrease in the volume of active blood-cell–producing bone marrow and to a pancytopenia. The remaining marrow becomes confined to small, often intensely active islands surrounded by fatty tissue. This fatty replacement is the sine qua non of true aplastic anemia.

The clinical manifestations are all directly related to the pancytopenia. The anemia may cause weakness, fatigue, and pallor; the granulocytopenia may cause fever and infections; and the thrombocytopenia may cause hemorrhages, hematomas, and petechiae. Hepatomegaly and splenomegaly are unusual findings in the early phase of the disease and their presence should lead to reevaluation of the diagnosis. However, after prolonged illness, recurrent infections may produce a reactive macrophage hyperplasia of the spleen, and transfusion hemosiderosis may lead to hepatomegaly and congestive splenomegaly.

The anemia is often macrocytic, and the reticulocytes are few in number but relatively immature. These findings reflect an accelerated bone marrow transit time and release, possibly caused by a high level of erythropoietin or by the crowded environment in the remaining bone marrow islands. Ferrokinetic studies reveal a reduced plasma iron turnover but this reduction may be difficult to appreciate, since the normal baseline value is quite low.

Of greater importance for the demonstration of a reduced rate of red cell production are the iron clearance time and the red cell utilization of iron. The reduced bone marrow mass can clear iron from plasma only slowly, giving extramedullary tissues such as liver or spleen extra time in which to compete with the marrow for circulating radio-active iron. The result is a prolonged iron clearance time and a low red cell iron utilization. This combination is characteristic for all anemias caused by a reduction in erythropoietic tissue and distinguishes them from anemias caused by ineffective red cell production. In the latter anemias, intramedullary destruction of nucleated red cells will also cause a low utilization of radioactive iron, but the iron clearance is short because of an abundance of erythropoietic bone marrow (Fig. 3–22). This distinction is of particular importance in establishing whether pancytopenia is caused by bone marrow hypoplasia or by ineffective cellular production. This latter condition has been called "aplastic anemia with a hyperplastic bone marrow," a confusing term for a condition that often is preleukemic and may be pathogenetically quite different from aplastic anemia.

Both plasma iron and erythropoietin concentrations are high in aplastic anemia, probably reflecting decreased utilization by a reduced bone marrow mass. The high plasma iron concentration may cause excessive tissue incorporation of iron and eventually hemosiderosis. Bone marrow preparations disclose many siderotic granules in the reticulum cells, but since maturation of the individual nucleated red cells is normal, siderotic granules in these cells are seen only rarely. The high erythropoietin titer in plasma and urine has made patients with aplastic anemia useful sources for the preparation of erythropoietin concentrates.

In some patients with aplastic anemia, particularly in children, there may be a substantial increase in the production of fetal hemoglobin. This challenging but still unexplained finding is of great potential interest, since it may provide a clue for the mechanism by which gamma chain production can be activated, a mechanism of potential use for patients with sickle cell anemia or Cooley's anemia.

Absolute granulocytopenia is always present in aplastic anemia and its severity will determine to a great extent the immediate prognosis. As a rough guide, an absolute granulocyte count of less than 200 per cu. mm. suggests imminent danger of infectious complications and demands some kind of a sheltered environment. In addition to an absolute granulocytopenia, there is often a reduction in the total number of lymphocytes. The reason for this reduction is not known but the functional significance is apparently of little importance, since immunoglobulin synthesis and delayed sensitivity reactions are usually intact.

Thrombocytopenia with its dramatic and visible hemorrhagic manifestations is also always part of the clinical picture of advanced aplastic anemia. Because of the insidious onset of this disease, it is difficult to assess the sequence by which the various cytopenias appear. However, during the recovery phase, thrombocytopoiesis is often the last

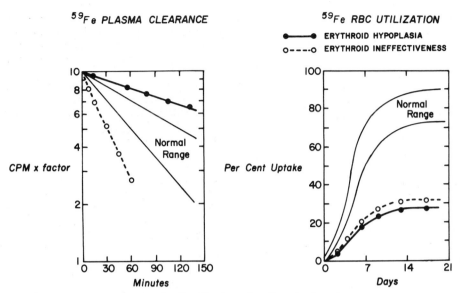

Figure 3–22 Plasma clearance and red cell utilization of radioactive iron in normals, patients with erythroid hypoplasia, and patients with ineffective red cell production. The clearance rate of ^{59}Fe injected intravenously at time 0 was determined by serial measurements of the radioactivity (C.P.M.) over a 3-hour period. The subsequent utilization of the ^{59}Fe for hemoglobin synthesis was estimated by measuring the total radioactivity in circulating red cells (Red cell mass × C.P.M.) and relating it in per cent to the total amount of ^{59}Fe injected. Although the utilization of ^{59}Fe is equally reduced in patients with erythroid hypoplasia or with erythroid ineffectiveness, the plasma clearance rate readily separates them from each other.

bone marrow function to recover and many patients may have thrombocytopenia for years after the other cytopenias have been corrected.

Etiology and Pathogenesis (Table 3–5). Numerous drugs, illnesses, and physical agents have the capacity to alter stem cell function presumably by interfering with intracellular metabolism.

TABLE 3–5 ETIOLOGIC CLASSIFICATION OF APLASTIC ANEMIA

I. Idiopathic
 A. *Constitutional* (Fanconi's anemia)
 B. *Acquired*

II. Secondary
 A. *Chemical and physical agents*
  Drugs
  Nonpharmacologic chemicals
  Radiation
 B. *Infectious*
  Viral (Hepatitis)
  Bacterial (Miliary TB)
 C. *Metabolic*
  Pancreatitis
  Pregnancy
 D. *Immunologic*
  Antibody
  Graft-vs.-host
 E. *Neoplastic*
  Myelophthisic anemia
 F. *Paroxysmal nocturnal hemoglobinuria*

However, these agents could also alter the stem cell microenvironment, and the relative importance of "seed" and "soil" in the pathogenesis of aplastic anemia is still not resolved. Although statistical and clinical cause-effect relationships between a specific agent or event and the development of aplastic anemia can be quite impressive, aplastic anemia is a disease in which the etiology can be only suspected, not established. No in-vitro test system is capable of duplicating the in-vivo events, and in-vivo tests in patients are too potentially dangerous to be justified. This makes the designation of an etiologic agent a question of judgment and clinical experience, hallowed but quite vulnerable criteria. In patients without exposure to a suggestive etiologic agent, the term "idiopathic" is used to conceal our ignorance. Obviously, even in these cases an etiologic agent must exist and may be present among the host of environmental toxins which have become part of our civilized existence.

Drugs and Chemicals. The drugs suspected of being potentially toxic for the hematopoietic stem cells have been listed in booklets published by the American Medical Association in 1965 and 1967 and include about 329 items. (See also review by Williams and co-workers, 1973). Table 3–6 lists those drugs with a strong etiologic relationship to aplastic anemia. It is a difficult list to interpret, since it does not give the actual incidence, the number of cases per number of patients receiving

TABLE 3–6 DRUGS LISTED BY A.M.A. AS BEING ASSOCIATED WITH THE DEVELOPMENT OF APLASTIC ANEMIA IN MORE THAN FIVE INSTANCES

	Number of Cases Receiving Drug Alone, or Drug in Combination with Nontoxic Drugs	Number of Cases Receiving Drug in Combination with Potentially Toxic Drug
Acetazolamide	3	7
Chloramphenicol	182	156
Chlordiazepoxide HCl	2	7
Chlorothiazide	2	13
Chlorpheniramine	2	15
Chlorpromazine	3	18
Chlorpropamide	4	2
Colchicine	2	3
Diphenylhydantoin sodium	3	21
Epinephrine	2	4
Gold salts	8	2
Mepazine	4	1
Meprobamate		15
Penicillin	4	91
Phenacetin	3	31
Phenantoin	9	14
Phenylbutazone	18	22
Potassium perchlorate	6	4
Primidone	2	6
Prochlorperazine	1	9
Pyrimethamine	2	3
Quinacrine HCl	3	2
Salicylamide	2	3
Streptomycin		31
Sulfadimethoxine	2	4
Sulfamethoxypyridazine	3	11
Sulfisoxazole	3	30
Sulfonamides	4	17
Tolbutamide	7	5
Trimethadione	2	4

the particular drug. However, it is possible to make a mental adjustment and realize that the incidence of aplastic anemia following treatment with aspirin or penicillin must be much lower than that following treatment with phenantoin, gold salts, or phenylbutazone. Furthermore, the incidence following treatment with the nitrobenzene compound chloramphenicol must be far higher than that following treatment with any other commonly used drug.

Many attempts have been made to relate potential toxicity to the presence of a benzene or nitrobenzene radical in the chemical structure of suspected drugs. Benzene itself is a major bone marrow toxin capable of inducing both aplastic anemia and leukemia, and in addition to chloramphenicol, many benzene-related chemicals such as trinitrotoluene, toluene, and the insecticides lindane and DDT have been strongly suspected of

inducing aplastic anemia. However, many drugs without the benzene radical also appear to be toxic to stem cells, and the common denominator may reside in an intermediate metabolic product rather than in the parent molecule.

Because of the high incidence of aplastic anemia in patients receiving chloramphenicol special efforts have been made to clarify the mechanism of the toxic action of this drug on the bone marrow. Although we talk about "high" incidence, it has to be emphasized that only one out of 10,000 to 20,000 treated patients develops aplastic anemia and that prospective metabolic studies are almost impossible. However, mild, reversible bone marrow suppression is observed in most treated patients, a suppression related to drug dosage and length of treatment. Clinically it can easily be recognized by a decrease in reticulocyte counts and an increase in serum iron concentration. Bone marrow examination reveals vacuolization of erythroid cells. After prolonged treatment vacuolization can be observed in other cellular elements as well, and granulocytopenia and thrombocytopenia may ensue. These effects were initially thought to be related to a suppressive action on the ribosomal protein synthesis similar to the action of chloramphenicol on the bacterial cells. However, in-vitro studies of bone marrow suspensions by Yunis and co-workers have suggested that in the mammalian cell chloramphenicol inhibits mitochondrial protein synthesis. Since many consider the mitochondria to be intracellular inclusions of plant origin with independent mechanisms for replication and metabolism, this finding could provide a link between the bacteriostatic and the bone marrow suppressive actions of chloramphenicol.

It is tempting to consider the suppressive action of the bone marrow as an early, still reversible manifestation of a stem cell injury which eventually leads to irreversible aplastic anemia. However, it seems more likely that patients who develop aplastic anemia have an abnormal response to the bone marrow suppressive effect of chloramphenicol. Not only is the regularly occurring suppression readily reversible even after prolonged treatment with large amounts of chloramphenicol, but many patients who develop aplastic anemia do so weeks or months after exposure to relatively small amounts of this drug. It has been proposed that the few unfortunate victims have an underlying genetic or acquired hypersensitivity to chloramphenicol. This could reside in the rate or extent of detoxification of the drug or in a specific stem cell abnormality. In-vitro studies of bone marrow from patients who have recovered from aplastic anemia or from their immediate relatives have suggested a greater than normal susceptibility to the suppressive action of chloramphenicol. However, we are still far from having established the pathogenetic mode of action of chloramphenicol or from having learned how to predict individual hypersensitivity to this or to other potentially toxic drugs.

Radiation. Bone marrow suppression is a well-recognized side-effect of the diagnostic and therapeutic use of radiation. Radiation energy, whether mediated by a direct hit of waves or particles or by the production of highly reactive free radicals, is capable of breaking molecular bonds in critical intracellular macromolecules. Although all cells can be injured by radiation energy, organ systems dependent on a rapid cellular turnover of nucleic acids are particularly vulnerable. These systems can be ranked, according to Cronkite and Bond, with regard to radiosensitivity as follows: (1) germinal cells of the testes, (2) hematopoietic cells, (3) intestinal cells, and (4) epidermal basal cells.

Brief exposure to radiation of high energy as in reactor accidents leads to extensive destruction of the bone marrow and intestine, and death is usually caused by acute granulocytopenia and thrombocytopenia and by intestinal ulcerations. If the patient should survive the acute effects the recovery is usually almost complete, since the dormant multipotential stem cells will have sustained very little radiation injury and are capable of bone marrow repopulation. In the aftermath of the atomic attacks on Nagasaki, for example, Kirschbaum and his Japanese co-workers found that aplastic anemia was observed in only a very small number of survivors.

Prolonged exposure to more moderate doses of radiation, on the other hand, may cause chronic bone marrow failure and aplastic anemia. This has been described in patients vigorously treated with external or internal total body radiation and in Martland's famous report on watch-dial painters who accidentally ingested paint containing radium with a long biologic half-life. It has also been suspected as a pathogenetic mechanism in aplastic anemia occurring in physicians or radiologists exposed to minimal amounts of radiation for many years, but as is the case for exposure to drugs and chemicals a definite cause-effect relationship can never be firmly established. The reason for defective bone marrow repopulation after chronic radiation exposure may reside in the fact that multipotential stem cells are activated and then share in the radiation injury. An alternative explanation for the development of aplastic anemia after chronic radiation has been provided by Knospe and co-workers; namely, that radiation-induced damage to the "endothelial stem cells" will change the structural microenvironment of the bone marrow and prevent bone marrow regeneration.

Immunologic Rejection. Aplastic anemia has been associated with a variety of seemingly unrelated diseases. Miliary tuberculosis has always been listed prominently among such disorders, but a critical evaluation of reported cases indicates that this association is rare indeed. Hepatitis with its many immunologic manifestations looms much larger as a possible etiologic event, and aplastic anemia associated with complement-sensitive red cells and nocturnal hemoglobinuria has been described so frequently by Lewis and Dacie in England and Vincent and de Gruchy in Australia that this combination ought to contain some clue to etiology or pathogenesis.

The most reasonable explanation is that an immunologic mechanism underlies the development of aplastic anemia. Support for this hypothesis is that aplastic anemia has been described after the transfusion of whole blood or bone marrow into immunologically deficient children. Miller has suggested that the disease in these unfortunate patients reflects a graft-versus-host immunologic rejection of either hematopoietic or structural stem cells. The therapeutic implication of such a concept would be to use immunosuppressive drugs, a most difficult decision to make because of the inherent bone marrow suppressive effect of currently used drugs. The effect of prednisone in aplastic anemia has unfortunately been too erratic to be of use in pathogenetic considerations and at present the possibility that aplastic anemia is another "autoimmune" disorder is merely a hypothesis.

Constitutional. Fanconi's anemia is a form of aplastic anemia which occurs as an inborn defect associated with other congenital abnormalities such as skin pigmentations, renal hypoplasia, absent thumb or radius, and microcephaly. Multiple abnormalities of the chromosomal pattern of lymphocytes and bone marrow cells have been described, but whether or not the basic disorder resides in the hematopoietic or the structural stem cells is no better known here than in the acquired cases. Of great interest, however, has been the demonstration by Shahidi and Diamond that the hypoplastic bone marrow in Fanconi's anemia appears to be quite responsive to the myelostimulatory effect of androgens. Many patients have been kept alive and well on a maintenance regimen of androgens, and these results have led to a revival of the therapeutic use of androgens in all cases of aplastic anemia. Androgens do enhance erythropoietin release, but this cannot explain their occasional effect on granulocyte and thrombocyte production and, as emphasized by Gardner and co-workers, they must have some direct or indirect action on the hematopoietic or the structural bone marrow stem cells.

The pathogenesis of cellular aplasia in a bone marrow injured by various toxins or illnesses has been clarified by recent successes with bone marrow transplantation. Until then, it was argued vigorously whether aplastic anemia was a disease of the "seed" or of the "soil", of hematopoietic stem cells or of structural, supporting cells. However, as reported by Storb, Thomas, and co-workers, the clear-cut "takes" of transplanted bone marrow cells leading in some cases to cures of aplastic anemia have shown that aplastic anemia is a disease of the hematopoietic stem cells. Although these cells are present and may form small and even large foci of hematopoietic cells, they are not capable of normal renewal and growth and can not reseed the fatty bony marrow stroma, as emphasized by Kansu and Erslev, this defect in proliferation is associated with defects in differentiation leading to the production of macrocytic red cells containing excessive fetal hemoglobin and being abnormally sensitive to the action of complement. The therapeutic implication is obviously to attempt to replace these abnormal stem cells with transfused normal stem cells. This has been accomplished with identical twins and with bone marrow from well-matched siblings, but is still not feasible between unrelated donor-recipient pairs.

Disorders of Unipotential Stem Cells

RENAL DISEASE. Anemia is a hallmark of chronic renal disease and is roughly proportional to the degree of renal failure as measured by urea or creatinine retention. Since the pathogenesis of the anemia and the uremia is related to the failure of many independent functions, it is actually surprising that the proportionality is as good as depicted in Figure 3–23. The two major failing functions are the renal excretory function and the renal endocrine function.

Failure of Renal Excretory Function

HEMOLYSIS. The red cell of patients with uremia frequently shows multiple tiny spicles (Fig. 3–24). The presence of this so-called burring has been related to the accumulation of toxic endproducts in the circulation and has been thought to be responsible for an impaired sodium-potassium pump activity and a shortened red cell life span. However, the correlation between azotemia and red cell life span is poor (Fig. 3–25), and when hemolysis occurs, it is often related more closely to changes in the microvasculature than to the degree of uremia. Indeed, extensive red cell fragmentation and hemolysis can be observed in patients with malignant vascular hypertension or with inflammatory vascular changes (hemolytic uremic syndrome) and with only mildly elevated BUN or creatinine concentrations. At present it seems most reasonable to relate the premature destruction of red cells in chronic renal disease to mechanical disruption of metabolically fragile red cells.

BLEEDING TENDENCY. As a manifestation of chronic renal disease, purpura is almost as characteristic as pallor. In addition to subcutaneous bleedings, gastrointestinal and uterine hemorrhage may cause a considerable loss of blood and increase the demands for an accelerated rate of red cell production. Iatrogenic blood loss should also not be forgotten. Patients with chronic renal disease are usually monitored by multiple laboratory tests and, if also hemodialyzed, may lose some blood in the dialysis coil. All in all, iron deficiency is one of the most common — but fortunately very treatable — problems in patients with chronic renal disease. The pathogenesis of the bleeding tendency is poorly understood, since thrombocytopenia and coagulation factor deficiency, when present, are rarely severe enough to be responsible for overt blood loss. Studies by Horowitz and co-workers, however, suggest that certain retention products may affect normal platelet function and cause an abnormal bleeding time, clot retraction, platelet adhesion, and platelet aggregation.

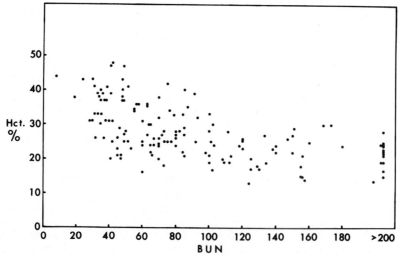

Figure 3–23   Relationship between hematocrit and BUN in 152 patients with various degrees of renal failure and uremia. (From Erslev, A. J.: Arch. intern. Med., *126*:774–780, 1970. Reprinted from Wesson, L. G. (ed.): Physiology of the Human Kidney, 1969, by permission of Grune & Stratton, Inc., New York.)

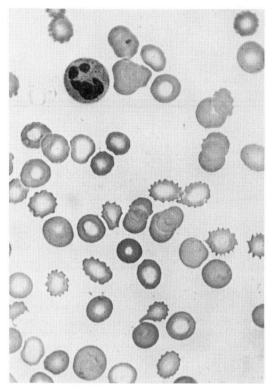

Figure 3–24 Burr cells in smear of blood from a patient with severe uremia.

The responsible toxic factor is believed to be a guanidino compound, and intensive dialysis has been found to reduce the bleeding tendency.

RESPONSIVENESS TO ERYTHROPOIETIN. In chronic renal failure there is both inadequate production of erythropoietin (see later) and decreased bone marrow response to erythropoietin (Fig. 3–26). The reason is not known, but the degree of responsiveness appears to be related to the severity of uremia. It seems probable that the improvement in erythropoietic function found after intensive dialysis is caused by an increased response to available erythropoietin rather than to an increased production of erythropoietin. Because of this refractory condition, it is anticipated that much more erythropoietin will be needed to abolish the anemia of chronic renal disease than is required for normal erythropoietic maintenance.

Failure of Renal Endocrine Function. The various effects of uremia on the rate of red cell destruction and production result in an increased demand for erythropoietin. This demand could easily be met by a normal but apparently not by an abnormal kidney. Impaired renal tissue is not capable of producing normal quantities of erythropoietin unless stimulated by intensive anemic hypoxia, and a balance between the rates of red cell destruction and red cell production is not achieved except at anemic levels. Under conditions of progressive kidney failure, the hypoxic stimulus needed to produce adequate amounts of renal erythropoietin becomes greater and the anemia more severe. However, even anephric individuals continue to manufacture red blood cells (Fig. 3–27). This residual erythropoietic activity appears to be generated by the release of extrarenal erythropoietin but the hemoglobin concentration which can be maintained in anephric patients is usually too low to be compatible with life and has to be augmented by transfusions.

CHRONIC DISORDERS. Although one of the most common of anemias, the anemia of chronic disorders is of relatively little clinical significance, since it is rarely severe enough to cause symptoms

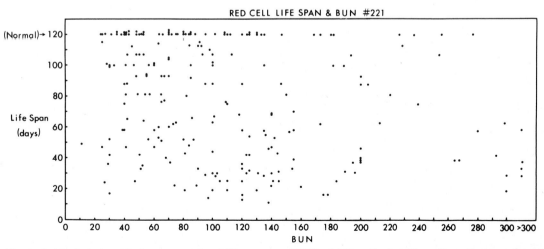

Figure 3–25 Relationship between red cell life span and BUN of 221 patients with various degrees of renal failure and uremia. (From Erslev, A. J.: Arch. Intern. Med., *126*:774, 1970. Copyright 1970, American Medical Association.)

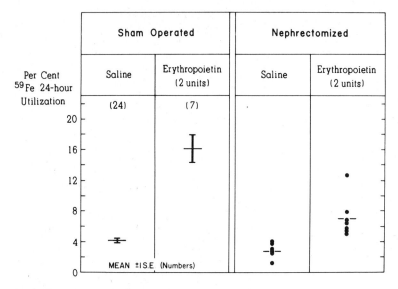

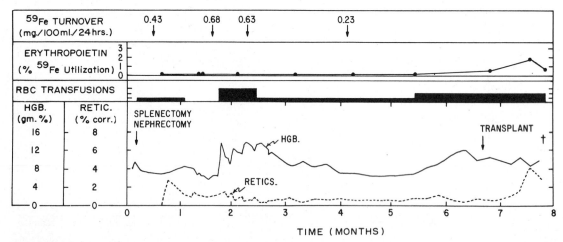

	Sham Operated		Nephrectomized	
Per Cent ^{59}Fe 24-hour Utilization	Saline	Erythropoietin (2 units)	Saline	Erythropoietin (2 units)

Figure 3–26 Erythropoietic response of normal and nephrectomized rats to the same amount of erythropoietin. On Day 0, the animals were transfused with 20 ml. per kg. of rat red cells. On Day 3, they were either nephrectomized or sham operated, and then given 2 units erythropoietin sc. On Day 4, ^{59}Fe was injected IV and its utilization determined 24 hours later.

or demand active transfusion therapy. On the other hand, it probably has been treated by more unneeded and ineffective hematinics than any other anemia, and the pathogenesis of this refractory anemia is still a fascinating enigma.

During the early part of this century, anemia was an invariable complication of many chronic debilitating infections, such as tuberculosis, osteomyelitis, or brucellosis, and it was known as anemia of chronic infection. With the change in the ecology of disease, it was realized that a similar anemia also occurred in patients with chronic, noninfectious diseases, such as rheumatoid arthritis, lymphomas, or disseminated carcinomas, and the anemia was given the noncommittal name of anemia of chronic disorders. It is characterized by a moderate reduction in hemoglobin concentra-

tion, a reduction in the level of both serum iron and iron-binding capacity, an increased amount of storage iron in the macrophages of the bone marrow, and a normal or elevated serum ferritin concentration.

The presence of decreased amounts of circulating iron, despite abundant iron stores, is probably caused by a defective iron release mechanism by the macrophages. The erythroid cells in the bone marrow apparently can handle available iron, and the utilization of radioactive iron is normal. However, the reutilization of iron is decreased (Fig. 3–28), indicating that hemoglobin iron, which normally is reutilized after being processed by the macrophages, is trapped in these cells and removed from the dynamic iron economy of the body. This relative iron deficiency is aggravated by a

Figure 3–27 Erythropoietic status of a patient who underwent nephrectomy and splenectomy seven months before a successful kidney transplantation. Although erythropoietin levels were unmeasurable, reticulocytes were produced throughout the anephric period.

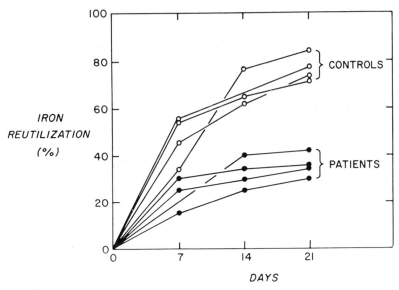

Figure 3–28 Reutilization of radioactive iron in normal individuals and in patients with anemia of chronic disease. Hemoglobin labeled with ^{59}Fe was injected intravenously and the combined process of hemoglobin sequestration, ^{59}Fe release and ^{59}Fe incorporation into new red cells (reutilization) was estimated by measuring the appearance of radioactivity in circulating red cells. (Redrawn from Haurani, F. I., Burke, W., and Martinez, E. J.: J. Lab. Clin. Med., *65*:560–570, 1965.)

moderate shortening of the red blood cell life span, resulting in a mild anemia. However, it has always been a puzzle why the anemia of chronic disorders does not display the morphologic characteristics of an iron deficiency anemia but is normocytic and normochromic, as if the basic defect resides in the stem cells. Recent studies by Ward and coworkers have suggested that there may indeed be an element of stem cell failure, since the serum level and the 24-hour excretion of erythropoietin are subnormal. No renal injury or abnormality can be held responsible for this defect, and studies so far have not shown any change in red cell oxygen affinity. Consequently, it is possible that the anemia of chronic disorders may reflect a primary defect in the oxygen sensing device or in the erythropoietin-producing cells. It is hoped that the unraveling of the pathogenesis of the anemia may provide us not only with means to correct the anemia but also with basic knowledge as to the relationship between erythropoietin production and iron metabolism.

ENDOCRINE DISORDERS

Pituitary and Thyroid Dysfunction. Pituitary and thyroid dysfunction or ablation are characteristically associated with a moderate normochromic, normocytic anemia. Although many attempts have been made to assign a specific erythropoietic effect to the thyroid, pituitary, or hypothalamic secretions, most current studies indicate that the anemia is an appropriate response to a decreased cellular demand for oxygen. The administration of thyroxin, triiodothyronine, or

desiccated thyroid will increase this demand, and the rate of red cell production will respond appropriately. It is questionable whether the administration of growth hormone, ACTH, or gonadal hormones are of additional benefit. In many cases of myxedema or other hypothyroid conditions, the anemia is somewhat atypical because of associated nutritional deficiencies. Malabsorption of B_{12} or folic acid may lead to a megaloblastic, macrocytic blood picture and the frequent uterine bleedings in hypothyroid females may lead to an iron-deficient, microcytic, hypochromic anemia. Even in hypothyroid men, the common achlorhydria may result in malabsorption of iron and an iron deficiency anemia.

Despite the erythropoietic effect of increased oxygen consumption induced by thyroid hormones, patients with hyperthyroidism or thyrotoxicosis are rarely polycythemic. This may be explained by the fact that thyroid hormones also increase cardiac output and tissue perfusion, making an increase in red cell mass less needed. Nevertheless, direct measurements by Muldowney and co-workers of red cell mass and plasma volume suggest that the absence of a high hematocrit in these conditions is caused by a concomitant increase in plasma volume, and that hyperthyroidism will cause true secondary polycythemia as defined by an increased red cell mass.

Gonadal Dysfunction. In normal mature men the hemoglobin concentration is about 1 to 2 grams higher than in normal females, whereas the male hemoglobin concentration in childhood, in advanced age, and in gonadal deficiency states is similar to that of females. This phenomenon has led to the assumption that physiologic excretions of androgens have an erythropoietic effect on the bone marrow. Conversely, it has been postulated that physiologic doses of estrogens cause a slight suppression of red cell production. Many experimental data on castrated animals have been marshaled to support these contentions, but unfortunately many studies were designed to prove rather than to test, and the erythropoietic effects of physiologic doses of gonadal hormones are still not quite clear. More impressive are the data indicating that androgens in pharmacologic doses can stimulate red cell production and even cause full-blown secondary polycythemia (Fig. 3–29). This effect may be mediated by a release of renal erythropoietin or by an enhanced effect of erythropoietin on the bone marrow or by both mechanisms as suggested by Shahidi.

Anemia of Pregnancy. Anemia of pregnancy is most often caused by an iron deficiency, and the routine use of iron in prenatal care is definitely in order. However, even under conditions of adequate iron intake, a mild anemia is present during the third trimester in almost all pregnant women. This anemia is normochromic and normocytic and unresponsive to any kind of treatment. Recent measurements of the red cell mass have shown it not to be caused by a lack of red cells but rather by an increase in plasma, a so-called dilution anemia. The red cell mass actually increases about 20 per cent during pregnancy, but the plasma volume increases even more. The physiologic effect of such an increase in blood volume is very advantageous for oxygen transport (Fig. 3–15), and despite the moderate decrease in hemoglobin concentration, the pregnant woman and her fetus are undoubtedly well provided with oxygen for their metabolic demands.

IMMUNOLOGIC DYSFUNCTION. Pure red cell aplasia is an unusual but dramatic disease characterized by severe anemia due to the isolated depletion of the erythroid tissue and is believed to be related to an immunologic dysfunction. The production and turnover of erythropoietin appear to be normal but the bone marrow response to this hormone is inadequate, as evidenced by the absence of proerythroblasts and other nucleated red blood cells despite high plasma titers of erythropoietin.

An acute, self-limited form of pure red cell aplasia has been reported following "virus" infections in patients with hereditary spherocytosis or other congenital hemolytic disorders. The predominance of reports dealing with such patients may be due to the fact that a brief period of erythroid aplasia in a patient with a short red cell life span will have a much more noticeable effect on the hemoglobin concentration than the same period of

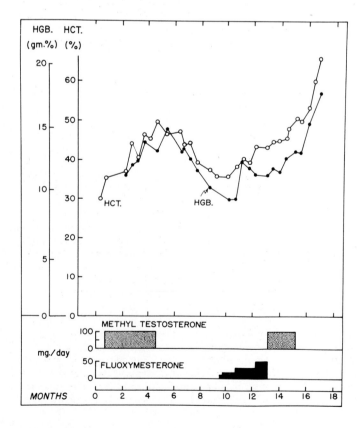

Figure 3–29 Erythropoietic response of a patient with myelofibrosis to various androgen preparations. (Redrawn from Gardner, F. H. and Pringle, J. C.: N. Engl. J. Med., *264*:103, 1961.)

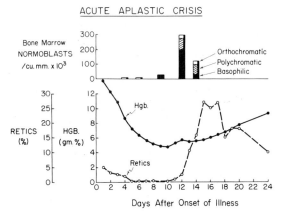

ACUTE APLASTIC CRISIS

Figure 3–30 Acute aplastic crisis following a brief febrile illness in a patient with hereditary spherocytosis. (Redrawn from Owren, P. A.: Blood, 3:231–248, 1948, by permission of Grune & Stratton, Inc., New York.)

aplasia would have if the red cell life span were normal (Fig. 3–30). Consequently, it is assumed that brief periods of asymptomatic erythroid aplasia may actually be quite common and if properly looked for found in many normals suffering from upper respiratory infections or viral gastroenteritis. The exact pathogenetic mechanism is unknown but it has been proposed that the erythroid cells or their immediate erythropoietin-sensitive progenitors are affected by a viral-related antibody.

Chronic pure red cell aplasia is a far more unusual disorder, but its relationship to thymic tumors has recently caused a flurry of interest regarding its pathogenesis.

Thymomas are present in about 30 to 50 per cent of cases, and although thymectomy is rarely of dramatic benefit, "spontaneous" recoveries have been described in patients who have undergone thymectomy. Since so-called autoimmune disorders are frequently associated with thymus abnormalities, it is of additional pathogenetic importance that prednisone may occasionally cause a striking reticulocyte response (Fig. 3–31) and that remissions may be induced by the therapeutic use of immunosuppressive drugs. Studies by Krantz and co-workers have demonstrated antibodies directed against erythroid bone marrow cells in the serum of some patients. These antibodies presumably coat and possibly reject the erythroid cells or the erythropoietin-responsive stem cells, and their presence could explain the development

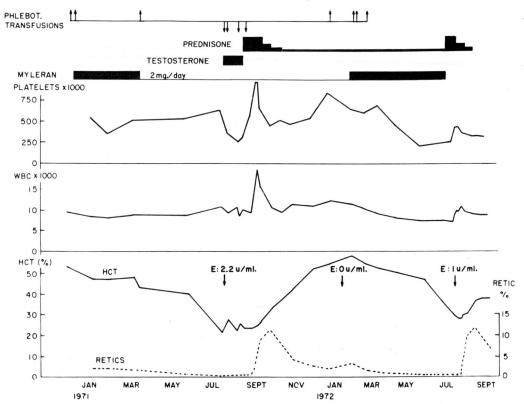

Figure 3–31 A patient with polycythemia vera, disseminated lupus erythematosus, and recurrent bouts of pure red cell aplasia. In each instance prednisone medication caused a striking increase in reticulocytes, followed by a return of the hematocrit to normal or even polycythemic values. (E = Erythropoietin).

of a pure red cell aplasia. The existence of antibodies directed against erythropoietin has also been reported, but since the erythropoietin titer is usually very high, these reports are difficult to accept. The cause-effect relationship of the autoantibodies to the thymic tumor is not clear, but it has been suggested that the tumor destroys normal thymic function and permits the survival of lymphocytic clones programmed to produce autoantibodies. Further studies of this fascinating disease may well lead to concepts of importance for the management not only of patients with pure red cell aplasia but also of patients with other autoimmune diseases.

Multiplication Disorders

Vitamin B_{12} and Folic Acid. The identification of vitamin B_{12} and folates as important anti-anemia principles ranks among modern medicine's greatest triumphs. The exemplary clinical investigations of Minot and Murphy and of Castle in the 1920s and 1930s were the first of a steady stream of basic and applied research accomplishments, the most recent of which has been the synthesis of vitamin B_{12} in the laboratory. Kass has recently recounted with rich pictorial detail the history of this fascinating chain of discoveries extending for

more than a century after Addison's clinical description of pernicious anemia in 1849.

B_{12} and folates participate as factors in a wide variety of biochemical reactions in the body. In some respects their biochemical reactions are interrelated. Their essential role in DNA synthesis explains why deficiencies of either or both lead to "megaloblastic anemia" and to disturbances in cell division not only in the marrow but in other proliferating cell populations, such as the gastrointestinal epithelium. Nervous tissue, which is not in a state of cellular proliferation, also has an important requirement for vitamin B_{12}.

Vitamin B_{12} (molecular weight 1355) is built asymmetrically around cobalt much like heme is built around iron. Cobalt, like iron, has six coordinate positions four of which are bound to nitrogen atoms in a planar tetrapyrrole corrin ring (Fig. 3–32). Below and almost perpendicular to the plane of the corrin ring, a benzimidazole nucleotide occupies the fifth coordinate position, also in a nitrogen linkage. The sixth position is ionic, and in "cyanocobalamin," the parent compound of the family of vitamin B_{12} relatives, it is occupied by cyanide. The presence of the cyanide ligand in this position, however, is an artifact of isolation. The physiologically active coenzyme forms of the vitamin contain either a methyl or a deoxyadenosyl

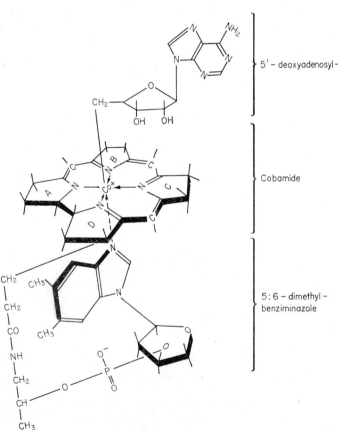

Figure 3–32 Structure of deoxyadenosyl cobalamin, a physiologically active form of vitamin B_{12}. (From Chanarin, I.: The Megaloblastic Anemias. F. A. Davis Co., Philadelphia, 1969, p. 16.)

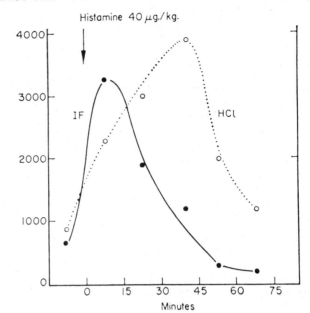

Intrinsic factor — units   HCl mEq.

Histamine 40 μg./kg.

Figure 3–33 Stimulation of gastric secretion of intrinsic factor (IF) and hydrochloric acid by histamine. (Redrawn from Arderman, S., et al.: Br. Med. J., 2:600, 1964.)

group in this position. Cyanocobalamin, as well as its relative hydroxycobalamin, is readily converted to these active forms within the body.

The absorption of vitamin B_{12} is dependent upon a unique mechanism unshared by any other essential nutrient. The parietal cells of the stomach produce, along with hydrochloric acid, a glycoprotein known as "intrinsic factor" (IF), which tightly and specifically binds B_{12}, the "extrinsic factor," after it has been ingested and is released from complexes in foodstuffs (Fig. 3–33). IF has a molecular weight of 60,000 and binds B_{12} on a mole-for-mole basis. The binding occurs with the benzimidazole nucleotide moiety of B_{12} and is independent of the specific chemical form of the vitamin. Dimers are formed when the vitamin is bound. It then travels down the length of the intestinal tract, protected in the IF complex from the degradative activities of digestive enzymes. Specific receptors on the surface of the microvilli of the terminal ileum take up the IF-B_{12} complex in a process dependent upon a pH of above 6.5 as well as upon divalent cations (calcium and/or magnesium((Fig. 3–34). It is still uncertain whether the entire complex enters the cell or whether IF is released back into the lumen after the vitamin is removed.

After a small dose of 1 μg of B_{12} about 60 to 80 per cent is absorbed. However, the proportion absorbed decreases as the amount of ingested B_{12} increases. About 1 to 5 μg. is absorbed from a dietary intake of 5 to 30 μg per day. A tiny amount of B_{12}, less than 1 per cent, is absorbed in an

IF-independent manner, but this is too small to be of physiologic significance. There is a substantial excretion of B_{12} from the biliary tract into the intestinal lumen, but this is efficiently reabsorbed in an IF-dependent enterohepatic circuit, and thus is not lost to the body economy.

In addition to IF, other specific vitamin B_{12} binding proteins are of importance to the body economy. A family of "R binders" (R for rapid electrophoretic mobility), found in plasma, saliva, milk, and other body fluids, share a common protein structure but differ in their carbohydrate content. Transcobalamin (TC) I and III are R-binders found in plasma. Most of the B_{12} present in plasma is attached to TC I and has a relatively slow rate of turnover according to Hall. TC III contains only a minor fraction of the plasma vitamin B_{12} and appears to arise from granulocytes largely as a result of in-vitro cell lysis. A third plasma binder, TC II, lacks carbohydrate and, like IF, differs in its protein make-up from the R-binders. TC II accounts for most of the unsaturated plasma vitamin B_{12} binding capacity and is responsible for binding newly absorbed vitamin B_{12} and rapidly transporting it to the tissues so its turnover rate is many times more rapid than that of TC I.

Much remains to be learned about the biologic roles of the vitamin B_{12} binding proteins. TC I seems to be dispensable since its congenital absence causes no clinically important abnormality. In contrast, congenital lack of TC II leads to megaloblastic anemia. Striking elevations of the plas-

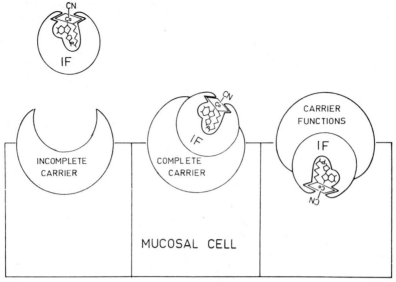

Figure 3–34 Mucosal absorption in the terminal ileum of vitamin B_{12} bound to intrinsic factor. (From Gräsbeck, R.: Scand. J. Clin. Lab. Invest., *19*:7 (Suppl. 95.), 1967. Universitetsforlaget, Oslo.)

ma R-binders and vitamin B_{12} levels are observed in patients with chronic myelogenous leukemia, other myeloproliferative syndromes, and in occasional patients with cancer.

Folic acid (pteroylmonoglutamic acid) consists of pteroic acid in combination with only one molecule of L-glutamic acid (Fig. 3–35). However, the term "folates" refers to a large family of related compounds containing as many as six or seven L-glutamic acid residues locked in gamma glutamyl polypeptide linkage. Most food folate is in the polyglutamate form and must be broken down in the intestine to the monoglutamate to permit efficient absorption. This is accomplished by the intestinal enzyme "conjugase" (Fig. 3–36).

Following its absorption, folic acid is reduced by the enzyme dihydrofolate reductase. The reduction is accomplished in two steps, each involving the addition of two hydrogen atoms to yield biologically active tetrahydrofolate (FH_4). Dihydrofolate reductase is inhibited by minute concentrations of the antifolate compound, methotrexate, an effective chemotherapeutic agent used in the treatment of neoplastic diseases.

Reduced folates, acting out their roles as agents of single carbon unit transfer, are methylated in a variety of ways. The active carbon may exist in one of several different chemical states (methyl, formyl, hydroxymethyl, methylene, methenyl, formimino), and it may be attached at several alternative sites on the parent FH_4 molecule (Fig. 3–35).

In addition to folic acid itself, the only other pharmacologically available folate is the N^5 formyl derivative, folinic acid (also called citrovorum factor, or Leucovorin). This agent is of use as an antidote for methotrexate toxicity, against which folic acid, the biologically inactive precursor of FH_4, is ineffective.

Plasma folate occurs almost entirely as the monoglutamate form of methyl FH_4, but following its uptake into cells the molecular size is once again increased by the enzymatic addition of multiple glutamic acid residues. This conversion (or reconversion) to the polyglutamate form markedly enhances coenzymatic activity. Thus, as reviewed by Hoffbrand, the intracellular pool of reduced and methylated polyglutamates is the principal source of folate biologic activity.

Although B_{12} and folates participate as cofactors in a number of biochemical reactions involving transfer of carbon or hydrogen atoms, their roles in DNA synthesis are of particular interest with respect to the pathogenesis of megaloblastic anemia. Patients with B_{12} deficiency show hematologic response to treatment with large doses of folic acid (although their neurologic symptoms may worsen). This clinical observation has for a long time aroused interest in the hypothesis that B_{12} and folates are interrelated in their roles as coenzymes in DNA synthesis. Several findings have shed some light on this interrelationship. Plasma levels of methyl FH_4 tend to be elevated in patients with B_{12} deficiency, while at the same time intracellular polyglutamate folates are decreased. This has suggested that B_{12} may play a role in cellular uptake of methyl FH_4 monoglutamate or in the conversion of monoglutamate to polyglutamate folate derivatives. However, the reciprocal changes in plasma and

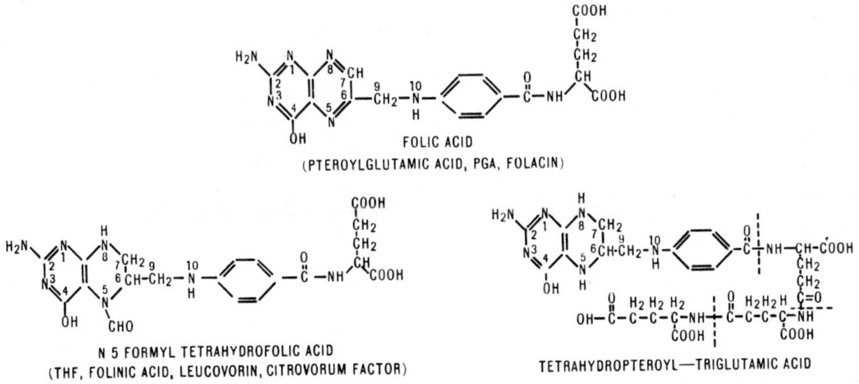

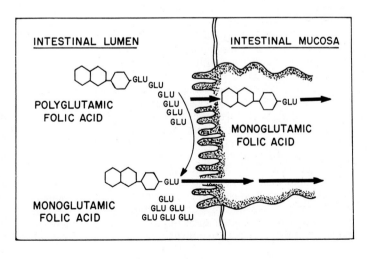

Figure 3–35 Structure of folic acid and its derivatives. Tetrahydrofolate is abbreviated here as THF and in the text as FH₄. (From Harris, J. W., and Kellermeyer, R. W.: The Red Cell. Harvard University Press, Cambridge, 1970, p. 395.)

Figure 3–36 Intestinal absorption of the folate derivatives in food, present largely in polyglutamate form. The site of action of the enzyme conjugase, which degrades the polyglutamate to the monoglutamate, is not known, but may actually be within the mucosal cell rather than in the intestinal lumen. Folate appears in the plasma as the reduced monoglutamate N₅ methyl tetrahydrofolate. (From Streiff, R. R.: J.A.M.A., *214*, 105, 1970. Copyright 1970 by the American Medical Association.)

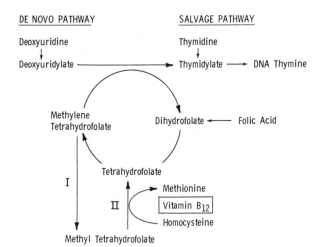

DE NOVO PATHWAY   SALVAGE PATHWAY

Figure 3–37 The methyl tetrahydrofolate "trap" hypothesis. Elevated plasma N_5 methyl tetrahydrofolate levels are observed in patients with vitamin B_{12} deficiency due to an inability to convert this, the major extracellular form, to tetrahydrofolate and other active coenzymic intracellular forms. Because of this lack of active intracellular folates (and specifically of $N_{5, 10}$ methylene tetrahydrofolate) there is a deficient conversion of deoxyuridylate to thymidylate and consequently also of DNA synthesis. The unutilized folate is "trapped" as N_5 methyl tetrahydrofolate. (Redrawn from Waxman, S., et al.: J. Clin. Invest., *48*, 284, 1969.)

intracellular folate levels may also be explained by the methyl FH_4 "trap" hypothesis, as explained in Figure 3–37.

The biochemical action of B_{12} in the nervous tissue is still controversial, but circumstantial evidence has pointed to its role in propionate metabolism (Fig. 3–38). Deoxyadenosyl cobalamin acts as co-factor in the rearrangement of active methylmalonate, formed as a result of carboxylation of propionate, to succinate. Indeed, increased urinary excretion of methylmalonate is a reliable indicator of B_{12} deficiency. An increase in the serum concentration as well as the urinary excretion is also seen in methylmalonic acidemia, a rare inherited defect of B_{12} conversion to its active deoxyadenosyl coenzyme form.

Although folate lack is not notable for the presence of neurologic sequelae, except inasmuch as other vitamin deficiencies may coexist, rare congenital deficiencies of the intermediary steps of folate metabolism may cause mental retardation and other neurologic problems early in infancy. This observation has stimulated interest in the possibility that folates are of importance in the normal development of the nervous tissue.

General Effects of Megaloblastic Anemia. The signs and symptoms are primarily related to the hematopoietic and gastrointestinal systems, although the neurologic system is also affected in B_{12} deficiency. The degree of anemia may be quite profound, but its onset is very slow and as a result it is amazingly well tolerated, unless congestive heart failure or angina pectoris supervenes. The sclerae are often slightly icteric, the tongue is usually atrophic and smooth, and splenomegaly may be present. There may be vague gastrointestinal complaints. The neurologic signs of B_{12} deficiencies include a spastic and incoordinate gait, paresthesias, and sometimes mental changes. Increased reflexes, Babinski signs, and loss of position and vibration sense are indicative of posterior

and lateral column demyelination (Fig. 3–39). Decreased reflexes and hypesthesia are signs of peripheral neuropathy, and altered behavior and impaired mentation may indicate cerebral involvement.

The deficiency affects all the proliferating hematopoietic elements, and therefore pancytopenia is commonly observed, but granulocytopenia and thrombocytopenia are usually not so severe that infectious susceptibility or hemorrhage results. The anemia is macrocytic, but wide variations of erythrocyte size on either side of the mean are characteristic, and indeed, some erythrocytes are microcytic. The presence of "macro-ovalocytes" is a particularly valuable morphologic sign. Mature segmented neutrophils have a greater than nor-

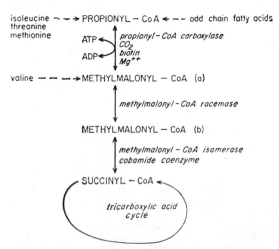

Figure 3–38 The role of vitamin B_{12} in propionate metabolism. The cobamide coenzyme is deoxyadenosyl cobalamin. (From Rosenberg, L. E., et al.: Science, *162*:805, 1968. Copyright 1968 by the American Association for the Advancement of Science.)

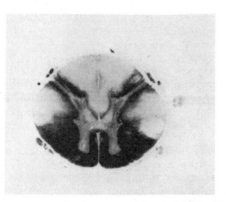

Figure 3–39 Degeneration of the posterior and lateral columns of the spinal cord in vitamin B$_{12}$ deficiency. (From Chanarin, I.: The Megaloblastic Anemias. Philadelphia, F. A. Davis Co., 1969, p. 576.)

mal mean number of lobes per nucleus; a few may contain as many as 7 or 8.

Not all macrocytic conditions are megaloblastic. An increase in mean corpuscular volume may be seen with reticulocytosis or if there is acquisition of excessive membrane surface area due to plasma lipid abnormalities (Table 3–7).

When the anemia is severe, megaloblastic erythroid precursors are found in the circulation, and a small proportion of mature erythrocytes contains nuclear remnants (Howell-Jolly bodies, Cabot's rings). The reticulocytes are not increased and polychromasia is not prominent. Distinctive morphologic changes are also seen in the gastrointestinal epithelial cells, but the diagnosis rests upon the finding of "megaloblastic" changes in the

bone marrow. This term was originally applied to erythroid precursors only, but today it is used to refer to changes in all three cell lines — granulocytic and megakaryocytic as well as erythroid. The entire erythroid line of maturation is altered to form a "megaloblastic series." There is the appearance of a "maturation arrest" because of the marked shift to the left, with large numbers of early erythroid precursors having intensely basophilic cytoplasm. The arrest in nuclear development is reflected in an abnormally finely divided and open pattern of the nuclear chromatin. Hemoglobin formation proceeds in the cytoplasm, however, and "nuclear-cytoplasmic dissociation" is observed. The entire series of cells is larger than normal, and mature cells emerge as macrocytic erythrocytes. The marrow granulocytic precursors also show distinctive changes, in particular large horseshoe- and C-shaped nuclear forms at the band stage of maturation. The marrow shows a marked over-all increase in cellularity.

The deficient marrow, driven by the stimulus of "poietins," reacts with a hypercellular proliferative response. However, the defect in nuclear development leads to intramedullary destruction of the blood cell precursors. Heme catabolism from the breakdown of erythroid precursors in the marrow is the major factor contributing to the signs of hemolysis — the elevated serum indirect bilirubin, the absence of plasma haptoglobin, and the elevation of serum lactic dehydrogenase to levels rarely seen even in the hemolytic anemias. Megaloblastic anemia is a classic example of the pathophysiology of ineffective erythropoiesis. The number of reticulocytes in the peripheral blood is not elevated despite intense erythroid hyperplasia

TABLE 3–7   SOME CAUSES OF MACROCYTIC ERYTHROCYTES

Impairment of DNA synthesis
Vitamin B$_{12}$ deficiency
Folate deficiency
Chemotherapy
Antimetabolites (e.g., 6-mercaptopurine, methotrexate)
Alkylating agents (e.g., cyclophosphamide)
Primary refractory anemias
Aplastic anemia
Sideroblastic anemia
Erythroleukemia and other myelogenous leukemia variants
Refractory megaloblastic anemias (acquired)
Rare hereditary blocks in DNA synthesis (e.g., orotic aciduria)

Reticulocytosis
Hemolytic anemia
Response to acute blood loss

Surface Membrane Excess
Liver disease
Obstructive jaundice
Post-splenectomy
Hereditary lecithin: cholesterol acyl transferase (LCAT) deficiency

in the marrow. The serum iron concentration is raised, and its rate of clearance from the circulation to the erythroid marrow is increased, with only small amounts appearing over subsequent days in the newly formed erythrocytes (Fig. 3–22). The amount of radioactive label appearing in the "early bilirubin" peak after administration of a tagged heme precursor is markedly increased (Fig. 3–69).

With treatment, the signs promptly revert to normal within several days: the serum iron concentration decreases and its utilization for the production of circulating erythrocytes becomes effective, the jaundice disappears, the elevated serum lactic dehydrogenase falls, and megaloblastic cells are no longer seen in the marrow. The reticulocyte count becomes elevated within three to four days, reaches a peak at 7 to 10 days, and then falls (Fig. 3–40). The reticulocyte response is the most reliable early sign of response, and in the more anemic individuals it may peak at 25 to 50 per cent. The neurologic symptoms of B_{12} lack are reversed, unless they have progressed to an advanced degree of severity. Pharmacologic doses of folic acid will produce a hematologic response in the B_{12}-deficient patient while worsening the neurologic complications. Presumably the folate causes a fall in serum B_{12} level, with a diversion of available B_{12} away from neural to hematopoietic tissue. Large doses of B_{12} will also give a hematologic response in the folate-deficient patient. Response to therapy is specific if the administered dose is limited to the range of the minimal daily requirement, about 1 μg. per day of B_{12} or 50 μg. per day of folate.

Vitamin B_{12} Deficiency

DIETARY LACK.   Inadequate intake is an exceptionally rare cause of B_{12} deficiency, since this vitamin is present in a wide variety of products of animal origin — meat, fish, eggs, butter, milk, and cheese — and the minimal daily requirement of 1 to 5 μg. is readily met unless a strict vegetarian diet is followed. Even then, the total body stores of 2000 to 5000 μg. are well conserved, with a loss of only 0.1 per cent per day of the total body pool, and the earliest signs of B_{12} deficiency are not seen until after 10 to 20 years on such a diet.

INTRINSIC FACTOR LACK.   The term "pernicious anemia" (PA) no longer seems appropriate, considering the fact that the condition can now be effectively cured. However, its historical roots are deep and it seems appropriate to continue to use this term but only for megaloblastic anemia caused by a lack of intrinsic factor.

Congenital PA is a rare autosomal recessive condition which is apparently clinically manifest only in the homozygous state. There is an isolated lack of IF without insufficiency of gastric acid or pepsin. Passively acquired B_{12} stores present at birth are exhausted in two or three years, and anemia then develops.

Adult PA is a disorder of mature and older adults. Genetic factors still not well defined play some role, since there is a significant intrafamilial occurrence as well as an ethnic predilection for individuals of northern and western European

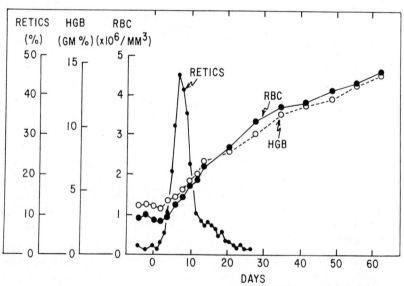

Figure 3–40 Hematologic response to treatment of vitamin B_{12} deficiency in a patient with pernicious anemia. (Redrawn from Castle, W. B. *In* Cecil and Loeb (eds.): A Textbook of Medicine. W. B. Saunders Co., Philadelphia, 1959, p. 1131.)

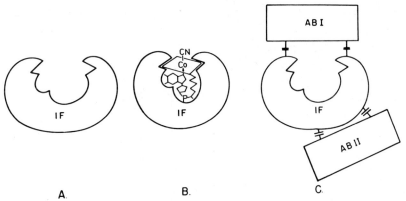

Figure 3–41 Anti-intrinsic factor antibodies of the blocking (AB I) and binding (AB II) types. (From Gräsbeck, R.: Progr. Hemat., 6:233–260, 1969. By permission of Grune & Stratton, Inc., New York.)

background. The absence of IF in the gastric juice is always found in association with atrophic gastritis, and there is accordingly a lack of gastric acidity and pepsin, even after stimulation with histamine. Atrophic gastritis is not uncommon in the general population, and its incidence increases with age. Why certain affected persons develop pernicious anemia is still uncertain, but the following evidence supports an autoimmune theory of pathogenesis:

(1) The histologic appearance of lymphocytic infiltration of the gastric mucosa suggests a local immunologic process.

(2) Antibodies which react against the cytoplasm of the gastric parietal cell are present in the serum of 90 per cent of patients with adult PA. A significant incidence of such antibodies is present, however, in patients who do not have PA. These include 60 per cent of all individuals with atrophic gastritis, 30 per cent of blood relatives of PA patients, and slightly less than 10 per cent of a control population. PA patients frequently have serum antibodies directed against parenchymal endocrine glands, most notably the acinar cells of the thyroid. Conversely, patients with primary myxedema and Hashimoto's thyroiditis have a 30 per cent incidence of antiparietal cell serum antibodies and a 12 per cent incidence of coexisting PA.

(3) About three fourths of PA patients have anti-IF antibodies in serum, saliva, and gastric juice. These are much more specific for PA and are rarely found in its absence. These antibodies are polyclonal and may be either IgG or IgA. They apparently react at two different sites on the IF molecule (Fig. 3–41). "Blocking" antibodies prevent the binding of B_{12} to IF, presumably by obstructing the site of attachment. "Binding" antibodies do not interfere with the attachment of B_{12} to IF, but they do impede absorption in the ileum.

Whether these various autoimmune phenomena associated with PA are cause or effect remains uncertain, but the properties of the anti-IF antibodies present in gastric secretions clearly suggest a role in its pathogenesis.

Total gastrectomy will predictably produce megaloblastic anemia after five or six years, but partial gastrectomy in most instances does not deplete IF sufficiently to lead to frank megaloblastosis. With the passage of years, however, an increasing proportion of partial gastrectomy patients develop low serum B_{12} levels, some of whom have mild megaloblastic changes in the marrow (Fig. 3–42). Iron deficiency is the commonest cause of postgastrectomy anemia, and its presence may mask concomitant megaloblastosis, the signs of which are brought out following iron repletion.

DECREASED ILEAL ABSORPTION. Ablation of the specific site of B_{12} absorption in the terminal ileum by surgical resection or by such diseases as regional ileitis, lymphoma, or tuberculosis leads to B_{12} deficiency without an associated lack of IF or of gastric acid. Certain drugs (neomycin, colchicine, para-amino salicylate) reportedly interfere with B_{12} absorption by mechanisms which remain obscure. The gastrointestinal epithelial changes of tropical sprue are extensive and commonly cause B_{12} deficiency, especially in chronic cases. The megaloblastic alterations of B_{12} or folate deficiency themselves cause sufficient epithelial change to interfere with ileal absorption. Indeed, patients with folate deficiency tend to have lower than normal serum concentrations of B_{12}, with spontaneous correction after folate repletion (Fig. 3–43). Poor absorption may also occur consequent to pancreatic insufficiency primarily because pancreatic enzymes cleave R-binder B_{12} complexes and make the vitamin available for attachment to IF. *Imerslund's syndrome* is a rare congenital deficiency of the receptor site in the terminal ileum causing megaloblastic anemia in children. IF secretion is normal. Renal structural abnormalities and proteinuria are also commonly present.

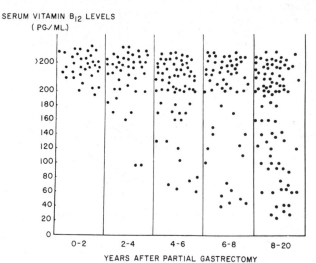

SERUM VITAMIN B$_{12}$ LEVELS
(PG./ML.)

YEARS AFTER PARTIAL GASTRECTOMY

Figure 3–42 Serum vitamin B$_{12}$ levels at various intervals after subtotal gastrectomy. Patients with B$_{12}$ deficiency megaloblastic anemia have values in the range of 0 to 100 pg. per ml. (Redrawn from Hines, J. D., et al.: Am. J. Med., *43*:555, 1967.)

DECREASED AVAILABILITY. Decreased serum B$_{12}$ levels and megaloblastic anemia are found in association with anatomic abnormalities of the gastrointestinal tract which lead to stasis and pooling of the luminal contents. Such "blind loop syndromes" — strictures, surgically created bypasses, fistulas, and large diverticula — have in common the presence of bacterial overgrowth along with steatorrhea. The anemia does not respond to orally administered B$_{12}$, but parenteral replacement is effective. Intrinsic factor is present in normal amounts, indicating that the IF-B$_{12}$ complex is unavailable for absorption in the terminal ileum. The finding that therapy with broad-spectrum antibiotics causes disappearance of the stigmata of B$_{12}$ lack provides strong evidence that bacterial utilization is responsible for the deficiency. A similar mechanism explains the megaloblastic anemia associated with the fish tapeworm (*Diphyllobothrium latum*). Infestation occurs because of eating improperly cooked fresh-water fish. The worms grow to great lengths in the intestinal tract and effectively compete with the host for available IF-B$_{12}$ complex. The disorder is especially common in Finland.

Folate Deficiency

DIETARY LACK. Poor nutrition — an unusual cause of B$_{12}$ deficiency — frequently gives rise to

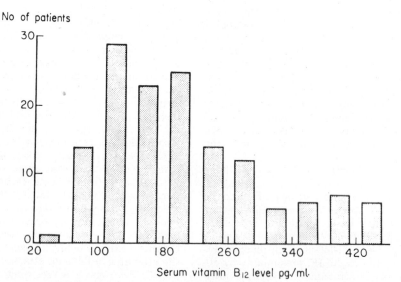

No of patients

Serum vitamin B$_{12}$ level pg./ml.

Figure 3–43 Serum vitamin B$_{12}$ levels in patients with megaloblastic anemia due to folate deficiency. The normal range of values is 200 to 800 pg. per ml. (Redrawn from Mollin, D. L., Waters, A. H., and Harriss, E., *in* 2 Europaisches Symposium, Hamburg, 1961, (H. C. Heinrich, ed.), Stuttgart, Enke. Reprinted in Chanarin, I.: The Megaloblastic Anemias. F. A. Davis Co., Philadelphia, 1969.)

folate depletion. The elderly recluse, the "tea and toast" faddist, and the alcoholic are prototypes of deficiency in the United States. In other countries, excessive cooking of food, often limited in amount and diversity, destroys labile folates and causes leeching out of the soluble folates in the cooking water. Newborns procure sufficient amounts even from deficient mothers, but develop megaloblastic anemia when they reach the two-year stage of rapid growth if they are raised on low folate diets, such as goat's milk or boiled milk. Folates are present in many different foodstuffs — leafy green vegetables, fruits, meats, eggs — and food intake must be severely limited in diversity in order to fall short of the minimal daily requirement of 50 μg. Lack of ascorbate, thiamine, and other essential nutrients often coexists. In alcoholics, poor diet is not the only factor, since ethanol seems to interfere with folate absorption, its intermediary metabolism, and its hepatic storage. It also exerts a direct toxic suppression on the bone marrow elements.

The sequence of events after limitation of folate intake has been studied experimentally by Herbert (Fig. 3–44). The serum folate concentration is the most sensitive indicator of deficiency, falling within a month of deficient intake. Red cell folate concentration is more stubbornly defended, but it also falls as megaloblastic anemia appears after three to four months of deficiency. Folate stores are neither as ample, relative to daily requirement, nor as avidly guarded as B_{12} stores.

The minimal daily requirement of folate increases during pregnancy to about 400 μg. Serum folate levels tend to fall as pregnancy proceeds to term. A diet that maintains body folate in a mar-ginal state of balance will prove inadequate in the face of such an increase in demands, and thus folate deficiency is the commonest cause of megaloblastic anemia of pregnancy. Conditions of increased cellular proliferation, such as hemolytic anemia, as well as thyrotoxicosis also raise the minimal requirement for folate.

MALABSORPTION. "Blind loop syndromes," which bring on B_{12} deficiency because of bacterial utilization, are not associated with folate lack. Possibly bacterial synthesis in the stagnant loop may actually add to the body's supply. On the other hand, gastrointestinal disorders affecting extensive areas of absorptive surface, with attendant malabsorption, frequently lead to folate deficiency. Gluten-sensitive enteropathy (non-tropical sprue) most severely affects the upper reaches of the bowel — the duodenum and jejunum — where folate absorption normally is maximal, sparing the terminal ileum along with B_{12} absorption in many instances. In tropical sprue, the involvement extends throughout the gut, affecting B_{12} as well as folate absorption. Folic acid therapy often improves the malabsorption along with the megaloblastic anemia in tropical sprue, but in non-tropical sprue improvement in gastrointestinal function is achieved by eliminating gluten from the diet. Oral therapy with folic acid — the monoglutamate form — is effective, suggesting that the polyglutamates of food are not absorbed as well.

Other gastrointestinal disorders with malabsorption are lymphoma, scleroderma, amyloidosis, Whipple's disease, and extensive surgical resection. In addition to deficiencies of folate and/or B_{12}, iron lack is also commonly present in malab-

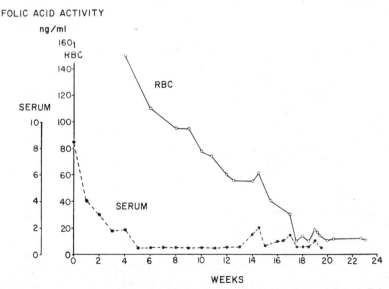

Figure 3–44 The fall in serum folate and red cell folate in a subject placed on a folate-deficient diet. (Redrawn from Herbert, V.: Trans. Am. Assoc. Physicians, 75:307, 1962.)

sorption syndromes, giving the picture of a combined deficiency anemia.

DRUGS. Patients on diphenylhydantoin therapy have a significant incidence of low serum folate levels and of megaloblastic anemia which responds readily to oral folic acid therapy. Estrogenic contraceptives occasionally have a similar side-effect. The notion that these agents interfere with the absorption of food folates by inhibiting intestinal conjugase activity has not yet withstood the test of scientific confirmation. Some evidence suggests that diphenylhydantoin may interfere with folate intermediary metabolism. The mechanism of megaloblastic anemia produced by the antimalarial pyrimethamine is more closely akin to that of methotrexate as a competitive inhibitor of folate metabolism.

Miscellaneous Megaloblastic Anemias. Therapy of neoplastic disease often leads to megaloblastic bone marrow and macrocytic red cells. Some of the cytotoxic agents in use which predictably inhibit nucleotide synthesis with secondary megaloblastic change are the antifolates (methotrexate), purine inhibitors (6-mercaptopurine, thioguanine, azathioprine), pyrimidine inhibitors (5-fluorouracil), and pentose analogues (cytosine arabinoside). *Primary refractory megaloblastic anemia* may represent a nuclear maturation defect of a myeloproliferative syndrome. When such a defect affects both the erythroid and granulocytic precursors with an increase in marrow myeloblasts it is known as *erythroleukemia (Di Guglielmo syndrome)*. In some proliferative disorders of the bone marrow, local shortages are brought on by the increased requirements of the abnormal proliferation, causing morphologic signs of deficiency in neighboring cells. *Hereditary orotic aciduria* is a rare megaloblastic anemia of childhood caused by an inherited block in pyrimidine synthesis.

Maturation Disorders of the Erythrocyte Cytoplasm

Hemoglobin Synthesis. The circulating erythrocyte is the most specialized of the body's cells — 95 per cent of its cytoplasm consists of the respiratory pigment hemoglobin packed into the cell interior at a concentration almost five times that of the proteins of the exterior plasma. The formation of hemoglobin begins at the earliest precursor stage of the developing erythroid cell and is completed when the anucleate reticulocyte matures to an erythrocyte. No additional hemoglobin is produced during the 120-day period of the erythrocyte's life span in the circulation. The biosynthesis of hemoglobin is a complex series of distinct but delicately coordinated biochemical events, so well balanced that component parts are brought together assembly-line fashion, without significant shortages or surpluses, to form the completed mol-

ecule. Heme is formed in a sequential series of enzymatically controlled reactions. Dissimilar polypeptide globin subunits under separate genetic control are assembled on polyribosomes. The finished molecule has two pairs of such subunits, each linked with its own prosthetic heme group into a tetrameric macromolecule.

GENERAL EFFECTS OF DISORDERS OF HEMOGLOBIN SYNTHESIS. Deficiency in the quantity of hemoglobin leads to microcytic, hypochromic anemia. The hemoglobin lack comes either from a lack of heme, as in iron deficiency, or from insufficient globin, to which the designation "thalassemia" is given. Qualitative abnormalities of the hemoglobin may alter the internal consistency of the erythrocyte cytoplasm and cause increased cell rigidity which leads to premature destruction and hemolysis. Abnormal hemoglobin oxygen affinity or oxidation state gives rise to cyanosis or erythrocytosis. Many abnormal hemoglobins produce no pathophysiologic abnormality because they function quite normally.

Porphyrin. Of all the tissues in the body, the erythroid marrow and the liver are the preeminent porphyrin producers. The synthesis begins on the mitochondria and requires energy. The intermediate steps take place in the cytosol and the process is completed once again on the mitochondria with the insertion of iron into the completed porphyrin molecule to form heme. The brightly colored finished product contains four pyrrole rings connected into a larger cyclic tetrapyrrole structure by methene bridges. Side chains are attached to the ring structure: 4 methyl, 2 vinyl, and 2 propionyl. The structure of heme is shown in Figure 3–45.

The biochemical steps in heme synthesis are outlined in Figure 3–46. Active succinate is joined to glycine to form delta-amino levulinic acid (ALA). This enzymatic step, controlled by ALA

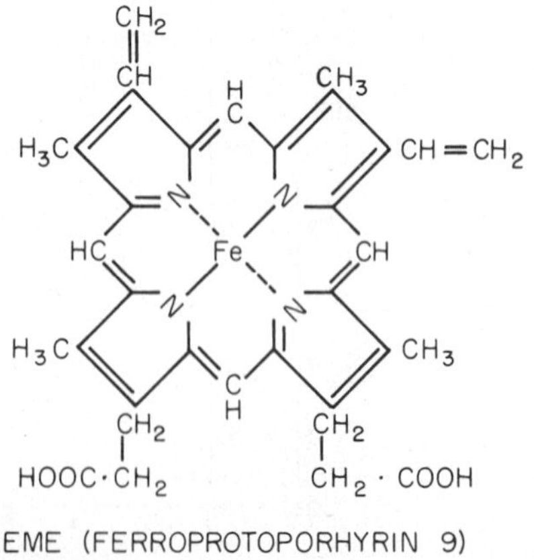

HEME (FERROPROTOPORHYRIN 9)

Figure 3–45 The structure of heme. (From Harris, J. W., and Kellermeyer, R. W.: The Red Cell. Harvard University Press, Cambridge, 1970, p. 3.)

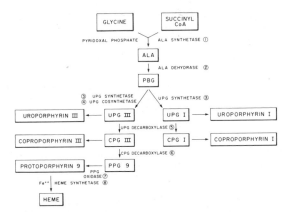

Figure 3–46 The synthesis of heme. Eight enzymatic steps are indicated. The initial step (1) is energy requiring, takes place on mitochondria, and uses pyridoxal phosphate as a co-factor. The final steps (6, 7, and 8) are also mitochondrial. The intermediate enzymes (2 through 5) are in the cytosol.

Demonstrated enzymatic deficiencies in hereditary porphyria are as follows: acute intermittent porphyria (3); erythropoietic porphyria (4); porphyria cutanea tarda (5); hereditary protoporphyria (8). Postulated defects, not proved, are: variegate porphyria (7 or 8); hereditary coproporphyria (6). In lead poisoning decreased activity of (2) and (8) are most pronounced, although (1) and (6) are also inhibited. As another example of "toxic" porphyria, the chemical compound hexachlorobenzene inhibits (5) and produces a clinical picture resembling porphyria cutanea tarda. The enzymatic lack in the various porphyria states is associated with induction of increased ALA synthetase activity due to the lack of feedback control and consequent overproduction of porphyrin precursors synthesized proximal to the site of the enzymatic block.

Abbreviations are as follows: ALA—δ amino levulinic acid; PBG—porphobilinogen; UPG—uroporphyrinogen; CPG—coproporphyrinogen; PPG—protoporphyrinogen.

synthetase, is both rate limiting and regulatory. It is subject to negative feedback inhibition and, as will be subsequently explained, in a variety of deficiencies of enzymes in the porphyrin synthetic pathway, the lack of end product causes deficient inhibition along with marked overproduction of precursors synthesized at sites above the block. Pyridoxal phosphate, the active form of the vitamin pyridoxine, is also required for this initial synthetic step.

Monopyrrole porphobilinogen rings are then formed by head-to-tail linkages of two ALA molecules. Four porphobilinogens in turn condense into the cyclic tetrapyrrole structure, which then undergoes progressive decarboxylation from uroporphyrinogen (containing 8 carboxyl side chains) to coproporphyrinogen (containing 4 carboxyl side chains) to protoporphyrinogen (containing 2 carboxyl side chains). Progressive decarboxylation is associated with an increased degree of insolubility which determines fecal as opposed to urinary excretion, the less soluble being predominantly fecal and the more soluble urinary (Table 3–8). Oxidation converts these colorless heme precursors into the brightly colored uroporphyrins, coproporphyrins, and protoporphyrins.

The porphyrins may exist in a variety of isomeric states depending on the position of the side chains, but only a limited number of isomers are of biologic significance. The uro- and copro- derivatives are found biologically only as the I and III isomers. In the formation of urobilinogen from porphobilinogen, a cosynthetase operating in conjunction with a synthetase directs the bulk of synthesis to the III isomer, which serves exclusively as heme precursor. In the absence of cosynthetase, uroporphyrinogen I is preferentially formed and this does not fulfill the requirements of heme synthesis. Following consecutive conversions from uroporphyrinogen III to coproporphyrinogen III to protoporphyrinogen 9 to protoporphyrin 9, four of the six coordinate positions of ferrous iron are chelated to the completed tetrapyrrole to form heme, ready for combination with globin or other apoproteins.

GENERAL EFFECTS OF DISORDERS OF PORPHYRIN SYNTHESIS. The porphyrias are caused by inherited or acquired blocks in the enzymatic steps governing heme synthesis, but the most pronounced consequence of the block is overproduction of the heme precursors above the site of the block. The liver is most commonly the major site of the defect with sparing of the erythroid cells ("hepatic porphyrias"), although in some conditions the erythroid tissue is affected. It is surprising that in those states affecting the erythroid cells heme synthesis is sufficient to meet almost completely the needs of hemoglobin synthesis, and hypochromia of the erythrocytes is either absent or minimal. Specific diagnosis is usually accomplished by quantification and characterization of the various heme precursors in the urine, feces, erythrocytes, and liver. The characteristics of the porphyrias are summarized in Table 3–9.

Pink or red urine may be observed if there is sufficient concentration of the colored derivatives uroporphyrin and/or coproporphyrin. The freshly passed urine is colorless, however, if the increase affects primarily colorless reduced precursors. In the case of protoporphyria the urine is normal; excretion is via the fecal route because of the insolubility of this derivative. Deposition of the colored derivatives in tissue slices is detected by observing the emission of red fluorescence upon exposure to ultraviolet light. Indeed cutaneous absorption of light in the 400 nm. wave length range produces photo-sensitive skin reactions with symptoms which range from mild itching and burning to erythema, edema, blistering, and even-

TABLE 3–8 NORMAL VALUES FOR PORPHYRINS AND PORPHYRIN PRECURSORS IN MAN

	Urine $\mu g./24$ hrs.	*Stool* $\mu g./gm.$ dry wt.	*Erythrocytes* $\mu g./100$ ml. cells
ALA	trace–2000	–	–
PBG	trace–1500	–	–
uroporphyrin	10–40	trace	trace
coproporphyrin	100–250	trace–50	0.5–1.5
protoporphyrin	0	trace–120	25–75

(Abbreviations as in Figure 3–46; From Marver and Schmid, 1972.)

tually even scarring and disfigurement involving exposed areas, such as the face and the backs of the hands. Damage to other tissues may also occur, as will be subsequently discussed.

INHERITED DISORDERS OF PORPHYRIN SYNTHESIS. *Acute intermittent porphyria* is an autosomal dominant hepatic disorder with onset in young adult life. The overproduction of ALA and porphobilinogen in the liver is associated with acute attacks of abdominal pain, polyneuropathy, and neuropsychiatric disturbance, sometimes with a fatal outcome, but with relative freedom from symptoms between episodes. In some instances the attacks are provoked by any of a variety of medications, such as barbiturates, estrogens, or sulfa drugs, which further increase ALA synthetase activity. Fasting also provokes attacks, while a high carbohydrate diet appears to be of value in their prevention. There have been reports by Dhar and co-workers that intravenously administered heme derivatives successfully terminate attacks by means of end production inhibition of ALA synthetase activity. It has still not been established if the increased porphyrin precursors are the direct cause of the neuropathic symptoms of the disease. Freshly passed urine is colorless, but may darken after several hours' standing owing to spontaneous oxidation of porphobilinogen to porphobilin. In addition to the classic acute intermittent porphyria, there are two variants, also autosomal dominant with late onset, "variegate porphyria" and "hereditary coproporphyria." These variants are distinguished by light sensitive skin, with more marked lesions in the variegate variety, and by the increased excretion of porphyrin precursors further along the pathway of synthesis in addition to ALA and urobilinogen, as described in Table 3–9. The acute attacks resemble those of acute intermittent porphyria.

Congenital erythropoietic porphyria is a rare but dramatic autosomal recessive condition in which the increase of uroporphyrin and coproporphyrin I isomers affects primarily the erythroid cells, but red staining of all the tissues and of the urine is prominent. The onset is usually in childhood. Photosensitivity is especially severe and there are signs of hemolysis along with splenomegaly.

Porphyria cutanea tarda, also an hepatic porphyria, presumably originates from a combination of inherited enzyme deficiency in addition to acquired factors essential for the expression of the clinical signs and symptoms, which typically do not begin until middle age, as reported by Kushner and co-workers. Among the acquired factors, alcoholism and liver disease and exposure to certain medications, especially estrogen, are commonly observed, but increased liver iron is always present, often along with elevation of the plasma iron concentration and increased saturation of the plasma iron binding protein. The excess liver iron is of pathogenetic importance since its removal by a series of phlebotomies ameliorates both the clinical and biochemical manifestations of the disorder (Figure 3–47). Although the primary deficiency involves uroporphyrinogen decarboxylase, cosynthetase also appears to be in some manner affected, since urinary uroporphyrin I excretion exceeds that of uroporphyrin III. Urine urobilinogen excretion may be normal, or if elevated is commensurate with the degree of liver dysfunction. In addition to the symptoms of liver disease, photosensitivity and red urine are usually present.

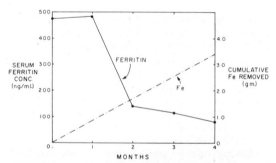

Figure 3–47 Decrease in serum ferritin concentration as iron stores were reduced by weekly phlebotomy in a patient with porphyria cutanea tarda. Initial liver biopsy documented markedly increased hepatocellular iron. The reduction in iron stores resulted in a marked decrease in the urinary porphyrin excretion (normal serum ferritin concentration 20 to 200 ng./ml.).

TABLE 3-9 CLASSIFICATION OF PORPHYRIAS

| Condition | Photo Sensitivity | Tissue Primarily Involved | | Biochemical Abnormalities Useful in Diagnosis (Abbrevs. in Fig. 3–46) |
		Erythroid	Hepatic	
Hereditary				
Acute intermittent porphyria	−	−	+	Increased urinary ALA and PBG.
Erythropoietic porphyria	+	+	−	Increased urinary and erythrocyte uroporphyrin I and coproporphyrin I.
Porphyria cutanea tarda	+	−	+	Increased urinary uroporphyrin I>III and coproporphyrin I and III. (Porphyrins also increased in liver, along with excess iron.)
Coproporphyria	+	−	+	Increased fecal and urinary coproporphyrin III. Increased urinary ALA and PBG during acute attacks.
Variegate porphyria	+	−	+	Increased fecal protoporphyrin 9 and coproporphyrin III. Increased urinary coproporphyrin III and, during acute attacks, ALA and PBG.
Protoporphyria	+	+	+	Increased erythrocyte and fecal protoporphyrin 9.
Acquired				
Lead poisoning	−	+	?	Increased urinary ALA and coproporphyrin III. Increased erythrocyte protoporphyrin 9.
Hexachlorobenzene toxicity	+	−	+	Increased urinary uroporphyrin I and III and coproporphyrin I and III.

Enzyme defects are listed in the legend to Figure 3–46. All inherited conditions are autosomal dominant, except erythropoietic porphyria which is autosomal recessive.

Hereditary protoporphyria is associated with high tissue concentrations of protoporphyrin 9 in both erythrocytes and liver. Symptoms may be entirely absent, but mild photosensitivity is often present from childhood. Cholelithiasis commonly occurs as a result of the high concentration of this relatively insoluble porphyrin in the bile. In some cases of long duration, chronic liver disease has developed. The excess porphyrin is excreted exclusively via the fecal route; the urine is normal. Mild anemia may be present, but there are no clinical signs of hemolysis, despite the fact that photohemolysis is demonstrable in vitro.

ACQUIRED DISORDERS OF PORPHYRIN SYNTHESIS. In *lead intoxication* several of the enzymes controlling heme synthesis are inhibited (Figure 3–46). Depression of ALA dehydrase activity is one of the earliest changes. Heme synthetase is also readily depressed as reviewed by Chisholm. Increases in urinary ALA and in erythrocyte protoporphyrin levels are accordingly observed early in the course of the disease. Urinary coproporphyrin III is also frequently increased, while urinary porphobilinogen is normal or only slightly increased. Photosensitivity is not a feature of lead toxicity because the increased intraerythrocytic protoporphyrin occurs as a zinc complex tightly bound to hemoglobin, in contrast to hereditary protoporphyria in which the protoporphyrin is loosely bound and passes out of the erythrocytes into the skin and other tissues, causing light sensitivity (Piomelli and co-workers). Increased amounts of ferritin and hemosiderin accumulate in the erythroid precursors because of the blocks in heme synthesis. The erythrocytes are slightly hypochromic and a significant proportion of them show punctate basophilic stippling due to the presence of aggregated incompletely degraded ribosomes. After having observed that hereditary deficiency of the red cell enzyme pyrimidine 5'-nucleotidase was associated with punctate basophilic stippling, Valentine and his co-workers found that this red cell enzyme was also low in patients with lead poisoning. Apparently this lack causes an impairment of ribosome ribonucleic acid degradation in reticulocytes. The anemia of lead toxicity is mild and the erythrocyte life span only slightly or moderately shortened. The neurologic symptoms are the most significant aspects of the disease — encephalopathy in the child and peripheral motor neuropathy in the adult. Abdominal pain as well as renal disease may also occur.

Toxic exposure to hexachlorobenzene mimics porphyria cutanea tarda. Affected individuals are photosensitive and have red urine. The resemblance is explained by the observation that the same enzyme, uroporphyrinogen decarboxylase, is depressed in both conditions. The original clinical observations, made following an outbreak in Turkey, have served to stimulate interest in experimental porphyria induced by this and other chemical agents.

Iron. NORMAL IRON METABOLISM. Iron, by far the most abundant heavy metal in the body is used chiefly for hemoglobin synthesis. About 1 mg. is required for each ml. of red cells produced, adding up to a daily need of 20 to 25 mg. for erythropoiesis. Almost all this iron is obtained through recycling and only about 5 per cent, or 1 mg. per day, is newly absorbed to balance losses incurred via fecal and urinary excretion and also in sweat and desquamated skin. The average menstruating female loses about twice this amount and so must absorb more to maintain balance. Menstrual loss of blood, however, is difficult to estimate and varies a great deal from woman to woman.

Absorption by the gastrointestinal epithelial cell is finely tuned to admit just enough iron to cover losses, without permitting either excess or deficiency of body iron to develop. Absorption normally admits about 5 to 10 per cent of a total dietary intake of 10 to 20 mg. per day. The physiologic signal between the size of the body iron

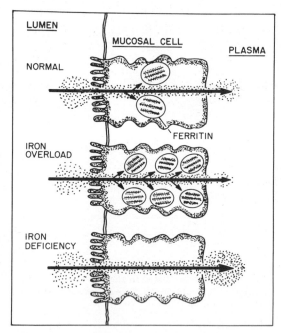

Figure 3–48 Regulation of iron absorption at the intestinal mucosa. Stippled dots represent iron molecules. Intracellular ferritin is symbolized by oval structures. The iron overloaded mucosal cell deposits more iron as ferritin, but admits relatively little into the plasma, while the iron deficient cell lowers its barrier to efficient transport of iron across into the plasma. Sloughing of mucosal cells into the intestinal lumen is a significant excretory route for iron, especially in states of iron overload. (Reprinted with permission of *Nutrition Today.* Copyright Summer, 1969, by Nutrition Today, Inc.)

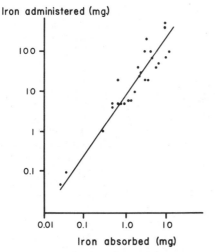

Iron administered (mg)

Figure 3–49 Augmentation of absolute amount of iron absorbed with increasing doses administered. (Redrawn from Bothwell, T. H., and Finch, C. A.: Iron Metabolism. Little, Brown & Co., Boston, 1962, p. 98.)

supply and the gastrointestinal mucosal cell is still only vaguely understood. The mucosal cell itself appears to act as a "ferrostat" by reflecting within its own cytoplasm the state of the body store of iron. A high concentration of cytoplasmic iron, present presumably almost entirely as ferritin, discourages further uptake, while an iron-poor intracellular environment encourages uptake into the cell and then on into the plasma for binding to transferrin (Fig. 3–48).

The absorption of iron is also increased in response to increased erythropoietic activity. The mucosal epithelial cells are in a constant state of renewal, proliferating from the crypts out toward the tips of the villi, where they are shed into the lumen. Such cellular loss is a significant source of iron excretion in the feces. The existence of a specialized iron transport protein within the mucosal cell remains open to question.

The barrier to excessive iron absorption set up by the mucosal cell is easily overcome, since increasing amounts of iron presented to the intestinal epithelial surface are met by additional increments of absorbed iron, although the proportion absorbed falls off (Fig. 3–49). The mucosal barrier is temporarily raised, however, by recently ingested iron, which decreases the absorption of a second dose given several hours later (Fig. 3–50).

The entire gastrointestinal tract has the capacity to absorb iron, but maximal activity is found in the duodenum and upper jejunum, probably because of the presence there of optimal conditions of pH and redox potential. Absorption occurs in the ferrous state, and ferric iron, which forms insoluble hydroxides at neutral and alkaline pH, must first be reduced before it is absorbed. For efficient reduction, an acid gastric juice is indispensable (Fig. 3–51). Chelation with low molecular weight compounds, such as fructose and amino acids, may also promote solubility preparatory to absorption. Whether the gastric juice itself contains special iron-chelating substances of either high or low molecular weight remains somewhat controversial. Dietary constituents such as phosphate and phytate render iron less soluble and thus less available for absorption. The concept that pancre-

Figure 3–50 The change in absorption of a test dose of radioactive iron at intervals after an initial loading dose of nonradioactive iron. (Redrawn from Stewart, W. B., et al.: J. Exper. Med., *92*:375, 1950.)

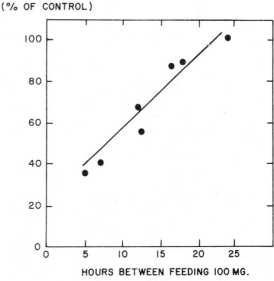

RADIOIRON ABSORPTION
(% OF CONTROL)

HOURS BETWEEN FEEDING 100 MG.
IRON AND RADIOIRON

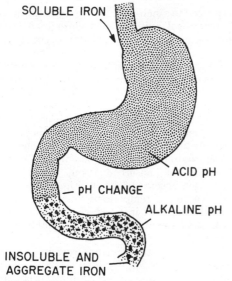

Figure 3–51 Relation of pH to the maximal site of iron absorption in the upper duodenum. (Reprinted with permission of *Nutrition Today.* Copyright Summer, 1969 by Nutrition Today, Inc.)

atic insufficiency, by reducing duodenal pH, causes increased iron absorption has been challenged. Food iron, in contrast to the inorganic ferrous form of medicinal iron, occurs as organic complexes, such as ferritin and myoglobin, much of it in the trivalent state. Some of the complexes are broken up and solubilized during acid digestion in the stomach, but the heme iron passes on and is readily absorbed intact into the mucosal epithelial cells, without dependence upon reducing systems and by a mechanism that is distinct from that for inorganic iron, as described by Weintraub and co-workers. The iron is stripped away from its complex with porphyrin only after cellular uptake. Myoglobin and hemoglobin are better nutritional sources of iron than ferritin and hemosiderin, which are not as well absorbed.

Effete red cells which have lived out their 120-day life span are taken up by the phagocytic macrophages, chiefly in the spleen, liver, and bone marrow. Inside these phagocytic cells the hemoglobin is broken down into its essential constituents, with an efficient salvage of the iron taken from degraded heme. This salvaged iron is packed in extremely high concentration inside apoferritin protein shells to form molecules of ferritin, each of which may contain up to 4000 atoms of iron (Fig. 3–52). Ferritin molecules, in turn, are compressed

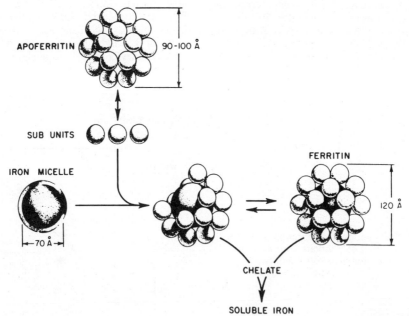

Figure 3–52 Structure of ferritin. A series of identical subunits is assembled to form a protein shell (apoferritin). An iron micelle, containing up to 4000 atoms of iron, is formed inside. Iron can be removed, leaving behind an intact apoferritin shell.

There are a series of isoferritins which differ depending on the tissue of origin. Thus, for example, ferritin extracted from macrophages differs from that found in erythroid cells or heart. Ferritin found in plasma also differs from that found in tissues, especially in its low iron content. It appears to originate predominantly from macrophages rather than parenchymal cells.

(Reprinted from Pape, L., et al.: Biochemistry, 7:606, 1968. Copyright 1968, American Chemical Society. Reprinted by permission of the copyright owner.)

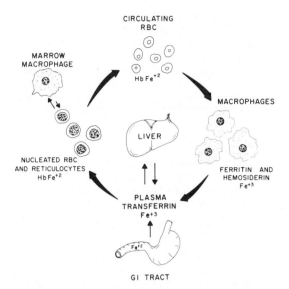

CIRCULATING
RBC

MARROW
MACROPHAGE

HbFe⁺²

MACROPHAGES

LIVER

NUCLEATED RBC
AND RETICULOCYTES
HbFe⁺²

FERRITIN AND
HEMOSIDERIN
Fe⁺³

PLASMA
TRANSFERRIN
Fe⁺³

Fe⁺²

GI TRACT

Figure 3–53 Metabolic pathways of iron. The bulk of body iron turnover goes to erythropoiesis in the marrow and is reutilized from hemoglobin degraded in macrophages located primarily in the liver, spleen, and marrow. Only a small proportion of the iron is newly absorbed from dietary sources to make up for excretory losses. Cell-to-cell interaction between erythroid precursors and macrophages takes place in the marrow with possible exchange of ferritin iron. The direction of this exchange is still uncertain, but most evidence suggests that marrow (and splenic) macrophages remove excess ferritin and hemosiderin iron from erythroid cells. Transferrin mediates iron transport from macrophages and the intestinal mucosa to immature erythroid cells. It also delivers iron to hepatic and other parenchymal cells, but at a much lesser rate.

into still larger amorphous aggregates of insoluble material called hemosiderin, which form granules visible by light microscopy. Thus it is as ferritin and hemosiderin, chiefly in macrophages, that the bulk of the reserve iron is stored. It is from these depots that iron recycles, fulfilling the continuing need for iron in the production of red cells (Fig. 3–53).

The storage iron most recently obtained from degraded heme is the first to be reutilized for hemoglobin synthesis; the chronologically more archaic iron depots may remain untouched for very long periods of time. In a normal adult with 2500-ml. red cell mass, 2500 mg. of iron circulates as hemoglobin while another 500 to 1500 mg. is present as storage iron. Although the vast bulk of the storage iron is found in macrophages, ferritin is detectable in many of the tissues of the body, including erythroblasts and the intestinal epithelial cells. Other significant pools of body iron are in myoglobin (130 mg.) and a variety of enzymes, such as the cytochromes, catalase, peroxidase, and many others (8 mg.).

Iron is taken from storage depots and transported back to erythroid precursors by a highly specialized plasma protein, transferrin. Stored in ferritin in the trivalent state, the iron is first reduced to the ferrous form for removal from the apoferritin shell, and then it is carried in the ferric state, up to two atoms per molecule of transferrin. The normal concentration of iron in the plasma is about 100 μg. per 100 ml., one third the total binding capacity of available transferrin. The total amount of iron in the transferrin pool, assuming that approximately half of it is intravascular and half extravascular, is about 4 to 5 mg. Although this transferrin-bound iron is only 1 per cent of that in the body, its metabolic rate of turnover is extremely rapid — 50 per cent of it is cleared from the intravascular space every 60 to 120 minutes. Transferrin molecules deliver their iron at the surface of the erythroid precursors and return empty to the macrophages to pick up another load (Fig. 3–54).

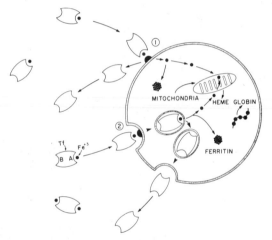

MITOCHONDRIA

HEME GLOBIN

Tf

Fe⁺³

B A

FERRITIN

Figure 3–54 Schematic representation of the delivery of iron to erythroid precursors. *A* and *B* indicate the two iron-binding sites on the transferrin molecule. Transferrin preferentially delivers its iron to receptors present on the surface of nucleated erythroid cells and on reticulocytes, but absent from mature erythrocytes (Aisen and Brown, 1977). The presence of an anion, physiologically probably bicarbonate, is necessary to establish the extraordinarily high affinity between transferrin and Fe⁺³; in its absence virtually no binding takes place. The cell frees iron from transferrin, possibly by removing the anion. Two mechanisms for delivery have been postulated. Pathway (1) envisions a receptor on the outer surface of the cell membrane. Pathway (2) pictures pinocytosis of the transferrin-iron complex, release of iron, and then ejection of the iron-free transferrin back to the plasma. Iron is transported within the cell to mitochondria for heme synthesis and is stored as ferritin and hemosiderin. Intracellular iron transport mechanisms have still not been elucidated.

Fletcher and Huehns have proposed a provocative, but still unproved, hypothesis stating that the two iron binding sites on the transferrin molecule, Site A and Site B, are unequal in their affinity for ferric iron and subserve different physiologic functions. Site A, they state, picks up iron at the intestinal mucosal cell and delivers it to receptors on immature erythroid cells (and the placenta). Site B preferentially gives up its iron to hepatocytes as well as to intestinal mucosal cells, the governors of the rate of iron absorption. The amount and distribution of iron on transferrin would then control its absorption as well as its distribution in the body. This remarkable hypothesis has had the merit of provoking a number of experimental tests, but the results so far have generally been at odds.

The rate of disappearance of radioactive iron from the plasma as well as its reappearance in the circulating red cells as newly produced labeled hemoglobin is a convenient method of measuring the functional state of erythropoiesis, as discussed by Ricketts and co-workers (Fig. 3–22). In hypoplastic conditions the utilization of iron is depressed, causing a rise in its plasma concentration along with a decrease in the rate at which it is cleared from the normal half-life of 1 to 2 hours to 3 to 4 hours or longer. In iron deficiency the clearance rate is more rapid than normal, as it is in conditions associated with increased proliferation of red cell precursors in the marrow, such as hemolytic anemia. Normally about 70 to 80 per cent of the tracer iron reappears in circulating erythrocytes within 10 days of administration, but this figure may approach zero in the absence of red cell production. The red cell utilization of tracer iron is also depressed in conditions such as thalassemia or megaloblastic anemia, in which the marrow is rich in proliferating erythroid precursor cells and in their requirement for iron, but owing to extensive intramedullary destruction of these cells, little of the radioiron reappears in circulating erythrocytes despite its rapid clearance from the plasma. A labile pool of storage iron contributes a minor slow component to the plasma radioiron disappearance curve.

IRON LACK

General Effects. The first change in the development of iron deficiency is the loss of storage iron from the macrophages of the spleen, liver, and bone marrow. The evaluation of marrow iron stores is a convenient method of assessing the state of the body iron stores; if they are preserved, iron deficiency can be excluded as the primary cause of anemia. After the stores of iron are used up, the plasma iron concentration falls, at the same time stimulating an increase in the synthesis of transferrin. The saturation of transferrin with iron thus falls from 30 per cent to values often below 10 per cent (Fig. 3–55). Plasma ferritin concentration is always depressed and distinguishes the hypoferremia of iron deficiency from

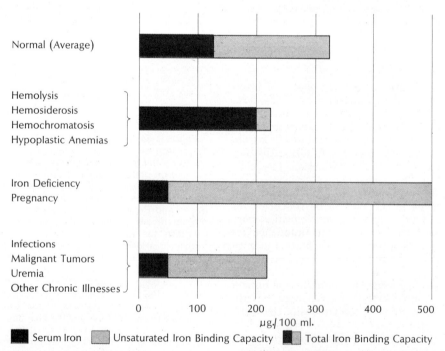

Figure 3–55 The changes in serum iron and iron binding capacity in various disorders. (From McIntyre, P.: Hosp. Pract., March, 1972, p. 101.)

that seen in association with the anemia of chronic disease, in which plasma ferritin is normal or elevated. Erythrocyte protoporphyrin levels are increased secondary to the intracellular deficit of sufficient iron for heme synthesis. Anemia is the last change to be observed. At first, the erythrocytes may be normocytic and normochromic and show only a few shape changes, but microcytic, hypochromic, and misshapen erythrocytes emerge as significant anemia develops. Even with only a moderate degree of anemia, the deficit in body iron is thus already advanced.

Whether iron deficiency without anemia causes significant symptoms remains a controversial issue. The activities of certain iron-containing enzymes decrease, but this change may not be of pathophysiologic significance. When anemia develops it is often well tolerated, except when there is acute blood loss or cardiovascular limitation. Changes in epithelial tissues complicate more protracted deficiency. There is inversion of the normal curvature of the fingernails ("spooning"), which also become more brittle; hair splits and breaks off; and a smooth red tongue reflects glossitis. Dysphagia with web formation in the upper esophagus rarely complicates iron lack of many years' duration. Atrophic gastritis with anacidity is frequently associated with iron deficiency, whether primarily the result of it (through secondary epithelial changes) or the cause of it (through impaired absorption of food iron) or both is not clear. Infants with iron deficiency anemia frequently have detectable occult blood in the feces without demonstrable gastrointestinal disease, presumably because of mucosal friability secondary to the deficient state. Mucosal changes secondary to iron deficiency in infants reportedly may be of sufficient magnitude to cause malabsorption. A moderately elevated platelet count is often seen in infants with iron deficiency anemia. Thrombocytosis in iron-deficient adults seems to be less prominent and more often explainable on the basis of reactive changes to hemorrhage, tumor, or other underlying disorders.

Pathogenesis. Iron deficiency always arises because of the inability of diet and absorption to keep pace with the increased requirements imposed either by the expansion of the red cell mass or by blood loss. The efficiency of absorption depends not only on the total amount of food iron but also on its form as well as on the dietary content of phosphate and phytate. Habitual eating of laundry starch or clay is commonly seen among iron-deficient patients of certain population groups. Such materials may have an adverse effect upon iron absorption, but of even greater importance is the fact that among such patients the dietary intake of good sources of iron, such as meat, is also often severely limited. A peculiar craving for ice may develop. Iron deficient children with pica may develop lead poisoning be-

cause they eat lead-containing paint. These unusual eating patterns appear to respond to the treatment of the iron deficiency.

The growth spurt of the 2-year-old and of the adolescent are common times for iron deficiency to appear. The well-nourished milk-fed infant is particularly prone because such a diet, while adequate in calories, is sorely lacking in iron. Iron deficiency is very rare at the time of birth, even if the mother is deficient. However, the rapid growth which follows premature birth requires iron supplementation during the first weeks of life to prevent the development of anemia. During pregnancy, the red cell mass expands by 20 per cent, which may require about 400 mg. of additional iron. The fetus requires about 280 mg., which is lost to the mother along with blood loss at childbirth. The losses of lactation are about equal to those which would have occurred from menstruation (Fig. 3–56).

The proper absorption of food iron being dependent upon a normal gastric milieu, anacidity acquired from either atrophic gastritis or from partial or total gastrectomy very commonly leads to iron deficiency anemia. Billroth type II procedures, which bypass the duodenum, are more commonly associated than those procedures which leave this site of maximal iron absorption intact. Rapid intestinal transit time may limit the time available for absorption. Excessive gastrointestinal blood loss contributes to iron depletion in those clinical situations which require gastric surgery, such as peptic ulcer. Iron lack coexists with other multiple deficiencies in the intestinal malabsorption syndromes, but if the duodenal surface is well preserved, sufficient iron may be absorbed to meet requirements.

Blood loss is the most important factor in the development of iron deficiency. Identification of its origin may bring to light the presence of unsuspected but significant underlying disease, such as carcinoma of the colon. Hiatus hernia, hemorrhagic gastritis, and peptic ulcer disease are particularly frequent causes of upper gastrointestinal bleeding. Chronic aspirin users develop iron deficiency anemia because of increased gastrointestinal blood loss with or without demonstrable underlying disease. Menorrhagia, sometimes associated with such underlying disease as uterine fibroids, is the most frequent cause in premenopausal females. Sources of urinary blood loss include renal tumors as well as the chronic hemoglobinuria and hemosiderinuria associated with chronic intravascular hemolysis. Vasculitis of the pulmonary vessels with chronic hemorrhage into the lungs will cause pulmonary macrophages to become iron-laden in *Goodpasture's syndrome*. However, iron is not efficiently reutilized from these cells and an iron-deficient bone marrow with microcytic, hypochromic anemia ensues.

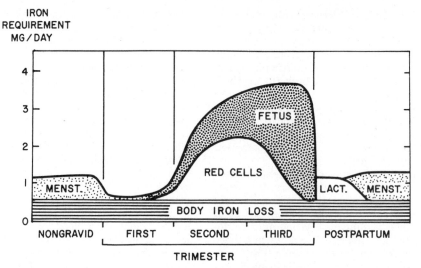

Figure 3-56   The change in iron requirement during pregnancy. (Redrawn from Bothwell, T. H., and Finch, C. A.: Iron Metabolism. Little, Brown & Co., Boston, 1962, p. 309.)

IRON EXCESS

General Effects.   The accumulation of excessive quantities of iron in the body ultimately originates from increased absorption or from parenteral administration as transfusions or as pharmacologic iron complexes. The capacity of the macrophages to gather the extra iron within their protective confines is immense, but ultimately the degree of transferrin saturation rises, its synthesis is inhibited, and the plasma iron concentration approaches 200 μg. per 100 ml. with near 100 per cent saturation of the iron-binding capacity (Fig. 3–55). As the transferrin saturation rises above 50 per cent parenchymal cells are no longer protected from pathologic iron uptake and damage occurs over the years to various organs, especially the liver, heart, pancreas, pituitary, and synovial tissues. Signs of chronic liver disease appear, along with those of heart failure, diabetes mellitus, and endocrine insufficiency. A characteristic form of arthropathy may develop. The term *hemochromatosis* is used to describe the disease which thus arises from such chronic iron overexposure. Grayish pigmentation of the skin is caused by deposition of melanin in the deeper layers of the epidermis. Deposits of iron are seen in the glandular structures of the skin.

Acute iron poisoning occurs chiefly in children who accidentally swallow an overdose of iron pills. Nausea, vomiting, and intestinal bleeding are soon followed by vascular collapse and shock, with a high likelihood of a fatal outcome.

The detection of iron overload would be best accomplished by the direct measurement of total body iron stores, but no satisfactory technique is available for this. A rise in the plasma iron concentration and transferrin saturation is associated with increased iron stores, but similar changes are seen secondary to altered bone marrow function, such as hypoplastic and megaloblastic anemia. Furthermore, the hypoferremic response to inflammation may depress an elevated plasma iron level and mask a state of iron overload.

A time-honored but cumbersome method of measuring iron stores uses quantitative phlebotomy carried out over many months to the point of early iron deficiency anemia, a sign that the iron stores initially present have been depleted. The total amount of hemoglobin iron removed, assuming 1 mg. Fe per ml. erythrocytes, is roughly equivalent to the iron stores initially present.

A "labile" intracellular pool of iron may be assessed by measuring the urinary excretion of iron for 24 hours after a single injection of the chelating agent desferrioxamine (DFOM). The normal excretes about 0.5 mg., whereas the iron-loaded patient may excrete up to 10 to 20 mg. This labile pool is thought to be physiologically chelated within cells to low molecular weight substances, since the other biologic forms of iron (ferritin, transferrin, heme) are not significantly available for DFOM chelation.

The concentration of ferritin in plasma may be extraordinarily high in iron-overloaded states, but normal values also are observed. The plasma ferritin level usually reflects the iron pool of the macrophages rather than that of the parenchymal cells, and thus normal levels may be seen in the face of parenchymal iron excess. Breakdown of normal hepatic or neoplastic parenchymal cells, however, may cause release of ferritin into the plasma. Thus, elevated plasma ferritin levels also occur in patients with acute or chronic liver disease, leukemia, or cancer. Plasma ferritin measurements may be useful in the detection of iron deficiency, of iron excess, or in following changes on body iron status (Fig. 3–47), but caution must be exercised in correctly interpreting the value.

Perhaps the most sensitive method for the early detection of iron overload is direct measurement on samples obtained by liver biopsy. Estimation is made microscopically after suitable staining or by chemical measurement. Although bone marrow iron content is invaluable in the detection of iron deficiency, it is less helpful in hemochromatosis, as discussed below.

Pathogenesis. An increase in the body content of iron in *primary hemochromatosis* occurs because of an inappropriate and as yet unexplained increase in iron absorption by the intestinal mucosal cells as reviewed in 1977 by Jacobs. An increase in liver iron, predominantly in the hepatocytes, may be the sole manifestation early in the course of the disease, but elevation of the plasma iron and increased saturation of transferrin is also often present initially (Edwards and associates, 1977). Iron loading in macrophages and elevation of the plasma ferritin occur later. In advanced stages the body may contain 30 to 40 grams of iron. The fact that macrophage and intestinal mucosal cell iron content do not appear increased early in the disease has led to the postulate that the primary defect may be a deficient rate of ferritin synthesis in these sites, with breakdown of the mucosal barrier against increased absorption, reduction of the normal protective storage function of the macrophages, and consequent iron loading of transferrin and of parenchymal cells, especially hepatic. Erythrocyte morphology is normal, and erythropoiesis is unaffected. Indeed, anemia is noteworthy for its absence. Although the disorder runs in families, its hereditary nature has been disputed. Excess dietary iron — usually in the form of certain beers and wines with high iron content, food cooked in iron utensils, or medicinal iron — leads to a similar disorder. Instances of apparent primary hemochromatosis which develop in patients with alcoholic cirrhosis presumably are related to the fact that a small proportion of such patients develop increased iron absorption secondary to the liver disease. The pathogenesis of this increase is obscure.

Iron overload due to chronic transfusion (transfusion hemosiderosis) contrasts with primary hemochromatosis inasmuch as iron loading occurs first in the macrophages and only later in the parenchymal cells. Plasma ferritin is elevated early in the course of the iron overload, and a rise in the plasma iron and transferrin saturation occurs later. The iron overload may be readily detected in bone marrow macrophages or circulating blood monocytes, which are not reliable parameters of iron overload in early primary hemochromatosis, although their iron content increases as the disease progresses.

Hemochromatosis also complicates disorders of erythropoiesis in which iron is not properly utilized for hemoglobin formation. The increased iron absorption is apparently related to the hyperplastic, although ineffective, erythropoiesis which characterizes these conditions. Red cell morphology is abnormal. The anemia is of any degree from minimal to severe. An excessive number of hemosiderin granules accumulates in the cytoplasm of erythroid precursor cells as well as in mature erythrocytes, where their presence becomes much more obvious after splenectomy. The term "sideroblast" is applied to any nucleated erythroid precursor which contains stainable iron granules. In normal marrow about 25 per cent of erythroid precursors are sideroblasts containing two or three small cytoplasmic granules. The number and size of such iron granules as well as the proportion of erythroid cells containing them increase in a number of states of increased erythropoiesis, including hemolytic anemia and megaloblastic anemia. However, in the marrow of certain iron-loading anemias there are seen a large number of "ringed sideroblasts," erythroid cells in which a necklace of iron granules surrounds the nucleus. To these conditions the term "sideroblastic anemia" is applied. The ringed configuration is presumably related to the fact that the iron accumulation is concentrated on the mitochondria, which cling to the nuclear membranes in the fixed and stained preparations.

The *sideroblastic anemias* are classified as primary or secondary, hereditary or acquired (Kushner, et al., 1971). Hypochromic, small, misshapen erythrocytes are often seen in the midst of a population of normocytic or even macrocytic cells. Hereditary sex-linked hypochromic anemia is usually first detected in young adult or adolescent males, whereas primary acquired sideroblastic anemia is seen in patients of either sex over the age of 60. Occasionally, with observation the latter condition will ultimately prove to be a secondary variety associated with a myeloproliferative syndrome culminating in acute myelogenous leukemia. The condition can also occur secondary to certain drugs (isoniazid, cycloserine, chloramphenicol), to lead poisoning, or to alcoholic excess, but reversibility averts the development of hemochromatosis. Rare ringed sideroblasts are occasionally seen in the marrow of patients with certain chronic diseases, such as rheumatoid arthritis or carcinoma, but hyperferremia and iron-loading do not complicate the picture.

Some of the sideroblastic anemias are pyridoxine-responsive, as described by Harris. The doses required are pharmacologic, and signs of pyridoxine deficiency are absent. Anemia is improved and the serum iron decreases. The response is not complete, although it is generally more satisfactory in the hereditary than in the primary acquired cases. The explanation of responsiveness may reside in a defect in conversion of pyridoxine to its active form, pyridoxal phosphate, which is required for the first step in heme synthesis on the mitochondria, upon which iron accumulates. Recent studies have provided some evidence for superior therapeutic efficacy of pyridoxal phosphate, but it would appear that the entire group of disorders is at present too heterogeneous to be properly analyzed until a more precise biochemical classification is achieved. Indeed, megaloblastic erythropoiesis and macrocytic erythrocytes are also sometimes observed along with a degree of folic acid responsiveness.

Hemochromatosis is a major cause of morbidity and mortality in thalassemia, a primary deficiency of globin synthesis. Erythroid cells are iron-loaded, but ringed sideroblasts are not prominent. Transfusional hemosiderosis contributes to the iron-load in thalassemia major, as well as in any anemia of sufficient severity to require chronic transfusion therapy.

Primary hemochromatosis is treated with removal of iron by repeated phlebotomy over a long period of time, until iron stores become depleted and the serum iron falls. This approach has also been used in hemochromatosis secondary to iron-loading erythrocyte disorders in which the anemia is mild. Another approach has been the use of iron chelating agents such as desferrioxamine. Recent observations by Propper and co-workers have shown enhanced efficacy of desferrioxamine given by continuous infusion rather than bolus injection. Iron chelators may be life-saving in the treatment of acute iron poisoning.

Globin

NORMAL STRUCTURE AND SYNTHESIS. The primary structure of the globin molecule as well as its production rate is under genetic control. Its specific amino acid sequence is governed by the triplet code of DNA bases passed down in the chromosomes from generation to generation. The rate at which globin polypeptide chains are synthesized is a function of the rate at which the DNA code is transcribed into messenger RNA. The sequence of translational events which follow modifies the production rate of the completed chains. These include the initiation and assembly on, and the release of the polypeptide chains from, the messenger RNA-polyribosome complex upon which the amino acids are joined together in proper sequence.

At least six genetic loci direct globin synthesis. The α and β chains of normal adult hemoglobin (HbA) are produced in matched amounts, but under the control of separate genes located far apart from one another on different chromosomes. The δ chain closely resembles the β chain, to which it is genetically linked on the same chromosome, but it is synthesized at only 1/40 the rate of β chains. Thus the concentration of Hb A_2 ($\alpha_2\delta_2$) in the normal adult is only about 2.5 per cent of the total hemoglobin. Alpha chains are synthesized from early embryonic life on, but are combined

with different chains according to the stage of development (Table 3–10). The ζ and ϵ globin chains are embryonic products produced during the first trimester of intrauterine development. Beyond the first trimester α and γ chain synthesis predominates in the formation of fetal hemoglo-

TABLE 3–10 SELECTED HEMOGLOBINS — THEIR STRUCTURES AND STRUCTURAL MUTATIONS

Normal Amino Acid Sequence	
HbA	$\alpha_2 \beta_2$
Hb A_2	$\alpha_2 \delta_2$
Hb F	$\alpha_2 \gamma_2$
Hb H	β_4
Hb Bart's	γ_4
Hb Portland	$\zeta_2\gamma_2$
Hb Gower-1	$\zeta_2\epsilon_2$
Hb Gower-2	$\alpha_2\epsilon_2$
Methemoglobinemia	
Hb M Boston	$\alpha^{58\ his\ \rightarrow\ tyr} \beta_2$
Hb M Iwate	$\alpha^{87\ his\ \rightarrow\ tyr} \beta_2$
Hb M Saskatoon	$\alpha_2 \beta_2^{63\ his\ \rightarrow\ tyr}$
Hb M Hyde Park	$\alpha_2 \beta_2^{92\ his\ \rightarrow\ tyr}$
Increased Oxygen Affinity with Erythrocytosis	
Hb Chesapeake	$\alpha_2^{92\ arg\ \rightarrow\ leu} \beta_2$
Hb Rainier	$\alpha_2 \beta_2^{145\ tyr\ \rightarrow\ his}$
Hb Hiroshima	$\alpha_2 \beta_2^{143\ his\ \rightarrow\ asp}$
Decreased Oxygen Affinity with Cyanosis	
Hb Kansas	$\alpha_2 \beta_2^{102\ asn\ \rightarrow\ thr}$
Unstable Hemoglobin with Hemolytic Anemia	
Hb Torino	$\alpha_2^{43\ phe\ \rightarrow\ val} \beta_2$
Hb Hammersmith	$\alpha_2 \beta_2^{42\ phe\ \rightarrow\ ser}$
Hb Zürich	$\alpha_2 \beta_2^{63\ his\ \rightarrow\ arg}$
Hb Tacoma	$\alpha_2 \beta_2^{30\ arg\ \rightarrow\ ser}$
Hb Philly	$\alpha_2 \beta_2^{35\ tyr\ \rightarrow\ phe}$
Hb Freiburg	$\alpha_2 \beta_2^{23\ val\ \rightarrow\ o}$
Hb Gun Hill	$\alpha_2 \beta_2^{93-97\ \rightarrow\ o}$
Hb Genova	$\alpha_2 \beta_2^{28\ leu\ \rightarrow\ pro}$
Hb Seattle	$\alpha_2 \beta_2^{76\ ala\ \rightarrow\ glu}$
"Exterior" Mutants	
Hb S	$\alpha_2 \beta_2^{6\ glu\ \rightarrow\ val}$
Hb C	$\alpha_2 \beta_2^{6\ glu\ \rightarrow\ lys}$
Hb E	$\alpha_2 \beta_2^{26\ glu\ \rightarrow\ lys}$
Hb C Harlem	$\alpha_2 \beta_2^{6\ glu\ \rightarrow\ val;}$ $^{73\ asp\ \rightarrow\ asn}$
Hb Korle-bu	$\alpha_2 \beta_2^{73\ asp\ \rightarrow\ asn}$
Hb G Accra	$\alpha_2 \beta_2^{79\ asp\ \rightarrow\ asn}$
Hb D Punjab	$\alpha_2 \beta_2^{121\ glu\ \rightarrow\ gln}$
Mutants with Low Synthetic Rate	
Hb Lepore	α_2 δ-β_2 (fusion gene)
Hb Constant Spring	$\alpha_2^{141\ \rightarrow\ 172} \beta_2$

Globin polypeptide subunits, each under the control of separate genes, are designated alpha (α), beta (β), gamma (γ), delta (δ), epsilon (ϵ), or zeta (ζ). The subscript refers to the number of subunits. The superscript indicates the mutation site.

bin, Hb F ($\alpha_2\gamma_2$), which makes up 75 to 90 per cent of the total hemoglobin at birth. Schroeder and co-workers have shown that at least two genetic loci govern the production of different types of γ chains, one with glycine at the 136 position Gγ, the other with alanine Aγ. Although the synthesis of adult type β chains is begun early in intrauterine development, predominance is not established until its synthetic rate sharply rises in the weeks just preceding birth. Hb A then gradually replaces Hb F in the circulating erythrocytes until the normal adult level of Hb F (<2 per cent) is attained, usually at about 6 months of age, although slight elevations may persist for two years (Fig. 3–57).

Thanks largely to the work of Perutz, the three-dimensional fine structure of the hemoglobin molecule is rather well understood. The α and β subunits, similar but not identical in size and shape, possess a complementariness of structure which causes them to spontaneously associate with each other and form a dimer which constitutes the basis of both the function of the molecule as an oxygen transporter and its physicochemical stability. Unpaired, the subunits not only are incapable of oxygen transport but are also excessively unstable. The stability of the dimer ($\alpha_1\beta_1$) comes from the extensive area of surface contact between the two subunits, involving 34 amino acid residues in the contact site. When two dimers come together to form the complete tetrameric configuration, an "asymmetric" contact point forms between the α chain of one dimer and the β chain of the other (Fig. 3–58). This asymmetric ($\alpha_1\beta_2$) contact area is somewhat less extensive, involving only 19 amino acid sites, but this region is important in the regulation of the normal sigmoid shape of the hemoglobin oxygen dissociation curve. It is at this point that the allosteric properties of hemoglobin, as it combines with its substrate oxygen, are modulated. The initial attachment of oxygen to the α chain heme causes its iron to "snap back" as if released from a position under tension. This signal

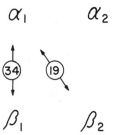

Figure 3–58 The α and β subunit contact regions in the hemoglobin molecule. The numbers of amino acids in the contact areas are indicated. (Redrawn from Weatherall, D. J., and Clegg, J. B.: the Thalassemia Syndromes. Blackwell Scientific Publications Ltd., Oxford, 1972, p. 17.)

then sends a "shock wave" through the molecule which increases the affinity of the β chain heme groups for oxygen atoms, producing the upward inflection of the oxygen dissociation curve and at the same time causing the β chains to move closer to another by 7 Å. The β chains shift back apart when oxygen is once again removed (Fig. 3–2). These intramolecular changes have led to the use of the terms "tense" (T) and "relaxed" (R) to describe the allosteric configurational states of deoxy- and oxyhemoglobin, respectively. The binding of low molecular weight phosphates, such as 2,3-diphosphoglycerate, takes place in the cleft between the two β chains when they are in the deoxy configuration, thus diminishing the oxygen affinity of the hemoglobin.

The globular subunit, which is divided into eight helical regions designated by the letters A through H, is physiologically submerged in an aqueous medium with which it blends because it carries all its hydrophilic groupings on its exterior surface. These include hydroxyl groups, such as those of serine and threonine, as well as polar carboxyl and amino groups. The molecular interior is arid and is lined with hydrophobic nonpolar groups. Each subunit has its heme group neatly tucked into a "heme pocket" which dips down from the molecular surface and is also completely lined with hydrophobic groups which exclude water from the region. The heme comes into contact at about 60 atomic sites with the surface of the pocket. The fifth coordinate position of the heme iron is bound to the "proximal histidine" residue (β^{92} and α^{87}). Molecular oxygen is carried between the sixth coordinate position of iron and the "distal histidine" (β^{63} and α^{58})(Fig. 3–1).

HEMOGLOBINOPATHY DUE TO STRUCTURAL DEFECTS (TABLE 3–10)

Nomenclature. In the years that followed the first description of sickle hemoglobin (Hb S) in 1949 it became evident that the letters in the alphabet would not be sufficient to accommodate

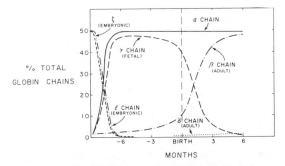

Figure 3–57 The change in globin chains during intrauterine development. (Redrawn from Bunn, H. F., Forget, B. G., and Ranney, H. M. Human Hemoglobins. W. B. Saunders Co., Philadelphia, 1977. p. 107.)

names for the large number of mutant hemoglobins being discovered. Family names and then place names were given as trivial expressions, to be followed by a specific designation of the amino acid substitution which characterized the abnormal hemoglobin. For example, "Hb Philly" was first observed in Philadelphia. It has normal α chains, but the β chains are affected by an inherited abnormality of the 35th amino acid from the N-terminal end of the β chains, at which phenylalanine is found in place of tyrosine (Fig. 3–59). This abnormal hemoglobin is thus designated $\alpha_2 \beta_2^{35tyr \to phe}$. Mutations of the β chain outnumber those of the α chain. Abnormal δ and γ chains have also been discovered. Many abnormal hemoglobins produce no abnormality in erythrocyte appearance or function and are not pathogenetic. Some are harmful only in the homozygous state, while others are lethal in the homozygous state and thus are only observed in heterozygous carriers.

Methemoglobinemia. A substitution of tyrosine for histidine at either the proximal or distal histidine residues of either the α or the β chains locks the heme iron into a trivalent state resistant to the action of the enzyme methemoglobin reductase, which has the responsibility of maintaining the iron atoms of hemoglobin in the ferrous state. The affected heme groups in half the molecule are incapable of oxygen transport while the unaffected pair of hemes retains the ability to combine reversibly with oxygen. In the α chain methemo-

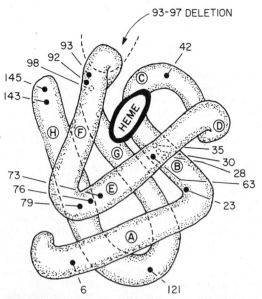

Figure 3–59 The β globin subunit. The letters *A* through *H* indicate the eight helical regions. The numbered positions indicate amino acid sites discussed in the text and in Table 3–10. (Redrawn from Giblett, E. R.: Genetic Markers in Human Blood. Blackwell Scientific Publications Ltd., Oxford, 1969.)

globinemias, the normal β partner has a somewhat decreased affinity for oxygen because of the absence of the "signal" which is normally sent across to the β chain from the α when it first combines with oxygen. In the β chain mutants, the oxygen affinity of the unaffected α subunit is more nearly normal. Inheritance is autosomal dominant and homozygosity is apparently lethal, in contrast to inherited deficiency of methemoglobin reductase, which is an autosomal recessive state. The methemoglobinemia of mutant hemoglobins is resistant to therapy while that occurring as a result of deficiency of the enzyme responds to treatment with such reducing agents as methylene blue or ascorbic acid.

High Affinity Hemoglobin With Erythrocytosis. Mutant hemoglobins which raise the hemoglobin oxygen affinity shift the oxygen dissociation curve to the left, impeding oxygen unloading at the tissues (Fig. 3–60). The erythropoietin response evokes a secondary form of polycythemia which is familial and benign and is unassociated with increases in the platelet or leukocyte count. The mutation sites affect either the area of $\alpha_1\beta_2$ subunit contact or the C-terminal ends of the β chains close to the cove where low molecular weight phosphates are bound. Mutants such as Hb Chesapeake, which are located at the $\alpha_1\beta_2$ contact, have a raised oxygen affinity along with a loss in the normal sigmoid contour of the oxygen dissociation curve, but their Bohr effect is preserved. In Hb Hiroshima and Hb Rainier, which affect the C-terminal region of the β subunits, the Bohr effect is impaired. These substitutions presumably raise oxygen affinity by interfering with low molecular weight phosphate binding and allosteric movements.

Low Affinity Hemoglobin With Cyanosis. Hb Kansas is a mutation at the $\alpha_1\beta_2$ contact which causes a lowered oxygen affinity (Fig. 3–60). Cyanosis is reversed if the patient is placed in an atmosphere of sufficiently high partial pressure of oxygen. Oxygen unloading is facilitated in the tissues, with a decreased stimulus to erythropoietin secretion causing a mild but "physiologic" anemia.

Unstable Hemoglobin With Congenital Heinz Body Hemolytic Anemia. Amino acid replacements which loosen the attachment of heme in its pocket or the dimeric association of the subunits at the $\alpha_1\beta_1$ contact region cause the mutant hemoglobin to be inordinately susceptible to oxidation. Water entry into normally hydrophobic regions is followed by conversion to methemoglobin and oxidation of the hemoglobin into insoluble lumps. These impede erythrocyte pliability and cause hemolysis. The intact spleen plucks these precipitates from the erythrocytes. After splenectomy, a large proportion of the circulating erythrocytes contain Heinz bodies, the term which is used to describe these intracellular inclusions of precipi-

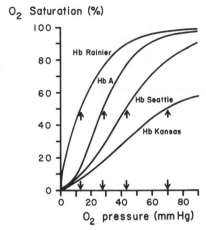

O₂ Saturation (%)

O₂ pressure (mm Hg)

Figure 3–60 Examples of hemoglobins with abnormal oxygen affinity. Arrows indicate P_{50}. (Reproduced with permission from "Abnormal Hemoglobins with High and Low Oxygen Affinity" by G. Stamatoyannopoulos, A. J. Bellingham, C. Lenfant and C. A. Finch, Annual Review of Medicine, Volume 22. Copyright © 1971 by Annual Reviews Inc. All rights reserved.)

tated hemoglobin. The replacement of one hydrophobic amino acid for another inside the heme pocket, as in Hb Torino, causes only mild hemolysis, but when a hydrophilic group is placed into the heme pocket lining, as in the case of serine in Hb Hammersmith, heme loss is marked and hemolysis severe. A gross deletion of a block of five amino acids adjacent to the proximal histidine residue in Hb Gun Hill produces gross molecular distortion with heme-deficient globin subunits and marked hemoglobin instability. Hb Zürich affects the distal histidine residue of the β chain, which is replaced by arginine. The polar group of arginine lies poised just outside the heme pocket and leads to very mild hemolysis unless the patient is given certain "oxidant" drugs, such as sulfonamides, which explosively provoke episodes of severe hemolysis. Hb Philly and Hb Tacoma are unstable because they affect the $\alpha_1\beta_1$ contact area. The globin subunit also cannot bear disruption of its helical regions without suffering molecular instability. The insertion of the hydroxyl group of proline into the B helix of the β chain in Hb Genova breaks up the regular helical structure and causes a gross alteration in molecular configuration with hemolysis.

The oxygen affinity of the unstable hemoglobins may be raised or lowered, with an effect on the level of hemoglobin at which the patient compensates. When the affinity is high, the erythropoietin response is greater and the degree of anemia less than in those mutants with a lowered affinity, in which compensation is achieved at a lower concentration of circulating hemoglobin. The severity of the hemolytic process obviously also determines the severity of the anemia.

Exterior Mutants. Mutants placed on the hydrophilic exterior of the molecule do not alter either the oxygen affinity or the oxidative stability of the molecule. Relatively few of the more than 50 variants described in this class of abnormal hemoglobins cause any significant signs. Two major exceptions are the most common structural hemoglobinopathies, Hb S and Hb C. Both these hemoglobins are substituted at the 6 position from the N-terminal end of the β chain, where glutamic acid is replaced by valine in the case of Hb S and by lysine in the case of Hb C. Hb E, prevalent in Southeast Asia, also has a lysine in place of glutamic acid, but the affected site is 26 from the N-terminus of the β chain.

Erythrocytes which contain Hb S undergo jagged distortion of their membranes under reduced partial pressure of oxygen, a phenomenon known as sickling (Fig. 3–61). The sickling is visualized by electron microscopy as a linear molecular stacking of hemoglobin molecules, the filaments intertwining into cable-like structures illustrated in Figure 3–62. The process is reversible, and as the oxygen tension is raised, the semisolid gelled hemoglobin liquefies once again, and the cell reassumes its normal biconcave shape. The reversibility of the process is a function of the allosteric shift of the β chains, the deoxy T configuration causing a "fit" between the β chains of one molecule and the α chains of the next, on to a linear stacking of molecule upon molecule. With reoxygenation, the β chains relax and move closer together and the complementariness between adjacent molecules is broken. The erythrocyte membrane may undergo irreversible deformation. The cell will then remain irreversibly sickled, even

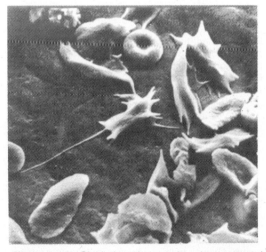

Figure 3–61 Sickled erythrocytes as demonstrated by scanning electron microscopy. (From Jensen, W. N., and Lessin, L. S.: Seminars Hematol., 7:409–426, 1970. By permission of Grune & Stratton, Inc., New York.)

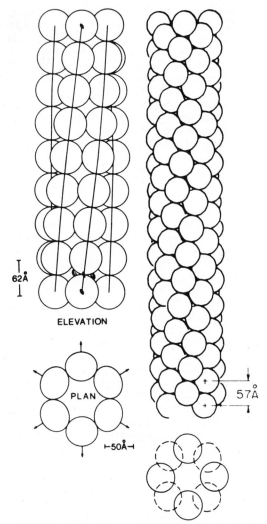

ELEVATION

62Å

PLAN

57Å

├─50Å─┤

Figure 3–62 Two currently proposed models of the deoxy Hb S fiber. To the left is the six-stranded model of Finch and to the right the eight-stranded fiber of Josephs. Both models picture a helical structure. (With permission from Finch, J. T., et al.: Proc. N.A.S. U.S.A., 70:718, 1973, and Josephs, R., et al.: J. Mol. Biol., 102:409, 1976. Copyright by Academic Press Inc. (London) Ltd.)

though the interior structure of the oxyhemoglobin S is not in the gelled state. Sickled erythrocytes seen in routine blood films prepared from blood of sickle cell anemia patients are examples of irreversibly sickled cells, or, as designated by workers in the field, "ISC's."

Murayama proposed that the substitution of valine with its hydrophobic side chain in place of glutamic acid with its exterior polar carboxyl group causes, in a sense, an interiorization of a portion of the molecular exterior. He suggested that a cyclic hydrophobic valine-to-valine bond forms between the 1 and 6 amino acid residues of

the β chain of Hb S. This changes the exterior molecular configuration and causes a key and lock arrangement between molecules when the β chains are in the deoxy configuration.

Further considerations of the orientation of tetramers of deoxy Hb S within the multistranded sickle fiber lead to the conclusion that there are many contact sites between the entrapped molecules in both horizontal and vertical planes, not just the one area of contact envisioned by Murayama at the site of the amino acid substitution. Wishner and co-workers have drawn up a model depicting a multiplicity of contact sites with an asymmetric placement of the hemoglobin tetramers within the fibers such that only one of the two substituted valines of deoxy Hb S tetramer is situated at a contact point (Fig. 3–63).

Wishner's model is based on studies of hemoglobin crystals, but it correlates in many respects with clinical observations made in individuals who have inherited another abnormal hemoglobin present in the red cells along with Hb S. For example, Hb C Harlem has two amino acid substitutions in its beta chains, one identical to that of Hb S and the other at the 73 position, where asparagine replaces aspartic acid. Despite the fact that this molecule is more abnormal than Hb S, its presence in patients also heterozygous for Hb S inhibits the sickling process. Another mutant, Hb Korle-bu, has the same property of inhibiting sickle fiber formation. Hb Korle-bu is characterized by the same substitution at position 73 of the beta chain as that found in the Hb C Harlem, but otherwise its structure is normal. From this observation one is led to the conclusion that position 73 of the beta chain is an important site of contact between hemoglobin tetramers in the sickle fiber, as in fact shown in Wishner's model. Analogous observations have been made by Bookchin and co-workers with a number of other mutant hemoglobins that interact with deoxy Hb S to affect the sickling process.

The presence of fetal hemoglobin together with Hb S also inhibits gelation. Newborn infants do not suffer from sickle cell disease. Symptoms only become manifest as the fetal hemoglobin is replaced by the adult type. Hb F levels are commonly raised in sickle cell anemia to values from 5 to 15 per cent, but the fact that it is heterogenously distributed among the erythrocytes explains why its level is not generally related to disease severity. However, those erythrocytes with higher Hb F content do survive longer in the circulation. In the doubly heterozygous condition of hereditary persistence of fetal hemoglobin and sickle trait, erythrocytes uniformly have 20 to 30 per cent Hb F mixed together with Hb S and the result is a benign condition.

On the other hand, Hb C rather strongly interacts with Hb S in the gelation and its presence in erythrocytes together with Hb S in equal pro-

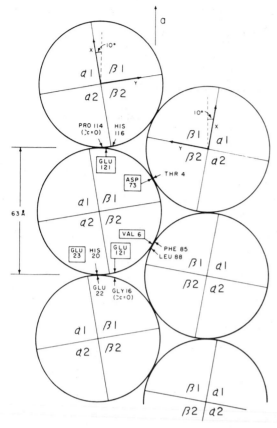

Figure 3–63 Intermolecular contact sites between deoxy Hb S molecules within fibers. The illustration is based on the results of x-ray crystallography of hemoglobin crystals and thus may not necessarily reflect physiologic conditions. (Wishner, B. C., et al.: J. Mol. Biol., *98*:179, 1975. Copyright by Academic Press Inc. (London) Ltd.)

tion. Acidosis, by shifting the oxygen dissociation curve to the right, promotes sickling, while alkalosis inhibits it. The gelation of deoxy Hb S is also highly dependent upon the intracellular hemoglobin concentration, which is raised as water moves out of erythrocytes during their movement through a hyperosmolar environment. As a result individuals with sickle cell trait or other sickle hemoglobinopathies may incur episodes of sickling within the renal medulla leading to infarction and painless hematuria. Low molecular weight phosphates (inorganic phosphate as well as 2,3-DPG) also promote sickling by decreasing the oxygen affinity of the hemoglobin.

Sickle cell anemia is usually a severe disease in which erythrocytic sickling causes chronic hemolytic anemia in a setting of vaso-occlusive phenomena which may affect any organ of the body. Periodic bouts of occlusion of the microvasculature in one or several parts of the body cause "painful crises," which at their worst produce prolonged excruciating pain, sometimes associated with fever. Major arteries and veins may also suffer occlusion. There is a serious susceptibility to infection. Organ damage is cumulative over the years, and death, if not from infection, may come unannounced from a major occlusion affecting a vital function, or it may come in more chronic fashion from gradual failure of any one of several organs, such as liver, kidney, or heart. The sickle variants, Hb SC disease and Hb S thalassemia, also suffer vaso-occlusive phenomena, but symptoms are usually milder. Carriers of sickle cell trait are asymptomatic except for an incidence of hematuria due to renal infarction.

Vascular changes occur in reaction to erythrocytic sickling. These changes are demonstrable in the kidney and are presumably etiologically related to a renal concentrating defect which cannot be reversed in adults despite exchange transfusion of normal for sickle erythrocytes. Vascular changes are also present in the eye, and retinal aneurysms leading to vitreous hemorrhage cause blindness, a complication particularly associated with Hb SC disease, as described by Condon and Serjeant in 1972.

Therapy over the years has been essentially symptomatic. Acidosis is treated, hydration ensured, and occasionally the sickled erythrocytes replaced by normal transfused cells as a temporary expedient. The search for a pharmacologic agent which would prevent sickling has been elusive. Methemoglobin as well as such liganded states of hemoglobin as carboxyhemoglobin and cyanmethemoglobin all assume the oxy R configuration and therefore do not sickle, but these altered states of hemoglobin do not function in oxygen transport. More recently it was discovered that treatment of Hb S erythrocytes with cyanate results in a carbamylation of the hemoglobin molecules which not only inhibits sickling but also

portions causes significant in-vivo sickling in the disorder known as Hb SC disease. Normal Hb A, which is found in a proportion of about 60:40 relative to that of Hb S in individuals who are carriers of sickle cell trait, also interacts with Hb S in the gelation, but to a much lesser degree. How other hemoglobins become intertwined with Hb S during deoxygenation is still not understood in molecular terms. Bunn and McDonough have observed that dimers of $\alpha^A\beta^A$ and $\alpha^A\beta^S$ combine to form the hybrid $\alpha_2^A\beta^A\beta^S$. Thus, hybridization of different hemoglobin types within the same erythrocyte may be the explanation.

Heterozygous carriers of the sickle cell trait show no abnormality of erythrocyte morphology, life span, or function, except under certain extenuating circumstances, such as severe hypoxia. At the tips of the papillae in the renal medulla a number of factors combine to produce an optimal environment for erythrocyte sickling. The region is hypoxic and acidotic, with a high salt concentra-

results in a marked improvement in the life span of the treated erythrocytes. Cyanate is an example of a class of antisickling agents which inhibit sickling by raising the oxygen affinity of the chemically altered hemoglobin (Fig. 3–64). Carbamylation, alkylation, amidination, and other chemical modifications of hemoglobin may also introduce new configurations at critical contact sites on the molecular surface, causing steric hindrance to fiber formation, much in the same manner that the mutant hemoglobins Hb C Harlem and Hb Korle-bu inhibit sickling. Among the growing list of chemicals which are being found to have significant in vitro antisickling effects, none has yet reached the stage of clinical usefulness in the prevention or reversal of sickling in patients.

Individuals homozygous for Hb C have a mild chronic hemolytic anemia associated with splenomegaly. The pathogenesis of the hemolysis apparently lies in the fact that this abnormal hemoglobin spontaneously crystallizes at a slightly lower concentration than Hb A, as described by Charache and associates. As red cells age in the circulation they undergo a measure of water loss, with concomitant increase in the intracorpuscular concentration of hemoglobin to values approaching 36 grams per 100 ml. Hb A does not begin to crystallize into an insoluble state until its concentration is over 40 grams per 100 ml., but Hb C begins to develop this change in physical state at the values physiologically approached during red cell aging in the circulation. At this point the cell becomes rigid and is subject to entrapment and destruction. The presence of this abnormal hemoglobin within erythrocytes causes a prominent tendency for the central deposition of a mass of hemoglobin into a "target cell" configuration. Intracellular crystals are readily demonstrable in vitro by suspending the erythrocytes in hypertonic saline, which raises intracorpuscular hemoglobin concentration, or in vivo after removal of the spleen. Heterozygotes have fewer target cells and do not show signs of significant hemolysis. The pathogenesis of Hb E disease presumably resembles that of Hb C.

Non-genetic Structural Alterations. As red cells age in the circulation glucose becomes attached to the N-terminal valines of one or both beta chains of hemoglobin in an irreversible ketoamine linkage. Older erythrocytes contain a higher level of glycosylated hemoglobin than young. The average value in normal individuals is about 7 per cent of the total hemoglobin. Several different glycosylated components are present, about one third hemoglobins A_{1a} and A_{1b}, and the remainder Hb A_{1c}. The oxygen affinity of the modified hemoglobin is increased because of impaired binding of 2,3 DPG at the blocked N-terminus. The level of glycosylated hemoglobin is approximately doubled in patients with diabetes mellitus. Following its level in diabetics may provide a more valid index of the adequacy of treatment

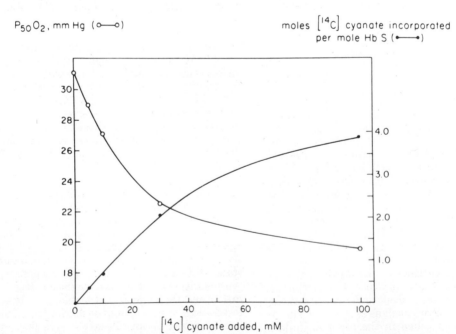

Figure 3–64   The increase in hemoglobin affinity after treatment of sickle cell anemia erythrocytes with cyanate, a possible mechanism for the inhibition of sickling. P_{50} is defined as the partial pressure of oxygen at which the hemoglobin is half saturated with oxygen. (Redrawn from deFuria, F. G., et al.: J. Clin. Invest., *51*:566, 1972.)

than serial blood sugar measurements according to Koenig and co-workers.

HEMOGLOBINOPATHY DUE TO QUANTITATIVE DEFECTS. The thalassemias are a heterogeneous group of disorders, usually inherited, characterized primarily by a deficiency in the rate of synthesis of specific globin chains. The deficit of one subunit may bring about an imbalance with surplus of another.

The structure-rate hypothesis as conceived by Itano in the 1950s postulated that the structure of an abnormal globin chain was an important factor which determined its synthetic rate. The fact that Hb S was synthesized at a slightly less efficient rate than Hb A provided support for this theory, but subsequent attempts to identify a mutant hemoglobin produced at a very low rate in thalassemic states were not successful, with the exception of two types of rare structural alterations which cause a marked slowing of their synthetic rate. One affects β chain production, and the other α. The first of these, Hb Lepore, is a globin chain which is a hybrid polypeptide consisting of a portion of the δ chain connected to a portion of the β chain to make a completed globin subunit of normal chain length which pairs with α chains in the completed tetrameric hemoglobin molecule. This hybrid globin subunit is the product of a fusion gene which presumably first originated in prior generations by a crossover occurring between homologous chromosomes slightly displaced during synapsis. Several different types of Lepore hemoglobins have been described, differing from one another in the proportion of the molecule which resembles the δ chain (Fig. 3–65). Protein synthesis is normally initiated at the N-terminal end of the molecule, which in the Lepore hemoglobins is always that of the δ portion of the chain, and thus its synthesis takes on the slow character of normal δ chain production. The deficit results in a β-thalassemia syndrome.

Hb Constant Spring, described by Milner and co-workers, is found in trace quantities in association with α-thalassemia states. In contrast to the normal α chain, which has 141 amino acids, this abnormal hemoglobin carries a defect in chain length which causes it to grow to an abnormal length of 172 amino acids, 31 too long. The pathogenetic basis of the defect appears to lie in the fact that at position 142 of the messenger RNA, where the triplet codon normally signals "terminate," a mutation signals instead for the insertion of a specific amino acid. Additional amino acids are then added until the next terminating codon is read from the messenger RNA strand at position 173. The defect in chain termination markedly slows its synthetic rate and causes an α-thalassemia syndrome.

However, these two examples notwithstanding, the basic pathogenesis of most of the thalassemia syndromes is not associated with the production of

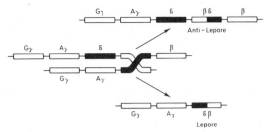

Figure 3–65 Hemoglobin Lepore, an example of a product of a fusion gene. Allelic chromosomes become misaligned. Crossover produces a fusion gene. Lepore hemoglobins resemble δ chain at their amino terminals and β chain at their C terminals. Anti-Lepore hemoglobins have the reciprocal structure, with β structure at their amino terminals. Several different Lepore hemoglobins have been described which differ from one another at the exact point of crossover. Also shown are the positions on the chromosome of the fetal globin genes Gγ and Aγ. (Wood, W. G., et al., 1977.)

structural abnormalities of the globin chain. In some instances messenger RNA is absent due to deletion of the genetic locus responsible for its transcription. In other cases, messenger RNA is transcribed at an abnormally low rate. In still other cases messenger RNA is transcribed in sufficient quantity but it does not function properly in translation. These diverse results at the basic scientific level parallel the heterogeneity observed clinically and permit the conclusion that a variety of underlying mechanisms cause low synthetic rates of proteins. According to Nienhuis and Benz, the protein synthetic mechanism itself operates normally in most cases of thalassemia.

Any one or combination of the genes directing globin chain synthesis may hypothetically be affected by a thalassemic lesion causing depressed production rates, but only those affecting the α or the β loci are important. The degree of depression of globin chain formation may be minimal, moderate, or virtually complete, but it is relatively consistent within the affected members of the same family.

In the heterozygous carrier state one member of the chromosome pair produces globin chains at a normal rate and the clinical condition is asymptomatic. Anemia is minimal or mild, the erythrocytes are microcytic and are often present in greater than normal numbers, and the erythrocyte morphology is abnormal. Some thalassemic carrier states are so minimal that they are completely silent and exhibit no abnormalities whatsoever. The depressed β chain production in the carrier state of β-thalassemia is reflected in an increased proportion of Hb A_2 to approximately twice the normal value, the shortage of β chains altering the ratio of β to δ chain production. A few also have slight elevations of Hb F to about 2 to 6 per cent of the total hemoglobin. Hb F is more elevated and the Hb A_2 normal in a less common strain of β-thalassemia trait, designated δ-β thalassemia because the genetic lesion appears to affect the δ locus along with the adjacent β, thus, keeping the proportionality of β and δ globin subunits normal while evoking an especially strong stimulus for γ chain production. In carriers of α-thalassemia trait the proportions of Hb A_2 and Hb F are not altered, since these hemoglobins, in common with Hb A, are all affected by the shortage of α chains. Table 3–11 summarizes the heterozygous thalassemias.

Homozygosity for β-thalassemia (Cooley's anemia) is associated with little or no capacity to produce β chains (and thus Hb A), because both alleles responsible for β chain synthesis are affected. Hb F becomes the major hemoglobin type produced, usually exceeding 50 per cent and often approaching 95 per cent of the total. The Hb A and the Hb F are contained in variable mixtures in the erythrocyte population. The better filled cells containing more Hb F have a more prolonged survival time than the more empty Hb F-poor cells. The pathogenesis of the severe hemolysis is explained by imbalanced production of α as compared to β chains. The surplus unpaired α chains are exceedingly unstable and precipitate readily within nucleated erythroid precursor cells, causing marked intramedullary destruction, i.e., ineffective erythropoiesis. Those cell lines which retain a greater capacity for γ chain production not only are better filled with hemoglobin but also have fewer surplus unpaired α chains and thus are less rapidly hemolyzed. The patients are severely anemic, are transfusion dependent beginning in early childhood, develop massive enlargement of the spleen and of the liver, show prominent signs of extramedullary hematopoiesis, and suffer physical disfigurement because of the bone deformity brought on by the extreme erythroid hyperplasia in the marrow. Iron overload ultimately causes failure of the heart or liver, along with diabetes mellitus. Some apparently homozygous patients have a much milder anemia because one or both of their inherited thalassemic genes are mild or minimal. Patients in such a state, designated as "thalassemia intermedia," are not transfusion dependent but over the years are apt to develop hemochromatosis.

Homozygosity for α-thalassemia-1, so far observed only in Oriental newborns with an erythroblastosis fetalis-like picture, is a lethal condition. Severe anemia is associated with nearly 100 per cent Hb Bart's (γ_4) which lacks α chains and therefore does not function in oxygen transport, its affinity for oxygen being too great. Death thus occurs before or soon after birth. Hemoglobin H disease is a milder form of α-thalassemia in a subject who carries one mild and one severe gene. It is associated with about 20 per cent Hb Bart's at birth. This is subsequently replaced by its adult counterpart Hb H (β_4), which also cannot function in oxygen transport. Hb H is the product of surplus β chains in the face of a shortage of α chains. Its degree of instability is not as marked as that of unpaired α chains, and it precipitates in more mature circulating erythrocytes, causing hemolytic anemia without the same degree of intramedullary erythroid cell destruction seen in Cooley's anemia. Newborn heterozygous carriers of α-thalassemia trait have slight increases in Hb Bart's in the cord blood, but this disappears with development, leaving no disturbance in the proportions of Hb A or Hb F in the adult erythrocytes. Examples of combinations of thalassemia genes are contained in Table 3–12.

Sophisticated techniques have been developed to diagnose sickle hemoglobinopathy and thalassemia in the fetus during early intrauterine life. Minute samples of fetal blood are obtained by amniocentesis or by direct fetoscopy. The pattern of globin chain synthesis is then characterized from the pattern of incorporation of radioactive amino acids. Since adult type globin chains are synthesized as minor components along with the predominant fetal type chains early in gestation, accurate diagnosis of beta chain hemoglobinopathy is possible. Kan and co-workers have brought the full force of high technology to bear on the problem of early intrauterine diagnosis of α-thalassemia-1. They used purified α chain mes-

TABLE 3–11   HETEROZYGOUS THALASSEMIA

Type	Hemoglobin A_2	Hemoglobin F	Abnormal Hemoglobin
Beta	Increased	Normal or slightly increased	Absent
Delta-beta	Normal	Increased	Absent
Lepore	Normal or decreased	Slightly increased	6–15% Lepore
Alpha	Normal	Normal	Absent in adults; 1–6% Bart's in cord blood
Constant Spring	Normal	Normal	1–2% Constant Spring

Thalassemia is subclassified according to the degree of the genetic deficit of β or α chains. β° is used to designate a more severe defect with absent β chain production. β^+ is milder. In analogous fashion, α–1 is more severe and α–2 milder.

TABLE 3–12 SOME EXAMPLES OF COMBINATIONS OF THALASSEMIA GENES

Type	Hemoglobin A₂	Hemoglobin F	Abnormal Hemoglobin
Homozygous beta	Normal, decreased, or increased	10–90% (usually above 35%)	Free alpha chain
Homozygous alpha-1*	Absent	Absent	80–90% Bart's; remainder H and Portland
Alpha-1 alpha-2	Decreased	Normal	3–30% H; 0–5% Bart's
Homozygous delta-beta	Absent	100%	None reported

*These values relate to the newborn. All other values are beyond the newborn period.

senger RNA to prepare synthetic "DNA probes." Hybridization experiments demonstrated deletion of the α chain genetic locus in DNA extracted from fetal fibroblasts cultured from amniotic fluid. These approaches are still experimental, however, and not yet ready for widespread clinical use.

HEMOGLOBINOPATHY: POPULATION GENETICS. Inherited abnormalities of globin chain structure or production rate sporadically affect individuals from all population groups, but by far the most frequently affected are those originating from tropical or subtropical regions. Incidence figures are highest in Africa, the Mediterranean Basin, the Near and Middle East, and Southeast Asia. Hb S reaches its highest frequency in Africa, where it affects 20 to 30 per cent or more of the Negro population in regions of West, Central, and East Africa. There is also a significant incidence in the Mediterranean countries and in localized regions of Arabia and India. Hb C has a peak prevalence of 10 to 20 per cent among West African Negroes in the region of Ghana. Hb E attains a comparable frequency in areas of Southeast Asia. The α- and β-thalassemia genes are relatively frequent throughout the entire "hemoglobinopathy belt," but Southeast Asia and regions of Greece and Italy have an especially high incidence.

Red Cell Survival Disorders

General Signs of Hemolysis. After a 4-month trip through the streams and bogs of the circulation, the normal erythrocyte ends its life span and is ingested by macrophages. Its death is heralded by cellular changes of aging: loss of surface membrane, decrease of cell water, and decline in activity of several enzyme systems. Premature disappearance of erythrocytes either by hemorrhagic loss from the circulatory compartment or by hemolysis may lead to anemia. Hemolysis occurs when the cell itself is intrinsically defective or when the milieu in which it is bathed contains noxious factors.

When the life span of the erythrocyte is only slightly shortened, the consequence may not be of significance. On the other hand, in severe hemolytic states a red cell life span of only 1/10 of 1/20 the normal period of 120 days severely strains the

capacity of the bone marrow to sustain erythroid cell production at a rate sufficient to maintain a circulating hemoglobin concentration compatible with health. The production of erythroid cells in the marrow is increased to meet the demands of increased erythrocyte turnover. This is reflected in hyperplasia of the erythroid precursor cells. Marrow normally occupied by fat is converted to hypercellular tissue. The proportion of erythroid to granulocytic precursors is increased. Young reticulocytes and sometimes nucleated erythroid cells are released into the circulation. The bone marrow is able to increase red cell production to a limited degree — about 6 to 8 times the normal rate. Therefore it is possible to compensate for shortened erythrocyte life spans that are 1/6 to 1/8 normal.

The hemolytic state is thus not necessarily associated with severe anemia. Indeed, the term "compensated hemolysis" is used to describe hemolytic states that are not associated with anemia at all. However, it is still not clear how the bone marrow, in the absence of the stimulus of anemic hypoxia, maintains a rate of red cell production high enough to compensate fully for the reduced erythrocyte life span.

Acute hemolysis causes a rapid reduction in red cell mass because the bone marrow is caught off guard; there is a four to five day delay before production is geared up in response to the anemia.

When chronic hemolysis is associated with anemia, the reduced red cell mass turning over at a faster rate represents the balance between production and destruction in a steady state condition. Limitations upon production may cause anemia even when the degree of erythrocyte hemolysis is moderate. Such limitation occurs secondary to other diseases, such as neoplastic or inflammatory states, or to deficiency of essential nutrients, especially iron and folate. The acute "aplastic crisis" is the most critical imbalance between production and destruction — erythroid precursors suddenly vanish from the marrow, the reticulocyte count drops, and soon after there is a rapid increase in the degree of anemia as the remaining short-lived erythrocytes, no longer being replenished from the marrow, disappear from the circulation. Fortunately, the period of aplasia of red cell formation, probably triggered by a minor infection, is usually short-lived, and recovery is the rule. Similar infections may well arrest erythropoiesis in normal individuals, but during the period of marrow arrest, the fall in blood count is imperceptible because of the longevity of normal erythrocytes.

In the Wright's stained peripheral blood film, reticulocytes are recognized as polychromatophilic macrocytes. Microspherocytes are small, round, densely stained erythrocytes seen in a variety of hemolytic states. Regular and irregular distortions of the erythrocyte membrane into spurs and burrs and the fracturing of erythrocytes into bits and pieces suggest metabolic or mechanical damage.

The biochemical signs of hemolysis are those of the release and breakdown of the pigment of the red cells. Erythrocyte destruction within the confines of the circulatory system ("intravascular hemolysis") causes leakage of hemoglobin directly into the plasma. Phagocytosis of intact erythrocytes or of erythrocyte fragments releases hemoglobin inside the phagocytic macrophages, where the heme is degraded to bilirubin ("extravascular hemolysis"). Hemolytic states are not exclusively intra- or extravascular, but when extensive cell damage causes the erythrocytes to "fall apart" in the circulation the signs of hemoglobin release into the plasma and urine are marked. Hemoglobin released from erythrocytes into the circulation is first bound to haptoglobin, a plasma protein with alpha-2 electrophoretic mobility (Fig. 3–66). The complex of hemoglobin with haptoglobin is then rapidly cleared from the plasma into the hepatocytes, promptly reducing the plasma concentration of haptoglobin to near absent levels.

Thus, a reduction of the plasma haptoglobin concentration (and of the alpha-2 fraction of the serum proteins) is often observed in hemolytic states, regardless of pathogenesis. Haptoglobin concentration, however, is subject to rather pronounced increases secondary to many inflammatory and neoplastic states, and its final level represents a balance between those factors promoting its synthesis and those producing its degradation, such as hemolysis. Haptoglobin normally is capable of binding hemoglobin to the extent of about 100 mg. per 100 ml. plasma. When the haptoglobin binding capacity is exceeded, hemoglobin is lost in the urine. Haptoglobin serves the purpose of conserving iron by preventing its loss in the urine as heme. Oxidized heme, split apart from its globin bond, may also be detected bound to hemopexin, a beta globulin of the plasma, as well as to albumin (as methemalbumin), giving the plasma a dirty brown color. Heme bound to hemopexin is also taken up into the hepatic parenchymal cells.

The detection of free hemoglobin in the plasma and urine indicates that the haptoglobin binding capacity has been exceeded and that the degree of intravascular hemolysis has been extensive. The free plasma hemoglobin, unattached to high molecular weight haptoglobin, is readily filtered through the glomerulus. Some passes through directly to produce urine benzidine positive for the presence of heme pigment. However, hemoglobin is also resorbed into the epithelial cells of the tubules, where its iron is removed and deposited within the cell as ferritin and hemosiderin. These iron-rich proteins are then sloughed with the normal loss of tubule epithelial cells into the urine, where they can be detected in the sediment by the Prussian blue reaction for iron (Fig. 3–67). Hemosiderinuria is a valuable sign that the patient either is suffering from intravascular hemolysis or has recently done so. After recovery from an acute intravascular hemolytic episode, the urine stain for hemosiderin will remain positive for some days after hemoglobinuria has stopped.

Jaundice is a common sign of hemolysis. Often the degree is subclinical and cannot be detected except by chemical measurement of the serum bilirubin concentration. The degree of jaundice is never intense; total serum bilirubin concentrations in excess of 6 mg. per 100 ml. suggest malfunction of the liver or of its biliary drainage system, since the capacity of the normal liver to process bilirubin is immense. Hemolytic jaundice involves primarily elevation of the unconjugated bilirubin (or indirect-reacting fraction). It circulates bound to plasma albumin and therefore is not lost in the urine. After its transport to the liver, bilirubin is processed by the hepatic cells and converted to the water-soluble diglucuronide derivative (direct-reacting, or conjugated), which is the major form excreted in the bile, as reviewed

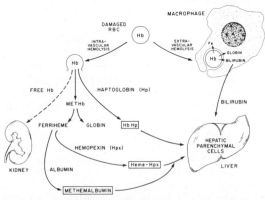

Figure 3–66 Extra- and intravascular disposal of erythrocytes. Intact erythrocytes and cell fragments are removed by extravascular uptake into phagocytic macrophages. Hemoglobin products leaked directly into the circulation are bound to several plasma proteins and redirected into hepatocytes. "Surplus" free hemoglobin is excreted in the urine.

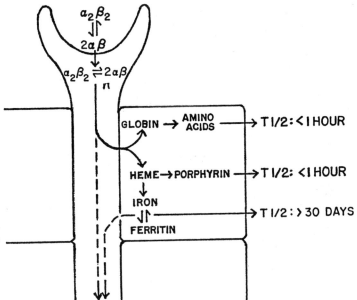

$$a_2\beta_2$$
$$\Updownarrow$$
$$2\alpha\beta$$

$$a_2\beta_2 \rightleftharpoons \frac{2\alpha\beta}{n}$$

GLOBIN → AMINO ACIDS → T 1/2 : < I HOUR

HEME → PORPHYRIN → T 1/2 : < I HOUR

IRON → T 1/2 : > 30 DAYS

FERRITIN

Figure 3–67 The renal handling of hemoglobin. Subunit dissociation into lower molecular weight components permits glomerular filtration. Some of the filtered hemoglobin is taken up into the epithelial cells of the tubules and degraded. The released iron is incorporated into ferritin and hemosiderin. Shedding of renal tubule cells causes persistence of hemosiderinuria for some time after hemoglobinuria has stopped. (From Bunn, H. F. and Jandl, J. H.: J. Exper. Med., *129*:925, 1969.)

by Schmid in 1972. A portion of this conjugated bilirubin is absorbed and undergoes enterohepatic circulation. Most of it is reduced by colonic bacteria to urobilinogen, which also has an enterohepatic circulation. In hemolysis the output of bile pigments into the intestinal tract is increased in direct proportion to the degree of heme degradation and thus to the extent of the hemolytic process. Measurement of the fecal urobilinogen excretion may be used to quantitate the extent of hemolysis as a function of heme degradation rate, but the procedure is too cumbersome for general use. Urine urobilinogen is likewise increased as a reflection of the increased enterohepatic circulation, but only a small proportion of the total is excreted by this route.

Bilirubin is produced in phagocytic cells throughout the body from degraded heme pigments of a variety of types, chief among which by far is hemoglobin. Phagocytes possess an efficient enzymatic mechanism which rapidly and voraciously strips away the iron for metabolic recycling, digests the globin into its constituent amino acids for re-entry into the body pool, and oxidizes the tetrapyrrole ringed structure of heme into biliverdin (Gemsa and co-workers, 1973). This conversion, mediated by heme oxidase, fractures open one of the four bridges (the alpha methene) that hold together the four pyrrole groups into a ringed tetrapyrrole structure. Carbon monoxide is produced in this reaction and is delivered to the lungs for respiratory excretion, one mole for each mole of heme degraded. Since there is almost no other source of endogenous carbon monoxide, measurement of its production rate accurately quantitates

the catabolism of heme compounds and thus also the rate of hemolysis (Fig. 3–68). Biliverdin, a green pigment, is reduced to bilirubin, which is then transferred from the phagocytic cells to the hepatic parenchymal cells for conjugation.

The load of heme pigments normally presented for degradation comes chiefly from dying senescent erythrocytes, but about 15 per cent is from other sources, some from the liver and some from the bone marrow (Fig. 3–69). The hepatic contribution may be increased in porphyria of hepatic origin or following the administration of certain drugs, as phenobarbital, which stimulate the endoplasmic reticulum along with heme synthesis. The bone marrow also produces heme which never reaches the safe haven of the circulating erythrocyte. This marrow heme, destined for early degradation, consists partly of hemoglobin shrouds which veil normoblast nuclei after their extrusion (Fig. 3–70), partly of defective normoblasts destroyed before they gain access to the circulation as mature erythrocytes, and possibly partly of heme which is never incorporated into hemoglobin but is "shunted" into an early catabolic demise. From the foregoing, it is apparent that hepatic or marrow defects can markedly affect the net pattern of heme degradation. The process of intramedullary hemolysis, i.e., ineffective erythropoiesis, so prominent in megaloblastic anemia and in homozygous β-thalassemia, may be the major contributor to heme catabolism and thus to the increased production of carbon monoxide and bilirubin associated with these disorders.

The measurement of red cell survival time would appear to be the most direct approach to the

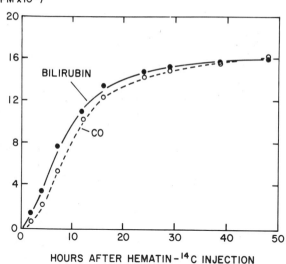

CUMULATIVE EXCRETION
(DPM x 10³)

Figure 3–68 Parallel appearance of radioactivity into bilirubin and carbon monoxide after administration of radioactive hematin. (Redrawn from Landaw, S. A., et al.: J. Clin. Invest., 49:914, 1970.)

diagnosis of hemolytic disorders, but this measurement presents a number of difficulties from practical as well as theoretical points of view. Not the least of these is the rather long time required, during which the patient should be in the steady state with regard to the maintenance of a constant red cell mass as well as to absence of significant loss of blood by hemorrhage. There are two basic approaches, both of which follow the behavior in the circulation of a tag on the erythrocytes. The first, called the cohort label, employs the use of a radioisotope which is administered and is then incorporated into a cohort of newly formed cells. Examples are isotopes of iron (e.g., ^{59}Fe) and of amino acids (e.g., glycine-2-^{14}C, ^{75}Se selenomethionine). Normally the cohort tag will appear in the peripheral blood erythrocytes and then rise to a plateau in about 10 days. This plateau is maintained until about 100 days, and at 120 days it reaches a maximum rate of decline as the cohort dies off. Mean erythrocyte survival time can be estimated from such curves, but this method is difficult to carry out and may be hampered by reutilization of these biologically active tags.

The second method, the population or random label, uses a nonphysiologic marker of a representative sample of the entire erythrocyte population. The sample should be uniformly tagged without difference or discrimination as to cell age, pathologic state, or any other cell variable, so that when it is reintroduced into the circulation, a clear picture is obtained of the rate of removal of the population of erythrocytes it represents. Normally a fixed number of erythrocytes reaches senescence and dies each day; the tag will represent this by a straight-line decline intercepting zero at 120 days, when the last of the tagged cells will have died off.

This is an age-dependent pattern of cell destruction. Many hemolytic states are characterized by random destruction of erythrocytes, without regard to their age. A fixed percentage of the remaining cells are destroyed per day; the tag disappears from the circulation at an exponential rate according to first order kinetics. The time required for disappearance of half the tag (the half-time or T/2) is the most conventional method of expressing erythrocyte survival time as measured with a population label.

No tags are ideal, but two of the best are diisopropylfluorophosphate (DF^{32}P) and sodium chromate (Na$_2$ ^{51}CrO$_4$). DF^{32}P attaches to red cell

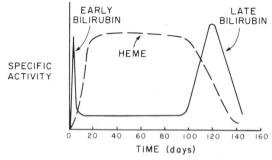

Figure 3–69 "Early" and "late" pathways of heme degradation into bilirubin. The graph illustrates in a normal subject the incorporation of a radioactive precursor of heme into circulating red cells (interrupted line) and into "early" and "late" bilirubin, the latter corresponding to completion of the life span of the labeled erythrocytes. Early bilirubin originates from both bone marrow and hepatic heme. It is markedly increased in conditions associated with ineffective erythropoiesis.

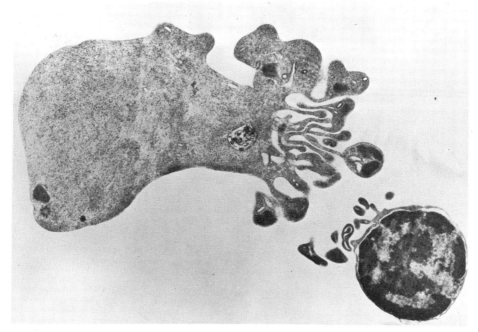

Figure 3–70 The extrusion from an erythroid precursor of a nucleus covered with a shroud of hemoglobin, leaving behind a reticulocyte containing mitochondria and ribosomes. (Reproduced from the Sandoz-Monograph, The Life Cycle of the Erythrocyte. M. Bessis, Basel, Switzerland, 1966.)

cholinesterase to form a tight bond which lasts for the duration of the erthrocyte's life span; its disappearance rate from the circulation yields a value quite close to the true life span, but the method is inconvenient. $Na_2{}^{51}CrO_4$ penetrates the red cell membrane and is reduced to the chromic state, and then the chromium tag forms a chelate with the β chain of hemoglobin. Its bond to proteins is not nearly so tight and it elutes from red cells at a rate of about 1 per cent per day, with significant differences in various disease states. Consequently, its disappearance rate from the circulation does not give a true measure of erythrocyte survival but rather a composite of this function minus the elution rate of the chromium. The normal half-time of ^{51}Cr-labeled erythrocytes is 25 to 35 days, a value considerably shorter than the physiologic half disappearance time of 60 days. Despite these patent disadvantages, ^{51}Cr has practical virtues and has gained widespread acceptance as a convenient method for the clinical assessment of erythrokinetics. Since ^{51}Cr is a strong gamma emitter, the accumulation of chromium-labeled red cells can be detected by external probes, and body surface counting is used to determine the degree of splenic participation in excessive red cell destruction.

Membrane Function and Energy Metabolism. The biochemistry of the erythrocyte has long been a subject of practical interest in the development of satisfactory methods of preserving shed blood in-

tended for transfusion therapy. This deceptively simple cell has also served as a model system in the basic investigation of glycolysis and of the structure and function of cell membranes. Along with the elucidation of the biochemical clock-works of the erythrocyte has come the definition in precise biochemical terms of a large number of different hemolytic states.

The red cell membrane consists of proteins embedded into lipids, chiefly phospholipids and cholesterol. The membrane proteins include the carbohydrate-rich blood group substances, a filamentous structural protein called spectrin, certain enzymes, and other proteins yet to be identified (Fig. 3–71). The membrane maintains a certain excess of surface area which, by dimpling into a biconcave shape, squeezes the hemoglobin into the peripheral ring of the doughnutlike cell. Weed and co-workers have shown that the preservation of this shape depends on energy expenditure. The extent of the surface area is subject to change; it normally decreases as the cell ages. However, mature erythrocytes, no longer able to synthesize lipid, may undergo volume changes through membrane interaction with the external environment. Rapid passive exchange of free cholesterol (but not esterified cholesterol) takes place between the membrane and the plasma. Phospholipid exchange also occurs, but at a much slower rate. The quantity of membrane free cholesterol can be manipulated by varying the free cholester-

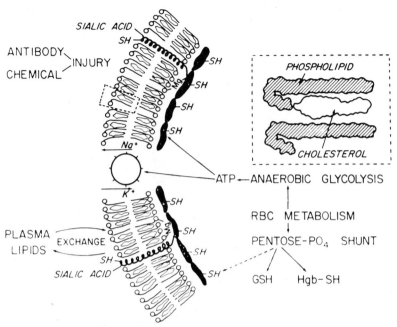

Figure 3–71 Diagrammatic representation of the erythrocyte membrane. (From Weed, R. I., and Reed, C. F.: Am. J. Med., *41*:681, 1966.)

ol content of the surrounding medium (Fig. 3–72). A high level will cause free cholesterol to accumulate in the membrane, thereby increasing its surface area. The increased surface-to-volume ratio confers upon the erythrocytes a greater distensibility in hypotonic media, i.e., their osmotic resistance is increased (Fig. 3–73). The redundant membrane of such cholesterol-replete cells produces a targeted appearance; the area of central pallor has a "bulls-eye" of hemoglobin deposited within. Conversely, suspension of erythrocytes in plasma or serum poor in free cholesterol will cause cholesterol loss from the membrane along with decreased osmotic resistance. Cooper has reported that other important factors such as the serum lipoproteins modify the plasma-membrane exchange.

A busy traffic hums through the pores of the erythrocyte membrane. Gas transport is high on the priority list in fulfillment of the cell's chief function. An active uptake of glucose is required to power the metabolic machinery. Of great interest — and still considerably a mystery — is the movement of electrolytes across the membrane. The pores, seemingly guarded by positively charged sentries (possibly calcium ions), freely allow anions to pass rapidly into the cell. Permeability to cations is quite another matter; cations diffuse across the membrane much more slowly. To oppose this slow, passive diffusion of cations, an active pumping mechanism in the membrane

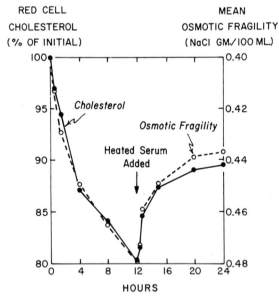

Figure 3–72 Free cholesterol exchanges between the serum and the erythrocyte membrane. After initial incubation with free cholesterol-poor serum, heated serum replete with free cholesterol was added. As the red cell cholesterol decreases, loss of membrane decreases the surface/volume ratio of the cell along with its osmotic resistance. Repletion of the red cell cholesterol reverses this change as the surface/volume ratio returns toward normal. (Redrawn from Cooper, R. A., and Jandl, J. H.: J. Clin. Invest., *48*:906, 1969.)

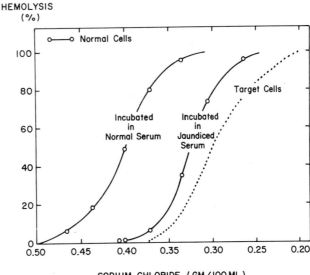

Figure 3–73 The erythrocyte membrane is affected by changes in its serum milieu. Osmotic resistance of normal erythrocytes increases when they are incubated in high free cholesterol serum from a patient with obstructive jaundice as compared to incubation in normal serum. The osmotic resistance of the patient's erythrocytes, which showed target cell formation, was likewise increased (dotted line). (Redrawn from Cooper, R. A., and Jandl, J. H.: J. Clin. Invest., 47:809, 1968.)

maintains concentration gradients of sodium and potassium. Sodium is actively extruded from the cell against a concentration gradient of 10 mEq. per liter inside the cell to 145 mEq. per liter in the extracellular plasma. Potassium is pumped into the cell against a concentration gradient from 4.5 mEq. per liter in the plasma to 100 mEq. per liter inside the cell. The active transport of cations requires ATP as an energy source; it consumes about 15 per cent of the erythrocyte ATP production. The membrane contains an ATPase to mediate its utilization there. Energy deprivation may therefore lead to a breakdown of the pumping mechanism, with serious consequences to the osmotic equilibrium of the cell.

The erythrocyte is the principal transporter of oxygen as fuel for the entire body. In addition to the high-energy phosphate bonds of ATP, it requires energy to perform biochemical reductions to protect its own parts from oxidative denaturation by this fuel. There are two major reducing systems. One, utilizing NADH, maintains the iron atoms of hemoglobin in the reduced state, a need imposed by the continuous slow conversion of hemoglobin to methemoglobin. The reduction is mediated by an enzyme, methemoglobin reductase (Jaffé and Hsieh, 1971). The other reducing system assumes responsibility for maintaining the cell's thiol groups — those of the membrane, the enzymes, and the hemoglobin — in the reduced state. This pathway is mediated through NADPH, which in turn ultimately works through maintaining glutathione in the reduced state.

Glucose is the sole source of energy. The mature erythrocyte consumes 90 per cent of its glucose through the anaerobic Embden-Meyerhof pathway, with conversion to lactate as the end-product and the net production of two moles of ATP and the reduction of two moles of NAD to NADH per mole of glucose (Fig. 3–74). Normally about 10 per cent of the glucose is consumed through the pentose phosphate pathway with the reduction of two moles of NADP to NADPH per mole of glucose. Under the influence of certain redox compounds (for example, methylene blue) the amount of glucose processed through this route is markedly increased, a factor of considerable importance in the pathophysiology of hemolysis in patients lacking key enzymes in this pathway.

Reticulocytes possess mitochondria and therefore have an active Krebs cycle for the oxidative metabolism of glucose, but this apparatus is lost as the reticulocyte matures.

A third pathway of glucose metabolism in the erythrocyte does not participate in energy generation, but rather sacrifices energy production to the cause of an important adaptive mechanism for changing hemoglobin oxygen affinity. This pathway (the Rapoport-Luebering shunt), controlled by diphosphoglycerate mutase (DPGM), generates 2,3-DPG, which binds to deoxyhemoglobin and reduces its affinity for oxygen. As more 2,3-DPG becomes bound, the free unbound pool becomes depleted, thus coaxing DPGM into detouring triose intermediates to replenish the pool. This detour costs the cell a loss of 2 moles of ATP per mole of glucose, but this loss does not appear to have any significant effect on fulfilling total energy requirements.

Classification of Hemolytic States. The seeds of premature erythrocyte destruction may lie either within the erythrocyte or outside in a hostile environment. Hemolytic states are thus readily categorized as "intrinsic" or "extrinsic" disorders, although some represent combinations of both. Most intrinsic defects are inherited; most extrin-

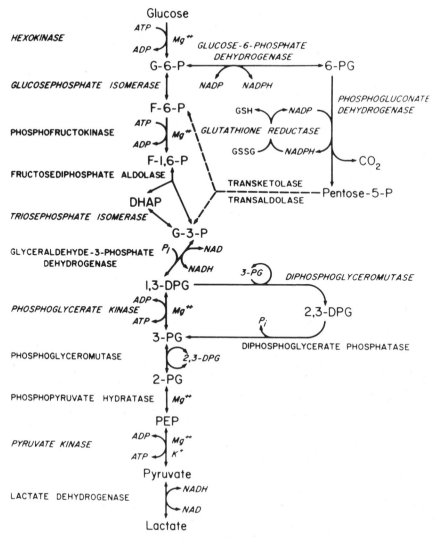

Figure 3–74 Glycolytic pathways in mature erythrocytes. (From Valentine, W. N.: Calif. Med., *108*:280, 1968.)

sic disorders are acquired. A classic experimental approach, no longer in common use, applied cross-transfusion techniques between the patient and a normal individual with compatible blood type. Erythrocytes from a patient with an intrinsic defect will exhibit a shortened survival time not only in the patient's own circulation but also in that of the normal recipient. Erythrocytes from a normal subject will survive as well in the patient's circulation as in his own. However, normal compatible erythrocytes will suffer a shortened survival time in the circulation of a patient with an extrinsic hemolytic disorder. Variations of this approach have also been applied to the study of combined disorders. Thus, tagged erythrocytes from a patient with glucose-6-phosphate dehydrogenase deficiency, an intrinsic drug-sensitive state, will survive quite normally in the circulation of a normal

compatible recipient until the offending drug is administered, which will cause hemolysis of the tagged abnormal erythrocytes but not of the normal person's own erythrocytes. The interaction of the intrinsically defective red cells of hereditary spherocytosis with the extrinsic splenic environment has been demonstrated by the observation that such erythrocytes, appropriately labeled, will exhibit a shortened survival in the bloodstream of a normal recipient with intact spleen (Fig. 3–75) but a normal survival time in a normal person lacking a spleen.

To establish that a hemolytic state exists, measurements of the reticulocyte count, the conjugated and unconjugated serum bilirubin, the serum haptoglobin, the plasma and urine hemoglobin, and the urine hemosiderin, along with careful morphologic examination of the peripheral blood and

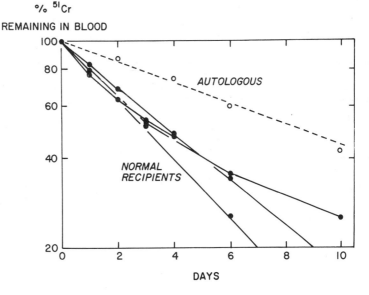

% ^{51}Cr
REMAINING IN BLOOD

AUTOLOGOUS

NORMAL
RECIPIENTS

DAYS

Figure 3–75 The survival of intrinsically defective ^{51}Cr-labeled erythrocytes from a patient with hereditary spherocytosis with intact spleen is even shorter in normal compatible recipients with intact spleen than in the patient. Survival time is normal in the absence of the spleen. (T/2 25–35 days.) (Redrawn from Wiley, J. S.: J. Clin. Invest., *49*:666, 1970.)

bone marrow should indicate its severity and point to the diagnosis. A second echelon of hemolytic tests may then pinpoint the precise cellular or extracellular pathophysiologic condition. These include osmotic fragility measured in a graded series of hypotonic NaCl solutions; the autohemolysis of erythrocytes incubated in vitro under sterile conditions; screening for enzyme defects; hemoglobin analysis; tests for immunologic factors, such as the Coombs antiglobulin, cold agglutinin, and cold hemolysin tests; and tests for the complement-sensitive erythrocytes of paroxysmal nocturnal hemoglobinuria (sucrose hemolysis and acid hemolysin tests). The morphology of the red cells or the clinical circumstances (such as the fact that the patient has cirrhosis or uremia) may alone readily yield the pathophysiologic classification.

Intrinsic Hemolytic Disorders. *Hereditary spherocytosis* (HS) is generally classified as a red cell membrane abnormality, but the molecular defect, inherited as an autosomal dominant trait, is not known (Weed, 1975). Its clinical expression is extraordinarily variable. At times it is first discovered incidentally in old age, but at the other extreme it may produce a severe hemolytic syndrome in the neonate or in early childhood. Many adults with HS maintain a state of completely compensated hemolysis. As with any chronic hemolytic disorder, there is a great likelihood that pigment gallstones will eventually develop. Spherocytosis is a prominent feature in the peripheral blood film along with polychromasia. Tests for autoimmune disorders are negative. The family study is typically positive. The autohemolysis and osmotic fragility tests, to be described, are abnormal. The enlarged spleen is the site of

the premature red cell destruction and its removal predictably restores the erythrocyte life span to almost normal, even though the intrinsic red cell defect remains.

Elegant investigations over the years have elucidated the cellular pathophysiology of HS. The membrane is leaky and allows sodium to enter the cells at a faster than normal rate. Osmotic balance is maintained at the cost of increased energy expenditure required to increase the pump rate of sodium out of the cell, a feat easily accomplished as long as an adequate supply of glucose is available to provide the necessary ATP. The circumstance, however, places the erythrocyte in a precarious state of dependence upon favorable surroundings; it is critically susceptible to glucose deprivation or other limitations on the availability of energy. If osmotic balance of the sodium ion cannot be maintained, water will enter the cell and cause it to swell and become a "macrospherocyte" and possibly eventually to rupture forth its contents.

This inability of the HS erythrocyte to withstand deprivation is demonstrated in the autohemolysis test. Whole blood is incubated at 37° C. under sterile conditions for 48 hours. The available glucose supply is sufficient to keep normal erythrocytes intact; less than 5 per cent will hemolyze. The HS erythrocyte consumes glucose at an increased rate. When the supply runs low, erythrocyte lysis is greatly increased, and 20 to 40 per cent autohemolysis is commonly observed. The addition of supplemental glucose prior to incubation has a salutary effect in reducing the degree of autohemolysis, sometimes to normal levels. Since lysis is produced by the osmotic imbalance between the cell interior and exterior, addition of impenetrable osmotically active agents, such as sucrose or ATP, to the plasma will also reduce autohemolysis.

In addition to increased cation permeability and glucose consumption, the cellular pathophysiology of HS is characterized by the loss of lipid materials from the membrane with a parallel loss of membrane surface area. The reduction in surface area without commensurate volume loss forces the biconcave erythrocytes to change into "microspherocytes" — small cells, densely stained, round, and lacking in central pallor. Since microspherocytes rather than macrospherocytes are the hallmarks of this and of other spherocytic hemolytic conditions, the loss of surface is probably the more important pathophysiologic event (Fig. 3–76). The microspherocyte contains its hemoglobin at a higher concentration than normal. Thus, the mean corpuscular hemoglobin concentration (MCHC) in HS frequently is elevated above 36 grams per 100 ml. Spherocytic erythrocytes (whether micro or macro) are exquisitely sensitive to osmotic lysis following suspension in hypotonic solutions of NaCl. Since as spheres they already have the minimum ratio of surface to volume, they can undergo no further volume expansion as water is taken into the cell. As the spherocyte attempts to swell further, the membrane pores distend and offer free permeability to cations soon to be followed by leakage of large molecules. The hemoglobin escapes from the cell interior into the surrounding medium, leaving behind the hollow "ghost."

The osmotic fragility test is always abnormal in HS, although at times it may be necessary to "bring out" the abnormality by first exposing the erythrocytes to glucose deprivation by a 24-hour in-vitro preincubation. The lipid-depleted microspherocytes represent a discrete subpopulation of especially osmotically fragile erythrocytes. These show up in the complete osmotic fragility test as a "fragile tail," some of them lysing even at a slight reduction of the NaCl concentration below 0.85

gram per 100 ml. The remaining nonspherocytic cells may exhibit normal osmotic fragility. But if the blood is incubated for 24 hours before being tested in graded concentrations of saline, the entire cell population will swell somewhat because of the cells' inability to maintain osmotic equilibrium. This limited degree of volume expansion produces spherodicity and increases osmotic susceptibility. Thus, the entire erythrocyte population in HS after 24 hours' incubation will show a marked shift toward increased fragility, much greater than that of normal red cells similarly treated.

Of crucial importance in the pathophysiology of hemolysis in HS is the unhappy interaction between the erythrocyte and the spleen. Removal of the spleen restores red cell life span to normal or near normal; all hemolytic manifestations are brought to a prompt halt, yet the cellular defect, along with the abnormal autohemolysis and osmotic fragility tests, remains. What is so unique about the splenic interior that these erythrocytes find so hostile to longevity? In many respects, the spleen subjects the red cells to the same stresses they undergo during sterile in-vitro incubation. The spleen is an organ of erythrostasis; erythrocytes linger in their passage through the splenic pulp. Plasma skimming concentrates erythrocytes to higher packed cell volumes. The splenic pulp has a lower glucose concentration and a more acid pH than the circulating blood. These factors place limitations upon glycolysis and cause lipid loss from the membrane surface. This damage may not be fatal to the erythrocyte during its first passage through the spleen, but with repeated passage the red cell becomes "conditioned," that is, it loses so much membrane surface area that it becomes a microspherocyte. This ball-like erythrocyte lacks the extreme pliability of the normal biconcave shape and it is finally retained in the splenic cords, unable to make the crossing through the finely fenestrated wall that separates the cords from the sinuses of the red pulp. The erythrocytes in the splenic cords must squeeze

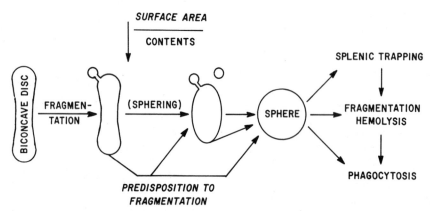

Figure 3–76 Microspherocyte formation. (From Weed, R. I., and Reed, C. F.: Am. J. Med., *41*:681, 1966.)

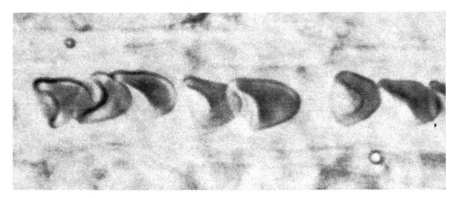

Figure 3–77 The pliability of normal erythrocytes as they move through small capillaries by assuming a parachute configuration. Rigid erythrocytes, such as microspherocytes, sickled erythrocytes, or erythrocytes containing Heinz bodies are subject to entrapment. (From Skalak, R., and Brånemark, P. I.: Science, *164*:717, 1969. Copyright 1969 by the American Association for the Advancement of Science.)

through this meshwork — past quality-conscious macrophages — to gain access into the splenic sinuses and on to drainage into the splenic vein. The small but plump spherocytes are detained, in the meantime suffering the ravages of the splenic environment to the point of outright cell destruction and phagocytosis. No other site in the body possesses such a finely tuned filtering mechanism as the spleen; it places the most stringent limitation upon rigid erythrocytes which cannot easily squeeze and twist through its small orifices (Fig. 3–77).

Hereditary elliptocytosis, an autosomal dominant condition about one fifth as common as HS, is just as obscure in terms of precise molecular genetics. The majority of erythrocytes have an elliptical shape. The diagnosis is clear from inspection of the peripheral blood film alone. Smaller numbers of elliptocytes are often present in the deficiency anemias, thalassemias, myeloproliferative syndromes, and other situations. The defect presumably resides in the membrane, but the pathogenesis of the shape change is not understood. About four fifths of cases exhibit little or no hemolysis. Those with clinical stigmata of hemolysis resemble HS in pathophysiology. Splenomegaly is also present and the hemolysis, as in HS, is corrected by splenectomy.

Paroxysmal nocturnal hemoglobinuria (PNH) is peculiar among the intrinsic red cell disorders in that it is acquired. Despite its rarity it has been intensively investigated, but a precise definition of its molecular basis is still lacking. At present PNH is considered to be an acquired defect of the red cell membrane that renders it pathologically sensitive to destruction by the complement system. This destruction is accomplished without the interposition of the antibodies which usually are required for the initiation of complement-related cell lysis. The onset may be at any age, and the disease usually has a chronic protracted course.

Its name is derived from the fact that intravascular hemolysis occurs at night, causing the first voided morning urine to be darkly colored by its hemoglobin content. In many cases, however, the nocturnal character is not prominent. Periods of exacerbation of the hemoglobinuria may follow infections, exercise, surgery, or other physical stresses. The most serious morbidity and mortality stem from a high incidence of intravascular thrombosis, chiefly venous and often involving the mesenteric and portal venous systems. Some patients become dependent on blood transfusion. Fortunately for them, normal compatible erythrocytes survive normally in their circulation.

The etiology of PNH is unknown. It bears an obscure relationship to aplastic anemia, both idiopathic and drug-induced. Interconversions from one syndrome to the other have been well documented. A few patients with PNH have developed acute leukemia, but this is decidedly a rare occurrence. Some exceptional cases of PNH have undergone complete and permanent remission. Along with the anemia and the elevated reticulocyte count and signs of intravascular hemolysis, the white cell and platelet counts are commonly reduced. Thus the disorder is "trilineage."

Although the red cell life span is shortened, the life span of the platelets is normal. Several odd cellular enzyme deficiencies are associated with PNH, including deficiency of granulocyte alkaline phosphatase and erythrocyte acetylcholinesterase, with unknown pathophysiologic significance.

The diagnosis usually is established by a positive stain of the urinary sediment for hemosiderin and a positive sucrose hemolysis test. The hemosiderinuria is a reflection of the predominantly intravascular nature of the hemolysis. Indeed urinary losses of iron, up to 20 mg. per day, frequently lead to iron deficiency, otherwise an uncommon complication of hemolytic anemia. The sucrose hemolysis test relies on the promotion of complement fixation to the PNH erythrocyte under the conditions of lowered ionic strength obtained when the cell-plasma suspension is diluted in an aqueous sucrose solution. The reason for using sucrose is to maintain osmotic balance, since the erythrocyte membrane is impermeable to it. Another simple screening test is the observation that gross hemolysis is present in the serum surrounding the retracted clot of freshly drawn PNH blood after 2 hours' incubation at 37° C.; autologous complement lyses the erythrocytes in vitro. The acid hemolysin (Ham) test utilizes still another property of complement activation, namely, its optimum at an acid pH of about 6.4. PNH erythrocytes suspended in fresh compatible complement-containing serum properly acidified will show lysis, absent when the serum is heated to 56° C. to inactivate complement. The hemolysis may be enhanced by the addition of crude bovine thrombin preparations (Crosby test), possibly because their heterophile antibody content promotes complement fixation.

The pathophysiologic basis of the disorder remains the subject of much speculation. There are two erythrocyte populations, one sensitive and the other insensitive (Fig. 3–78). The sensitive population, perhaps the offspring of stem cells with a somatic mutation or a self-perpetuating drug-induced change, undergoes hemolysis. The insensitive population has a more normal cell life span. Götze and Müller-Eberhard have reported that

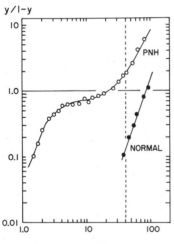

Figure 3–78 Complement sensitivity of normal and PNH erythrocytes. Two cell populations are evident in PNH. In some patients a third population of intermediate sensitivity can be demonstrated. Complement concentration is shown on the horizontal axis and the proportion of lysed to unlysed erythrocytes on the vertical. (Redrawn from Rosse, W. F., et al.: J. Exper. Med., 123:969, 1966.)

properdin and the related serum proteins of the "alternate pathway" are able to fix C3 directly onto the PNH cell, without the usual prior attachment of C1, C4, and C2. The "membrane attack" unit, C5-9, then proceeds to pierce the erythrocyte membrane and bring on intravascular hemolysis.

Intrinsic enzyme deficiency of the erythrocytes may cause either overt hemolysis or hemolytic susceptibility under adverse environmental circumstances. Dacie recognized that a group of hereditary hemolytic disorders could be set apart from hereditary spherocytosis, which they otherwise resembled clinically. Their distinguishing features were the presence of few, if any, spherocytes in the peripheral blood and either a less favorable or no response to splenectomy. He also soon recognized that the "hereditary nonspherocytic hemolytic anemias" did not form a homogeneous group, and he classified them as Type I or Type II according to the results of the autohemolysis test. Type I showed a modestly positive test with correction by the addition of glucose. Type II showed marked autohemolysis without correction by the addition of glucose. The subsequent development of methods for the assay of red cell enzymes has led to the discovery of a large number of deficiencies which appear to explain the etiology of many of the hereditary nonspherocytic hemolytic anemias. Hemolysis has been attributed to deficiency of hexokinase, glucose phosphate isomerase, triose phosphate isomerase, diphosphoglyceromutase, phosphoglycerate kinase, glutathione reductase, pyruvate kinase, and glucose-6-phosphate dehydrogenase, among others. Only the two most common — pyruvate kinase and glucose-6-phosphate dehydrogenase deficiency — will be discussed here.

Pyruvate kinase deficiency, itself a rare disorder, ranks second only to G-6-PD deficiency in frequency among the red cell enzymopathies. The clinical severity is extremely variable, even within a given family. Inherited as an autosomal recessive, the disorder produces hemolysis only in the homozygous state. The heterozygote is hematologically normal, but demonstrates about half the normal enzyme activity. Most patients have splenomegaly. Splenectomy may produce some improvement if the anemia is severe, but the benefit is not nearly as predictable nor as great as it is in hereditary spherocytosis. The postsplenectomy changes in the peripheral blood also contrast with those in HS. In the latter the reticulocyte count promptly declines to near-normal levels within a week as the hemolysis is halted, while patients with PK deficiency often demonstrate a paradoxical rise in reticulocyte count along with the rise in hemoglobin concentration after splenectomy. This clinical observation has suggested that, as in paroxysmal nocturnal hemoglobinuria, the young erythrocyte population is particularly susceptible to hemolysis. In PK deficiency, the destruction of reticulocytes is in the spleen, whereas in PNH it is primarily intravascular.

Pyruvate kinase stands astride an important ATP generating step, the conversion of phosphoenol pyruvate to pyruvate. Deficiency thus leads to impairment of the erythrocyte's ability to provide an adequate supply of energy in the form of ATP necessary to power the membrane cation pump as well as other glycolytic reactions. PK-deficient erythrocytes exhibit a positive autohemolysis test of the Type II variety; adding glucose does not correct the positive test because of failure to utilize glucose. The reason for the inordinate susceptibility of reticulocytes to PK deficiency is not entirely clear, but their high energy requirement presumably narrows their margin for survival in the circulation of the spleen. Reticulocytes derive their energy primarily through the high ATP generating capacity of the oxidative Krebs cycle, which is lost as the reticulocyte matures. The conditions in the spleen — low glucose concentration, low pH, hemoconcentration, plus the delay of the passage of reticulocytes owing to their excessive stickiness in comparison with mature erythrocytes — all lead to a lower safety factor, especially when the mitochondria are in the process of being lost. Although, as with many enzymes, PK concentrations are higher in young than in old red cells, the activity is not high enough to prevent the cell damage which then subsequently leads to cell destruction in both the liver and spleen.

PK deficiency can be caused by a variety of different molecular defects, as is the rule in hereditary disorders. Some represent qualitative structural defects of the enzyme which lead to low activity; others presumably are a quantitative lack of a structurally normal enzyme. In either circumstance the result is a lack in enzyme function.

Glucose-6-phosphate dehydrogenase (G-6-PD) deficiency is by far the most common red cell enzyme abnormality, as discussed by Motulsky. A sex-linked condition, it affects 11 per cent of American black males. In Mediterranean regions it affects about 1 in 1000, but in certain isolated populations it has higher frequencies, affecting up to 50 per cent of male Kurdish Jews, for example. Over 100 genetic variants have already been discovered. From the clinical point of view, three major categories are recognized:

(1) Chronic hereditary non-spherocytic hemolytic anemia is a rare condition that occurs sporadically among various ethnic groups, including Northern European, and represents a variety of differing molecular genetic defects of the enzyme.

(2) The "Mediterranean" variety is one in which the loss of enzyme activity is profound (about 1 per cent of normal) but does not produce clinically significant hemolysis until the erythrocyte is exposed to an extrinsic stress, usually of an oxidative nature, to which the erythrocyte, unable to regenerate reduced glutathione, cannot respond in self defense. The extrinsic stresses include certain drugs as well as such acquired illness as hepatitis and other infections, acidosis, and uremia. Certain deficient individuals in this group are sensitive to fava beans, a sensitivity which may be so severe that it can lead to fatal hemolysis. Genetic factors apparently set these fava bean-susceptible patients apart from the others.

(3) The "Negro" variety resembles the Mediterranean variety but is less severe, deficient males having about 10 to 15 per cent of the normal G-6-PD activity. The affected individual also is hematologically normal until exposed to one of the extrinsic stresses mentioned previously (with the exception of fava beans).

Inheritance is sex-linked, and significant hemolytic episodes are thus observed among affected males and the relatively rare homozygous females. The identification of heterozygous females is not always possible because of the wide range of enzyme levels found in this group, many falling within the normal range, and hemolytic reactions are usually so mild that they pass unnoticed. Beutler and co-workers showed that random inactivation of the X chromosome in the female leads to a dual red cell population, some erythrocytes carrying the normal X chromosome and others in the affected heterozygote carrying the G-6-PD-deficient one. The mean enzyme level will depend upon the relative proportions of normal and deficient erythrocytes. Tests which utilize intact erythrocytes rather than cell lysates may thus be more successful in detecting female heterozygotes.

The two most common types — the "Mediterranean" and the "Negro" — form relatively homogeneous genetic groupings. In the normal black population there are two electrophoretic types of G-6-PD which differ in only one amino acid site on the molecule. The faster migrating type is designated A and the slower B. Thus, nondeficient normal black males possess either A or B (approximately 18 per cent carry A), while the female may be homozygous AA or BB or heterozygous AB. The deficient enzyme in the black has the same electrophoretic mobility as the A type and it is therefore called A⁻. Caucasians, including the Mediterraneans, have only the B type of G-6-PD, and the Mediterranean type of G-6-PD deficiency is called B⁻ (Fig. 3–79).

The clinical severity of the drug-induced hemolysis varies from a clinically inapparent episode to a life-threatening event in an individual who may experience flank and abdominal pains, faintness from shock, and dark-colored urine from massive intravascular hemolysis. The antimalarials such as primaquine, pamaquine, and quinine are the

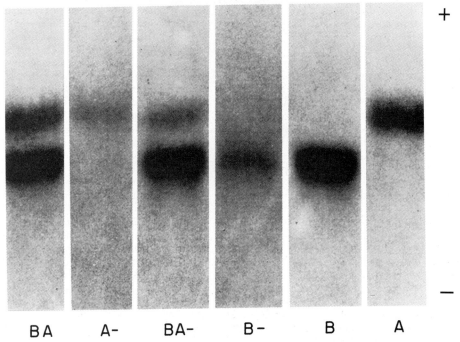

+

BA   A-   BA-   B-   B   A

—

Figure 3–79 Genetic types of G-6-PD deficiency identified by electrophoresis. BA is a normal Negro female heterozygote and BA– is a deficient Negro female heterozygote. The other patterns demonstrate normal and deficient male phenotypes. (From Giblett, E. R.: Genetic Markers in Human Blood. Blackwell Scientific Publications Ltd., Oxford, 1969.)

best known offenders, but sulfonamides, nitrofurans, analgesics, sulfones, and vitamin K derivatives are also frequently implicated. The hemolysis begins within 1 to 3 days of drug exposure, preferentially affecting the more aged erythrocytes because their level of enzyme is lower than that in the young cells. The initial change is a rapid drop in hemoglobin concentration in the peripheral blood. A reticulocyte elevation is observed 4 to 5 days later. After 7 to 10 days the patient enters into a phase of "drug resistance" during which the anemia becomes less pronounced and the patient appears to develop a tolerance to the drug (Fig. 3–80). The explanation for this apparent tolerance is that the younger erythrocytes have a higher enzyme level than the older ones and thus are somewhat better able to cope with the oxidative stress.

Some drugs act directly as oxidants, but most of the chemical agents which provoke oxidative hemolysis do so by interacting with oxyhemoglobin to cause the release of peroxide and other active states of oxygen. The normal erythrocyte meets this oxidative challenge by increasing the rate of glycolysis through the pentose phosphate pathway to maintain NADPH and glutathione in the reduced form. Reduced glutathione, through the good offices of glutathione peroxidase, rapidly detoxifies peroxide. The G-6-PD deficient erythrocyte cannot respond in this fashion. Its hemoglo-

bin is denatured into insoluble Heinz bodies attached to the inner membrane (Fig. 3–81). Between the increased rigidity caused by these inclusions and the direct oxidative damage wrought on the membrane and other cell constituents, hemolysis ensues. Some chemical agents, phenylhydrazine for example, are so potent they cause oxidative hemolysis in normal people. In addition to the potency of the agent and its dose, the genetic type of G-6-PD deficiency also determines the severity of the hemolysis. Pharmacogenetic differences in the population are sometimes important in determining whether or not oxidative hemolysis occurs. One person may metabolize a drug to a harmless intermediate, while another may convert the same agent to a by-product with toxic oxidative properties.

Direct enzyme assay is commonly used to establish the diagnosis of the G-6-PD–deficient state, but the result is affected by the average age of the red cell population. Thus, immediately following a hemolytic episode the levels may be nearly normal unless a correction is made for the mean cell age by the simultaneous measurement of another nonaffected enzyme such as hexokinase which also has a higher concentration in young than in old red cells. A number of simple screening tests have been devised, two of the more common in clinical use being the methemoglobin reduction test and the fluorescent spot test. The methemo-

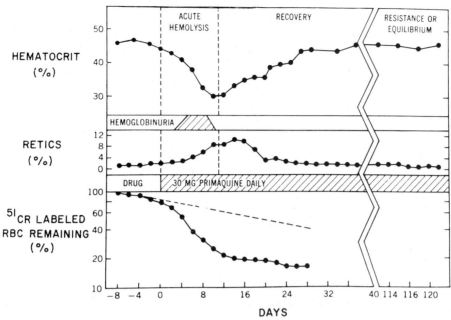

Figure 3–80 Drug-induced hemolysis in a male with G-6-PD deficiency. A period of hemolytic anemia is followed by compensation at higher hematocrit and relative drug resistance due to higher enzyme levels in the young population of erythrocytes. (Redrawn from Alving, A. S., et al.: Bull. WHO, 22:621, 1960.)

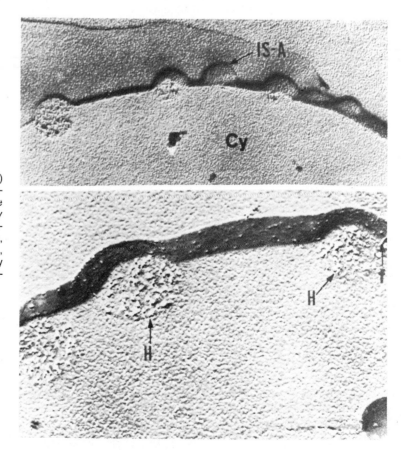

Figure 3–81 Heinz bodies (*H*) attached to the erythrocyte membrane demonstrated by freeze etching electron microscopy. *Cy* = cytoplasm; *IS-A* = intramembrane surface A. (From Lessin, L. S., et al.: Arch. Intern. Med., 129:306, 1972. Copyright 1972 by the American Medical Association.)

globin reduction test takes advantage of the fact that methylene blue establishes a redox bridge between the pentose phosphate pathway and methemoglobin reduction with NADPH as hydrogen donor. Intracellular hemoglobin is first converted to methemoglobin by incubation with sodium nitrite. After addition of methylene blue, normal erythrocytes rapidly reduce the methemoglobin and change color from brown to red. G-6-PD–deficient erythrocytes, unable to increase glycolysis through the pentose phosphate pathway, remain the chocolate-brown color of methemoglobin. The fluorescent spot test is based on the reduction by lysate of NADP to NADPH, which fluoresces under ultraviolet light. G-6-PD–deficient erythrocytes, unable to accomplish this reduction, fail to produce fluorescence in the spot.

Intrinsic hemolysis may result from the presence of *abnormal hemoglobin.* As already discussed in detail, some abnormal hemoglobins are so unstable to oxidative stresses that they undergo spontaneous precipitation into insoluble deposits in the red cell, even in the presence of a normal enzymatic machinery. Some are drug sensitive, and in this respect resemble G-6-PD deficiency. The selective destruction of newly formed erythroid cells in homozygous β-thalassemia is reminiscent of a similar preferential susceptibility of young cells in paroxysmal nocturnal hemoglobinuria and in pyruvate kinase deficiency, but the pathogenetic mechanism is quite distinctive for each of these disorders. Sickle cell anemia, the most common of the hemoglobin diseases, results not from oxidative instability but from a physicochemical alteration of the hemoglobin which produces rigid erythrocytes. The final common pathway in the intrinsic hemoglobin disorders is membrane damage and reduction in cell pliability to the point of entrapment and destruction.

Extrinsic Hemolytic Disorders. Hemolytic conditions are caused by a wide variety of extrinsic physical and chemical factors. Extensive burns cause thermal damage to the erythrocyte membrane, with fragmentation, spherocytosis, and acute hemolysis. Acute poisoning with arsenate or copper or drowning (with hypotonic hemolysis) are other examples of acute hemolytic syndromes in patients suffering severe medical emergencies. Infections produce hemolysis indirectly, as in hypersplenism secondary to miliary tuberculosis or subacute bacterial endocarditis, or by direct invasion of the erythrocyte, as in the case of malaria or bartonellosis. In *Clostridium welchii* septicemia, the organism secretes a phospholipase which attacks the phospholipid backbone of the red cell membrane. The high oxygen tensions used in hyperbaric therapy cause hemolysis by peroxidation of membrane lipids. Chemical hemolysis by phenylhydrazine was once used therapeutically to reduce the red cell mass in patients with polycythemia. This agent, still commonly used to produce

hemolytic anemia experimentally in animals, causes a "Heinz body anemia" in normal erythrocytes quite similar to that observed in G-6-PD–deficient individuals given drugs to which they are sensitive.

The types of extrinsic hemolysis of greatest clinical interest from the pathogenetic point of view are those caused by mechanical damage and those which are the result of plasma factors.

Mechanical hemolysis is vividly illustrated by *march hemoglobinuria,* so called because it was observed in soldiers after the exertion of a long march (Davidson, 1969). The hemolysis is intravascular but benign and self-limited. The mechanical damage to the red cells occurs during the physical impact of the soles of the feet on hard surfaces. Ingeniously simple experiments have shown that it can be prevented among track athletes by placing shock absorbing material in the footwear or by running on soft grass instead of hard asphalt or concrete. The syndrome has even been seen in karate fighters, the damage in this instance coming from the palms of the hands as well as the soles of the feet.

Mechanical hemolysis also occurs because of damage to erythrocytes from physical impacts within the circulation. High pressure turbulence behind a stenotic aortic valve may cause mild cardiac hemolysis even in the unoperated patient. Modern cardiovascular surgery has contributed an important iatrogenic variety of *"traumatic" hemolysis* from red cell damage in the heart after insertion of prosthetic devices, as discussed by Marsh and Lewis. Its presence indicates an abnormal turbulence of blood or an exposed plastic surface not yet covered with endothelium. Examples of underlying causes are a loosened stitch at the base of a valve prosthesis through which a high-pressure jet of blood squirts; a bare Teflon patch used to close a septal defect upon which a regurgitant jet of blood strikes; and "ball variance," a late cause of postoperative hemolysis due to improper valve closure from slow swelling and distortion of the plastic ball. Technical improvements such as the use of a metal ball have reduced the frequency of postoperative traumatic hemolysis. Cardiac hemolysis is intravascular. When it is severe the loss of iron in the urine from the chronic hemoglobinuria and hemosiderinuria leads to iron deficiency and compromises the ability of the bone marrow to compensate for the reduced red cell life span.

Traumatic cardiac hemolysis has been aptly called the "Waring blender syndrome" because the morphologic alterations of the red cells suggest that they have been chopped by the whirling blades of this kitchen apparatus. They are sheared into bits and pieces, and display pointed and triangular forms, "helmet" shapes, and other distorted contours (Fig. 3–82). Microspherocytes and polychromasia are also present.

These morphologic changes are also a charac-

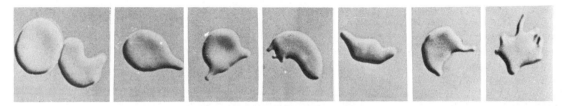

Figure 3–82 Irregular distortion of erythrocytes demonstrated by interference microscopy. (Reproduced from the Sandoz-Monograph, The Life Cycle of the Erythrocyte. Basel, Switzerland, Bessis, M., 1966.)

teristic feature of another group of hemolytic disorders which have in common an occlusive process of the microvasculature and hence have been called by Brain the *"microangiopathic hemolytic anemias."* The fragmentation has been reproduced experimentally in vitro by forcing red cells through a fibrin meshwork and in vivo by inducing intravascular coagulation in animals with injections of endotoxin or thrombin (Fig. 3–83). The clinical counterparts of these experiments are those conditions characterized by a thromboocclusive process in the small vessels, including the various disseminated intravascular coagulation syndromes, hemolytic uremic syndromes, and thrombotic thrombocytopenic purpura. Fragmentation hemolysis has also been encountered in patients with malignant hypertension or disseminated carcinoma.

Of the plasma factors that adversely effect erythrocyte survival time, antibodies against red cell antigens have received the most scrutiny. Much remains to be learned about the effects of non-immune plasma factors. The role of plasma lipids and lipoproteins in the hemolytic anemia of cirrhosis however warrants special consideration.

Anemia in cirrhosis is the result of a combination of factors — blood loss, iron and/or folate lack,

and hypersplenism. Even in the absence of these complicating factors, the erythrocyte life span is slightly to moderately reduced. Macrocytosis is a common feature of hepatocellular disease, often in association with target cells. The increased erythrocyte volume comes from accumulation of excessive lipid in the erythrocyte membrane, free cholesterol to a greater degree than phospholipid. The passive exchange between plasma and red cell membrane favors uptake into the latter because impairment of cholesterol esterification in liver disease leads to a relative increase in plasma free cholesterol at the expense of cholesterol esters. Indeed, inherited deficiency of the cholesterol esterifying enzyme, lecithyl cholesterol acyl transferase (LCAT), also causes macrocytosis with target cells. The increased levels of plasma free cholesterol secondary to obstruction of the biliary tract affect erythrocytes in a similar way. Marked hemolysis is not a feature of these forms of target cell anemia.

The *"spur cell"* anemia of cirrhosis is a more severe form of hemolysis. Its name is derived from the pointed thorny projections which protrude from the red cells (Fig. 3–84). This hemolytic disorder is seen in association with fulminating hepatocellular disease and is apparently a more extreme form of membrane accumulation of free

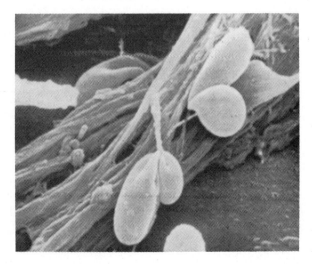

Figure 3–83 Erythrocyte fragmentation on fibrin strands. (From Bull, B. S., and Kuhn, I. N.: Blood, *35*:104–111, 1970, by permission of Grune & Stratton, Inc., New York.)

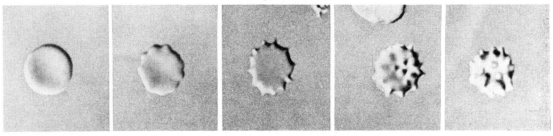

Figure 3–84   Regular distortion of an erythrocyte to form an acanthocyte. (Reproduced from the Sandoz-Monograph, The Life Cycle of the Erythrocyte. Basel, Switzerland, Bessis, M., 1966.)

cholesterol in excess of phospholipid. Plasma lipoproteins with abnormally high ratios of free cholesterol to phospholipid are important in its pathogenesis. The spur cells are susceptible to entrapment in the enlarged spleen commonly present in cirrhosis. Normal compatible erythrocytes transfused into affected patients soon acquire the membrane defect. Serum from patients with these disorders when added in vitro to normal compatible erythrocytes will produce macrocytosis and targeting or spur cell formation, as the case may be.

Hereditary acanthocytosis is characterized by absence of plasma beta-lipoproteins together with hypolipidemia and abnormal erythrocytes which closely resemble spur cells but are called "acanthocytes." The degree of hemolysis is mild. Acanthocytosis is occasionally seen in individuals after splenectomy who are otherwise hematologically normal. Spiculated erythrocytes are also seen. The pathogenesis of the erythrocyte shape change in these disorders remains unexplained.

Immune hemolysis may take place when antibodies present in the circulation react with antigens on the red cell surface. Hidden behind this deceptively simple theme lie the countless complexities of antigens, antibodies, and complement. *Isoimmune hemolysis* is the result of immunologic reactions between antibodies and antigens which reflect differences between individuals. Examples of isoimmune hemolysis include hemolytic transfusion reactions and immunohemolytic disease of the newborn, i.e., erythroblastosis fetalis. ABO incompatible erythrocytes are destroyed by "natural" isoantibodies normally present in the plasma. "Irregular" isoantibodies are produced only as a result of previous antigenic exposure, usually from transfusion or pregnancy. An autoantibody produced within a given individual with specificity directed against that individual's own autologous erythrocyte antigens brings on *autoimmune hemolytic anemia.*

The "natural" isoantibodies of the ABO system are predominantly IgM immunoglobulins with potent complement fixing ability. Isoimmume hemolytic reactions due to accidental transfusion of ABO incompatible erythrocytes are abrupt and

life-threatening. The degree of complement fixation is extensive and provokes prompt intravascular hemolysis with hemoglobinemia and hemoglobinuria. Hypotension, disseminated intravascular coagulation, and acute renal failure are common complications.

"Irregular" antibodies directed against other red cell antigens, such as those of the Rh locus (CcDEe), are usually IgG immunoglobulins with a lesser propensity to fix complement. Their activity is maximal at 37°C. Demonstration of their presence requires the Coombs test. They are "warm" "incomplete" antibodies as distinct from the isoantibodies of the ABO system, which agglutinate erythrocytes in saline suspension at room temperature and therefore are "complete". Hemolysis secondary to irregular antibodies is less brisk and may be relatively more extravascular.

The Coombs test is central to the evaluation of immunohemolytic states. It is designed to detect either immunoglobulin or complement components coated on the erythrocyte surface. Coombs reagent, or "antiglobulin serum", is an antiserum raised in animals injected with these human plasma protein constituents. This antiserum when incubated with erythrocytes coated with immunoglobulin or with complement causes them to clump together. In general antiglobulin serum of broad specificity is used, sensitive to the presence either of immunoglobin or complement. Antiglobulin serum of more restricted specificity will distinguish immunoglobulin from complement on the erythrocyte surface. The term "gamma" Coombs refers to identification of immunoglobulin and "non-gamma" to the demonstration of complement. In experimental work, antiglobulin serum of even greater specificity permits identification of immunoglobulin subclasses. The "direct" Coombs test is performed on washed erythrocytes suspected of being coated in the circulation. The "indirect" test detects antibodies present in serum by first reacting the serum in vitro with erythrocytes and then testing these washed erythrocytes as described above.

Isoimmune hemolytic disease of the newborn is caused by the passage of 7S IgG antibodies across the placental barrier from the maternal into the fetal circulation, where they proceed to combine with antigens present on fetal erythrocytes. Although most of the natural isoantibodies of the ABO system are IgM antibodies too large to cross the placenta, some natural ABO isoantibodies are IgG and can cause erythroblastosis even during the first pregnancy. The usual incompatibility pairing is maternal type O and fetal type A or B. The hemolysis is generally mild and often requires no treatment. The antibody coating on the fetal erythrocyte may be so sparse that the Coombs test is negative.

Transplacental hemorrhage of fetal erythrocytes containing an antigen absent on the maternal red cell surface may raise the production of an irregular isoantibody in the maternal circulation, harmless to the mother but potentially detrimental to fetal erythrocytes once it crosses the placental barrier. Most significant is the D antigen of the Rh locus, although other antigens are occasionally responsible. ("Rh positive" indicates presence of the D antigen, "Rh negative" its absence.) Erythroblastosis fetalis due to Rh incompatibility causes severe hemolysis. The direct Coombs test on fetal erythrocytes is always positive. Hemorrhage of fetal erythrocytes into the maternal circulation is an event which most often occurs near term or at the time of labor and delivery. They can be demonstrated by a simple slide elution test which depends on the resistance of fetal hemoglobin to acid elution. Because of this requirement for prior immunization, first borns are usually spared, assuming that the mother has not been accidentally sensitized by previous transfusion of Rh incompatible cells.

A number of natural factors operate to reduce the incidence of Rh incompatibility neonatal he-

molytic disease. One of these is the dependence on prior occurrence of feto-maternal hemorrhage. Another is "ABO cancellation." If incompatibility within the ABO system coexists with Rh incompatibility, the rapid removal of the fetal erythrocytes by the natural isoantibodies anti A and/or anti B prevents active maternal immunization to the foreign Rh antigen on the fetal erythrocyte.

Following on this observation, it was reasoned that rapid removal of Rh incompatible fetal erythrocytes from the maternal circulation by the passive administration to the mother of a human gamma globulin preparation, hyperimmune with respect to its anti D titer, would prevent active maternal sensitization. This has indeed proved to be the case, and current practice calls for the routine prophylactic use of such gamma globulin preparations shortly after delivery in all Rh negative mothers at risk. Since this form of preventive therapy has been introduced, the incidence of Rh incompatibility neonatal hemolytic disease has decreased dramatically (Fig. 3–85). This remarkable reduction in cases deserves to rank among the major therapeutic achievements of recent years.

Kernicterus is the most dread complication of neonatal hemolytic disease, provided the infant survives the initial crisis. Lipid-soluble unconjugated bilirubin, present in excess of the plasma albumin binding capacity, is taken up into the nervous tissue, causing toxic damage. Therapeutic strategy is aimed at preventing the build-up of unconjugated bilirubin. This has traditionally been accomplished by exchange transfusion. More recent efforts have explored the use of albumin infusion, of pharmacologic agents such as phenobarbital to stimulate the hepatic enzymes to increase the rate of bilirubin conjugation in the

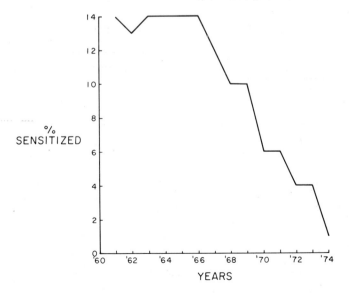

Figure 3–85 Following the routine prophylactic administration of anti Rh hyperimmune gamma globulin to mothers at risk, there has been a dramatic decrease in the incidence of erythroblastosis fetalis due to Rh incompatibility. The vertical axis represents the proportion of the Rh negative mothers sensitized to Rh. Clinical trials began in 1964 and routine use started in 1968. (Redrawn, by permission, from Freda, V. J., et al.: New England Journal of Medicine, 292:1014, 1975.)

%
SENSITIZED

YEARS

immature fetal liver, and exposure to light which appears to convert the bilirubin to less toxic derivatives.

The *autoimmune hemolytic anemias* are classified as "warm antibody" or "cold antibody" types. Warm antibody is an IgG immunoglobulin with maximal activity at 37°C. Its presence on the red cell is demonstrated by a positive Coombs test. It may or may not fix complement. Many of the warm antibodies have a specificity for the "core" antigen of the Rh locus. They react with all Rh phenotypes but not with the rare type Rh null, presumably a genetic deletion of the entire Rh locus.

Cold reactive autoantibody has increased activity as the temperature is reduced; the highest titer is at 4°C. It is demonstrated by the cold agglutinin test. In this simple procedure, dilutions of the patient's serum are mixed with normal type-compatible erythrocytes and incubated overnight at 4°C. The greatest dilution at which agglutination occurs is recorded. Titers greater than 1:64 are abnormal. Clinical hemolysis is associated with titers in excess of 1:1000, and they usually are considerably higher, some times as high as several million. The cold antibody, with one exception noted below, is an IgM immunoglobulin. It usually has specificity for the I antigen present on most adult erythrocytes, but absent on fetal erythrocytes which have the i antigen. Cord blood erythrocytes are thus usually not agglutinated by cold reactive antibody. A few cold antibodies have specificity for the i rather than the I antigen. Curiously, the reason for the cold reactivity of this class of antibodies does not appear to be a function of the antibody but rather of the Ii antigens. These presumably move to more accessible positions at the membrane surface as the temperature is reduced. Conversely, as the temperature is again increased the antigen sinks down into the more fluid lipid membrane, the immune complex is broken, and the antibody is released (Pruzanski and Shumak, 1977). However, the complement component, fixed by the cold antibodies to the membrane surface, remains and is responsible for the positive direct Coombs test usually observed in cold antibody hemolytic anemia (Table 3–13).

Warm antibody autoimmune hemolytic anemia is the most common of the immunohemolytic anemias. It affects all age groups. The onset may be insidious or acute, with fever, weakness, flank and abdominal pain. The spleen is commonly enlarged and the patient slightly jaundiced. The peripheral blood film shows microspherocytes mixed together with polychromatophilic macrocytes. It is distinguished from hereditary spherocytosis by the positive Coombs test. The autohemolysis test gives variable results. Osmotic fragility testing may show a "fragile tail" because of the population of osmotically susceptible microspherocytes.

Cold antibody autoimmune hemolytic anemia is almost always of the cold agglutinin type. It may occur in acute and self-limited form during the recovery phase of certain infections, most notably mycoplasma pneumonia and infectious mononucleosis. A chronic variety occurring usually in older patients is associated with a monoclonal autoantibody — and often with a monoclonal M-component on serum protein electrophoresis. This "idiopathic" condition is presumably "paraneoplastic" and closely related to the lymphoproliferative diseases. The degree of hemolysis is often mild in chronic cold agglutinin disease, even when the titer is very high. Exposed parts of the body — the fingers, toes, ears, and nose — may suffer the consequences of reduced temperatures with vaso-obstructive signs such as Raynaud-like symptoms or local tissue necrosis. The "thermal amplitude" refers to antibody activity as a function of temperature. The activity decreases as the temperature increases and usually no activity is present above 32°C. Spontaneous agglutination of anticoagulated blood at room temperature may cause technical errors in the laboratory unless precautions are taken to maintain the blood at temperatures above 32°C. Autoagglutination, along with spherocytosis, is a dominant feature of the peripheral blood film. The marrow is often infiltrated with lymphocytes in the idiopathic chronic variety.

Paroxysmal cold hemoglobinuria is a very rare acquired immunohemolytic anemia caused by an IgG cold reactive autoantibody demonstrated by the Donath-Landsteiner test. The antibody is bound at 4°C. and complement is fixed. Agglutination is not present, but as the sample is warmed complement induced hemolysis takes place. Acute hemolytic episodes are provoked by exposure to cold. Signs of intravascular hemolysis are marked. Some cases are idiopathic, while others are related to infections, especially syphilis.

The pathogenesis of the hemolysis in autoimmune hemolytic anemia has posed apparent paradoxes. For example, a strongly positive Coombs test may be associated with an absence of clinical

TABLE 3–13   LABORATORY DIAGNOSIS OF AUTOIMMUNE HEMOLYTIC ANEMIA

	Routine Coombs Test	"Gamma" Coombs Test	"Non-gamma" Coombs Test	Cold agglutinin Test
Warm type	+	+	+ or −	−
Cold agglutinin type	+	−	+	+

hemolysis on the one hand, while on the other an occasional case of acquired autoimmune hemolytic anemia may be discovered with a negative Coombs test. Some explanations for these apparent contradictions between laboratory tests and clinical events have in large measure been provided by new information about the subclasses of immunoglobulins and their relationships to complement fixation and to specific receptors on the surface of macrophages.

It stands to reason that the density of the antibody coating on the red cell is a major determinant of the severity of hemolysis, as Rosse and others have demonstrated (Fig. 3–86). About 500 IgG molecules per erythrocyte are necessary to produce a positive Coombs test. For a given antibody the greater this number the shorter the red cell life span. However, reduced erythrocyte life span may also be present at values less than 500.

The process of complement fixation is directly a function of the density of antibodies on the red cell surface. In order for the first component of complement to be fixed, two IgG molecules must achieve a certain critical distance apart from each other (250-400 Å). Low-density IgG coatings are thus not likely to fix complement. On the other hand, the pentameric IgM contains within its intrinsic structure five potential immunoglobulin binding sites. Since these five "feet" fall within the critical distance, IgM on the cell surface invariably fixes complement. If the antigenic sites on the red cell surface are spaced too far apart to permit the corresponding IgG antibodies to be placed within the critical distance, then complement fixation cannot take place. Such is the case with the Rh

antigens; immunohemolytic disease due to Rh antibodies lacks complement on the cell surface (Logue and Rosse, 1976).

The immunoglobulin subclasses do not fix complement equally well. In addition to IgM, IgG$_3$ and IgG$_1$ are active. IgG$_2$ has only weak activity. IgG$_4$, IgA, and IgE do not fix complement at all. Thus, the specific subclass to which the autoantibody belongs, along with its concentration, is important as a hemolytic determinant.

The specific details of the complement system have been clearly depicted by Müller-Eberhard. The "recognition unit" (C$_1$ qrs) is followed by "the activation unit" (C$_{4, 2, 3}$) which in turn may develop a "membrane attack unit" (C$_{5-9}$). An immense amount of C$_1$ must be fixed to bring on the membrane attack unit to punch holes through the cell surface and cause direct hemolysis. This usually does not occur in autoimmune hemolytic anemia. If complement fixation is achieved, it ordinarily is arrested at the level of the activation unit, which leaves C$_3$b on the cell surface. However, this component can also bring about cell damage by interaction with macrophages.

Macrophages have at least two specific receptors on their surfaces, one for the Fc fragment of IgG and the other for the C$_3$b component of complement. Once again the subclasses of IgG are important; receptor activity is greatest for IgG$_3$ and IgG$_1$ and absent for IgG$_4$ and IgA, in parallel to the complement fixing activity of these immunoglobulin types. Immunoglobulin and/or C$_3$b on the erythrocyte surface brings the coated erythrocyte into close juxtaposition to macrophages at these receptor sites. At the interface the macrophage proceeds about its work, gnawing bits and pieces

Figure 3–86 The relation between IgG density on the erythrocyte membrane and the degree of anemia in nonsplenectomized patients with warm antibody autoimmune hemolytic anemia. The measurement of membrane antibody density employs a sensitive technque of first reacting the coated erythrocytes with anti-human gamma globulin and then measuring complement fixation on the doubly coated cells. (Redrawn from Rosse, W. F.: J. Clin. Invest., 50:734, 1971.)

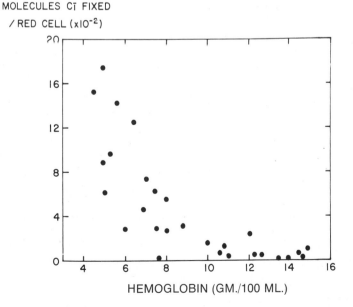

MOLECULES C̄1 FIXED / RED CELL (x10^{-2})

HEMOGLOBIN (GM./100 ML.)

away from the cell surface. Lost surface causes spherocytosis culminating in the eventual entrapment and engulfment of the entire erythrocyte. These events are depicted diagrammatically in Fig. 3–87. Erythrocyte fragmentation at the cell-cell interface has been vividly documented by electron microscopy (Fig. 3–88).

Other variables also affect the severity of the hemolysis. One of these is the state of activation of macrophages. Another is C_3 inactivator. This ingredient of the complement system cleaves C_3b on the erythrocyte surface, leaving behind a fragment called C_3d. This is still detectable in the Coombs test, but its presence on the cell surface protects against further phagocytosis, thus limiting hemolysis (Jaffe and coworkers, 1976). In fact, C_3 inactivator appears to be able to release the C_3b coated erythrocyte from the grasp of the hepatic macrophage and allow it once again to circulate without further damage (Fig. 3–87).

Thus the lack of correlation between the results of routine clinical tests and clinical phenomena has become more understandable. The reason why IgG_4 or IgA do not produce hemolysis is clear; neither fix complement and neither bind to macrophages. Conversely an erythrocyte coated with both IgG_3 and C_3b is rapidly destroyed since both

moieties bring about lethal contacts with macrophage receptors.

What determines splenic as against hepatic hemolysis? In warm antibody hemolytic disease the IgG coating on the erythrocyte is often unaccompanied by complement and splenic macrophages are the preferred site of destruction. Hence splenectomy is often successful as a definitive means of therapy if glucocorticoids cannot adequately control the hemolysis. On the other hand, cold agglutinin hemolytic disease is predominantly hepatic, probably because C_3b on the erythrocyte surface favors interaction with the hepatic Kupfer cells. Splenectomy is usually unsuccessful and glucocorticoids of less benefit than in warm antibody hemolytic disease. By similar reasoning resistance of warm antibody hemolytic anemia to these therapeutic measures may be related to class and concentration of antibody and to complement fixation.

Glucocorticoids act primarily by blocking macrophage–erythrocyte interactions and inhibiting phagocytosis. Only later do they cause autoantibody concentrations to fall. Other immunosuppressive modalities have also been used in the treatment of resistant cases.

How does an autoantibody come to be produced

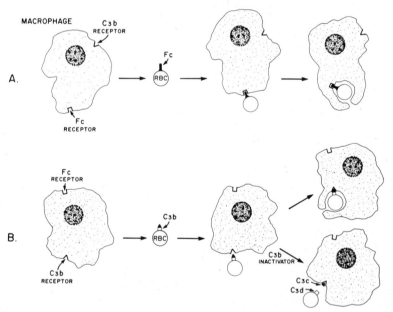

Figure 3–87 The role of macrophage surface receptors in immune hemolytic anemia, illustrated diagrammatically. Macrophages have separate receptors for immunoglobulins and for complement. The immunoglobulin receptors have a restricted specificity for the Fc fragment of the subclasses IgG_1 and IgG_3. The other immunoglobulins do not bind to macrophages. The complement receptor is specific for the C_3b component.

A. An IgG coated erythrocyte is attached to a macrophage. Erythrocyte fragmentation and/or outright engulfment follows.

B. A C_3b coated erythrocyte is attached to a macrophage. Phagocytosis may follow, as in A, or C_3b inactivator may cleave C_3b and cause release of the erythrocyte from the clutches of the macrophage. C_3d is left behind on the erythrocyte. This surface coating renders the erythrocyte resistant to further phagocytic damage.

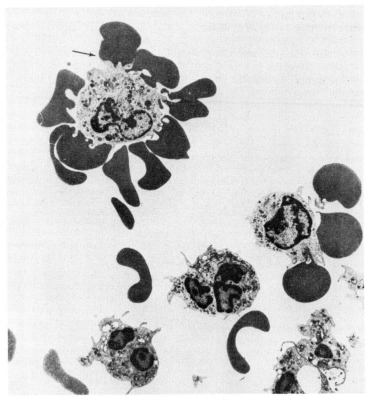

Figure 3–88 The adherence of IgG coated erythrocytes to macrophages, with fragmentation of small pieces of the erythrocyte membrane at the cell to cell interface. (From Abramson, N., et al.: J. Exper. Med., *132*:1191, 1970.)

in violation of the principle of immune self recognition and tolerance to autologous antigens? Hypotheses for this phenomenon as a pathogenetic factor in a variety of disease states have been put forth: (1) There is a shared antigenicity between an exogenous inciting antigen and an autologous antigen which brings on the immune attack upon the autologous tissue. (2) "Forbidden clones" of immunocytes emerge, perhaps due to lack of proper immunologic "suppressor" or "surveillance" activity, and these produce antibodies against autologous antigen. (3) A subtle change takes place in autologous antigen, rendering it immunogenic.

What is clear is that a large proportion of autoimmune hemolytic anemias occur in association with altered states of immunity. Acute self-limited syndromes appear in the recovery phase from certain infections while the immune response is taking place. Others occur in association with immune deficiency syndromes, such as agammaglobulinemia and a variety of chronic lymphoproliferative disorders, especially chronic lymphatic leukemia, lymphocytic lymphoma, and Hodgkin's disease. They also complicate the course of other autoimmune disorders, such as disseminated lupus erythematosus and ulcerative colitis. Many however remain unexplained and are designated "idiopathic."

Coombs-positive immunohemolytic anemias also occur as adverse reactions to certain medications, and a consideration of these may provide some further insight into pathogenetic mechanisms. They fall into three classes:

(1) The "haptene" (or penicillin) type. The serum of the patient contains antipenicillin antibodies of the 7S type. Penicillin, if given in very high doses, is soaked up into the erythrocyte membrane. The antipenicillin antibodies are not directed against red cell antigens but do bind to the penicillin in the membrane, giving rise to a positive "gamma" Coombs test and to hemolysis.

(2) The "immune complex" (or "innocent bystander") type. IgM antibody is formed to the drug (quinidine, quinine, stibophen) which is associated with an unidentified serum protein as carrier. The antibody then reacts with the antigen to form an immune complex, which attaches to the red cell membrane and fixes complement. The antibody may then be detached, leaving complement behind. The "non-gamma" Coombs test is positive because of the complement coat. The red cell is considered the innocent bystander. The mechan-

ism is the same as that of quinidine thrombo-cytopenia, except that the latter is characterized by the production of a 7S IgG antibody.

(3) The true autoimmune (or alphamethyldopa) type. In a time- and dose-dependent manner, the drug induces the formation of an antibody specifically directed against a normal red cell anti-

gen, usually of the Rh complex. The autoimmune state persists for months after discontinuation of the drug, gradually subsiding without additional treatment. This drug-related form of autoimmunity suggests a possible pathogenesis of other types of autoimmune states by undefined exogenous agents.

REFERENCES

Abramson, N., LoBuglio, A. F., Jandl, J. H., and Cotran, R. S.: The interaction between human monocytes and red cells. Binding characteristics. J. Exp. Med., *132*:1191, 1970.

Adamson, J. W., Fialkow, P. J., Murphy, S., Prechal, J. F., and Steinman, L.: Polycythemia vera: stem cell and probable clonal origin of the disease. N. Engl. J. Med., *295*:913, 1976.

Aisen, P., and Brown, E. B.: The iron binding function of transferrin in iron metabolism. Seminars Hematol. *14*, 31, 1977.

Alving, A. S., Johnson, C. F., Tarlov, A. R., Brewer, G. J., Kellermeyer, R. W., and Carson, P. E.: Mitigation of the haemolytic effect of primaquine and enhancement of its action against exoerythrocytic forms of the Chesson strain of plasmodium vivax by intermittent regimens of drug administration. Bull. WHO, *22*:621, 1960.

Arderman, S., Chanarin, I., and Doyle, J. C.: Studies on secretion of gastric intrinsic factor in man. Br. Med. J., *2*:600, 1964.

Bert, P.: La pression barométrique. Masson, Paris, 1878.

Bessis, M.: Life Cycle of the Erythrocyte. Sandoz Monographs, 1966.

Beutler, E., Yeh, M., and Fairbanks, V. F.: The normal human female as a mosaic of X-chromosome activity: Studies using the gene for G-6-PD deficiency as a marker. Proc. Nat. Acad. Sci., U.S.A., *48*:9, 1962.

Bookchin, R. M., and Nagel, R. L.: Interaction between hemoglobins: sickling and related phenomena. Seminars Hematol. *11*:577, 1974.

Bothwell, T. H., and Finch, C. A.: Iron Metabolism. Little, Brown & Co., Boston, 1962.

Brain, M. C.,: Microangiopathic hemolytic anemia. Ann. Rev. Med., *21*:133, 1970.

Brown, S. M., Gilbert, H. S., Krauss, S., and Wasserman, L. R.: Relative polycythemia: a non-existant disease. Am. J. Med., *50*:200, 1971.

Bull, B. S., and Kuhn, I. N.: The production of schistocytes by fibrin strands (a scanning electron microscopic study). Blood, *35*:104, 1970.

Bunn, H. F., Forget, B. G., and Ranney, H. M.: Human Hemoglobins. W. B. Saunders Co., Philadelphia, 1977.

Bunn, H. F., and Jandl, J. H.: The renal handling of hemoglobin. II. Catabolism. J. Exp. Med., *129*:925, 1969.

Castle, W. B.: Current concepts of pernicious anemia. Am. J. Med., *48*:541, 1970.

Chanarin, I.: The Megaloblastic Anemias. F. A. Davis Co., Philadelphia, 1969.

Charache, S., Conley, C. L., Waugh, D. E., Ugoretz, R. J., and Spurrell, J. R.: Pathogenesis of hemolytic anemia in homozygous hemoglobin C disease. J. Clin. Invest., *46*:1795, 1967.

Chisholm, J. J., Jr.: The continued hazard of lead poisoning. Hosp. Pract., *8*:11, 127, 1973.

Chodos, R. B., Wells, R., Jr., and Chaffee, W. R.: A study of ferrokinetics and red cell survival in congestive heart failure. Am. J. Med., *36*:553, 1964.

Condon, P. I., and Serjeant, G. R.: Ocular findings in homozygous sickle cell anemia in Jamaica. Am. J. Ophthalmol., *73*:533, 1972.

Cooper, R. A.: Abnormalities of cell membrane fluidity in the pathogenesis of disease. N. Engl. J. Med., *297*:371, 1977.

Cooper, R. A., and Jandl, J. H.: Bile salts and cholesterol in the pathogenesis of target cells in obstructive jaundice. J. Clin. Invest., *47*:809, 1968.

Cooper, R. A., and Jandl, J. H.: The selective and conjoint loss of red cell lipids. J. Clin. Invest., *48*:906, 1969.

Cronkite, E. P., and Bond, V. P.: Radiation Injury in Man. Charles C Thomas, Springfield, Illinois, 1960.

Davidson, R. J. L.: March or exertional hemoglobinuria. Seminars Hematol., *6*:150, 1969.

deFuria, F. G., Miller, D. R., Cerami, A., et al.: The effects of cyanate in vitro on red blood cell metabolism and function in sickle cell anemia. J. Clin. Invest., *51*:566, 1972.

Dhar, G. J., Bossenmaier, I., Petryka, Z. J., Cardinal, R., and Watson, C. J.: Effects of hemetin in hepatic porphyria. Further studies. Ann. Int. Med., *83*:20, 1975.

Donohue, D. M., Reiff, R. H., Hanson, M. L., Betson, Y., and Finch, C. A.: Quantitative measurements of the erythrocytic and granulocytic cells of the marrow and blood. J. Clin. Invest., *37*:1571, 1958.

Edwards, C. Q., Carroll, M., Bray, P., and Cartwright, G. R.: Hereditary hemochromatosis. Diagnosis in siblings and children. N. Engl. J. Med., *297*, 7, 1977.

Erbe, R. W.: Inborn errors of folate metabolism. N. Engl. J. Med., *293*, 753, 1975.

Erslev, A. J.: Humoral regulation of red cell production. Blood, *8*:349, 1953.

Erslev, A. J.: The role of erythropoietin in the control of red cell production. Medicine, *43*:661, 1964.

Erslev, A. J.: Anemia of chronic renal disease. Arch. Intern. Med., *126*:774, 1970.

Erslev, A. J.: The renal biogenesis of erythropoietin. Am. J. Med., *58*:25, 1975.

Filmanowicz, E., and Gurney, C. W.: Studies on erythropoiesis. XVI. Response to a single dose of erythropoietin in polycythemic mouse. J. Lab. Clin. Med., *57*:65, 1961.

Finch, C. A.: Iron metabolism. Nutrition Today, Summer, 1969, p. 2.

Finch, C. A., Harker, L. A., and Cook, J. D.: Kinetics of the formed elements of human blood. Blood, *50*:699, 1977.

Finch, C. A., and Lenfant, C.: Oxygen transport in man. N. Engl. J. Med., *286*:407, 1972.

Finch, J. T., Perutz, M. F., Bertles, J. F., and Döbler, J.: Structure of sickled erythrocytes and of sickle cell hemoglobin fibers. Proc. Nat. Acad. Sci., U.S.A., *70*, 718, 1973.

Freda, V. J., Gorman, J. G., Pollack, W., and Bowe, E.: Prevention of Rh hemolytic disease — 10 years' clinical experience with Rh immune globulin. N. Engl. J. Med., *292*, 1014, 1975.

Gallo, R. C., Fraimow, W., Cathcart, R. T., and Erslev, A. J.: Erythropoietic response in chronic pulmonary disease. Arch. Intern. Med., *113*:559, 1964.

Gardner, F. H., Nathan, D. G., Piomelli, S., and Cummins, F. J.: The erythrocythaemic effects of androgen. Brit. J. Haematol., *14*:611, 1968.

Gardner, F. H., and Pringle, J. C., Jr.: Androgens and erythropoiesis. II. Treatment of myeloid metaplasia. N. Engl. J. Med., *264*:103, 1961.

Gemsa, D., Woo, C. H., Fudenberg, H. H., and Schmid, R.: Erythrocyte catabolism by macrophages in vitro. The effect of hydrocortisone on erythrophagocytosis and on the induction of heme oxygenase. J. Clin. Invest., *52*, 812, 1973.

Giblett, E. R.: Genetic Markers in Human Blood. Oxford, Blackwell Scientific Publications Ltd., 1969, p. 349.

Gidari, A. S., and Levere, R. D.: Enzymatic formation and cellular regulation of heme synthesis. Seminars Hematol., *14*, 145, 1977.

Gilette, P., Manning, J. M., and Cerami, A.: Increased survival of sickle cell erythrocytes after treatment in vitro with sodium cyanate. Proc. Nat. Acad. Sci., *68*:2791, 1971.

Gordon, A. S., Cooper, G. W., and Zanjani, E. D.: The kidney and erythropoiesis. Seminars Hematol., *4*:337, 1967.

Götze, O., and Müller-Eberhard, H. J.: Paroxysmal nocturnal hemoglobinuria. Hemolysis initiated by the C3 activator system. N. Engl. J. Med., 286:180, 1972.

Granick, S., and Levere, R.: Heme synthesis in erythroid cells. Progr. Hematol., 4:1, 1964.

Gräsbeck, R.: Intrinsic factor and the transcobalamins with reflections on the general function and evolution of soluble transport proteins. Scand. J. Clin. Lab. Invest., 19:(Suppl. 95), 1967.

Gräsbeck, R.: Intrinsic factor and other vitamin B_{12} transport proteins. Progr. Hematol., 6:233, 1969.

Hall, C. A.: Transcobalamins I and II as natural transport proteins of vitamin B_{12}. J. Clin. Invest., 56, 1125, 1975.

Harris, J. W.: Notes and comments on pyridoxine responsive anemia and the role of erythrocyte mitochondria in iron metabolism. Medicine, 43:803, 1964.

Harris, J. W., and Kellermeyer, R. W.: The Red Cell. Cambridge, Harvard University Press, 1970.

Haurani, F. I., Burke, W., and Martinez, E. J.: Defective reutilization of iron in the anemia of inflammation. J. Lab. Clin. Med., 65:560, 1965.

Herbert, V.: Experimental nutritional folate deficiency in man. Trans. Am. Assoc. Physicians, 75:307, 1962.

Hershko, C., Cook, J. D., and Finch, C. A.: Storage iron kinetics. II. The uptake of hemoglobin by hepatic parenchymal cells. J. Lab. Clin. Med., 80, 624, 1972.

Hillman, R. S., and Finch, C. A.: Erythropoiesis: normal and abnormal. Seminars Hematol., 4:327, 1967.

Hines, J. D., Hoffbrand, A. V., and Mollin, D. L.: The hematologic complications following partial gastrectomy. Am. J. Med., 43:555, 1967.

Hoffbrand, A. V.: Synthesis and breakdown of natural folates (folate polyglutamates). Progr. Hematol., 9, 85, 1975.

Horowitz, H. J., Stein, J. M., Cohen, B. D., and White, J. M.: Further studies on the platelet-inhibitory effect of guanidinosuccinic acid and its role in uremic bleeding. Am. J. Med., 49:336, 1970.

Hurtado, A.: Acclimatization to high altitudes. In Weihe, W. H. (Ed.): Physiological Effects of High Altitude. Pergamon Press, New York, 1964, p. 1.

Itano, H. A.: The human hemoglobins; their properties and genetic control. Adv. Protein Chem., 12:216, 1957.

Jacobs, A.: Iron balance and its disorders. Proc. Roy. Soc. Med., 63:1215, 1970.

Jacobs, A.: Iron overload — clinical and pathologic aspects. Seminars Hematol., 14, 89, 1977.

Jacobson, L. O., Goldwasser, E., Fried, W., and Plzak, L.: Role of the kidney in erythropoiesis. Nature (London), 179:633, 1957.

Jaffe, C. J., Atkinson, J. P., and Frank, M. M.: The role of complement in the clearance of cold agglutinin sensitized erythrocytes in man. J. Clin. Invest., 58, 942, 1976.

Jaffé, E. R., and Hsieh, H. S.: DPNH dependent methemoglobin reductase deficiency and hereditary methemoglobinemia. Seminars Hematol., 8:417, 1971.

Jensen, W. N., and Lessin, L. S.: Membrane alterations associated with hemoglobinopathies. Seminars Hematol., 7:409, 1970.

Josephs, R., Jarosch, H. S., and Edelstein, S. J.: Polymorphism of sickle cell hemoglobin fibers. J. Mol. Biol., 102, 409, 1976.

Jourdanet, D.: De l'anémie des altitudes et de l'anémie en général dans ses rapports avec la pression de l'atmosphére. Braillere, Paris, 1863.

Kan, Y. W., Golbus, M. S., Trecartin, R. F., et al.: Prenatal diagnosis of β thalassemia and sickle cell anemia. Lancet, i:269, 1977.

Kansu, E., and Erslev, A. J.: Aplastic anemia with "hot pockets". Scand. J. Haematol., 17:326, 1976.

Kass, L. S.: Pernicious Anemia. W. B. Saunders Co., Philadelphia, 1976.

Kirschbaum, J. D., Matsno, T., Sato, K., Ishimarn, M., Tsucchmoto, T., and Ishimarn, T.: A study of aplastic anemia in an autopsy series with special reference to atomic bomb survivors in Hiroshima and Nagasaki. Blood, 38:17, 1971.

Knospe, W. H., Blom, J., and Crosby, W. H.: Regeneration of locally irradiated bone marrow. II. Induction of regeneration in permanently aplastic medullary cavities. Blood, 31:400, 1968.

Koenig, R. J., Peterson, C. M., Jones, R. L., et al.: Correlation of glucose regulation and hemoglobin A_{1c} in diabetes mellitus. N. Engl. J. Med., 295, 417, 1976.

Krantz, S. B., and Kuo, V.: Studies on red cell aplasia. II. Report of a second patient with an antibody to erythroblast nuclei and a remission after immunosuppressive therapy. Blood, 34:1, 1969.

Kushner, J. P., Barbuto, A. J., and Lee, G. R.: An inherited enzymatic defect in porphyria cutanea tarda. Decreased uroporphyrinogen decarboxylase activity. J. Clin. Invest., 58, 1089, 1976.

Kushner, J. P., Lee, G. R., Wintrobe, M. M., and Cartwright, G. E.: Idiopathic refractory sideroblastic anemia. Clinical and laboratory investigation of 17 patients and review of the literature. Medicine, 50:139, 1971.

Landaw, S. A., Callahan, E. W., Jr., and Schmid, R.: Catabolism of heme in vivo: comparison of the simultaneous production of bilirubin and carbon monoxide. J. Clin. Invest., 49:914, 1970.

Leblond, P. F., Chamberlain, J. K., and Weed, R. J.: Scanning electron microscopy of erythropoietin — stimulated bone marrow. Blood Cells, 1:639, 1975.

Lessin, L. S., and Bessis, M.: Morphology of the erythron. In Williams, W. J., et al. (Eds.): Hematology, 2nd Ed. McGraw-Hill Book Co., New York, 1977, p. 103.

Lessin, L. S., Jensen, W. N., and Klug, P.: Ultrastructure of the normal and hemoglobinopathic red blood cell membrane. Arch. Intern. Med., 129:306, 1972.

Lewis, S. M., and Dacie, J. V.: The aplastic anemia: Paroxysmal nocturnal hemoglobinuria syndrome. Br. J. Haematol., 13:236, 1967.

Lipschitz, D. A., Cook, J. D., and Finch, C. A.: A clinical evaluation of serum ferritin as an index of iron stores. N. Engl. J. Med., 290, 1213, 1974.

Logue, G., and Rosse, W.: Immunologic mechanisms in autoimmune hemolytic disease. Seminars Hematol., 13, 277, 1976.

Marks, P. A., and Rifkind, R. A.: Protein synthesis in erythropoiesis. Science, 175:955, 1972.

Marsh, G. W., and Lewis, S. M.: Cardiac hemolytic anemia. Seminars Hematol., 6:133, 1969.

Martland, H. S.: The occurrence of malignancy in radioactive persons. Am. J. Cancer, 15:2435, 1931.

Marver, H. S., and Schmid, R.: The Porphyrias. In Stanbury, J. B., Wyngaarden, J. B., and Frederickson, D. S. (eds.): The Metabolic Basis of Inherited Disease. McGraw-Hill, New York, 1972, p. 1087.

McIntyre, P.: Radioactive tracers in hematologic disease. Hosp. Pract., 7:3, 99, 1972.

Metcalfe, J., Dhindsa, D. S., Edwards, M. J., and Mordjinis, A.: Decreased oxygen affinity of blood for oxygen in patients with low-output heart failure. Circ. Res., 25:47, 1969.

Miller, M. E.: Thymic dysplasia ("Swiss agammaglobulinemia"). I. Graft vs. host reaction following bone marrow transfusion. J. Pediatr., 70:730, 1967.

Milner, P. F., Clegg, J. B., and Weatherall, D. J.: Hemoglobin H disease due to a unique hemoglobin variant with an elongated alpha-chain. Lancet, 1:729, 1971.

Modan, B., and Lilienfeld, A. M.: Polycythemia vera and leukemia — the role of radiation treatment. A study of 1,222 patients. Medicine, 44:305, 1965.

Mollin, D. L., Waters, A. H., and Harriss, E.: Clinical aspects of the metabolic inter-relationships between folic acid and vitamin B_{12}. Vitamin B_{12} and intrinsic factor, 2. In Heinrich, H. C. (Ed.): Europaisches Symposion, Hamburg. Stuttgart, Enke, 1961, p. 737.

Morley, A., and Stohlman, F., Jr.: Erythropoiesis in the dog: the periodic nature of the steady state. Science, 165:1025, 1969.

Motulsky, A. G.: Hemolysis in glucose-6-phosphate dehydrogenase deficiency. Fed. Proc., 31:1286, 1972.

Muirhead, H., Cox, J. M., Mazzarella, L., and Perutz, M. F.: Structure and function of haemoglobin III. A three-dimensional Fourier synthesis of human deoxyhaemoglobin at 5.5 A resolution. J. Mol. Biol., 13:646, 1965.

Muldowney, F. P., Crooks, J., and Wayne, E. F.: The total red cell mass in thyrotoxicosis and myxoedema. Clin. Sci., *16*:309, 1957.

Müller-Eberhard, H. J.: Chemistry and Function of the complement system. Hosp. Pract., *12*:8, 33, 1977.

Murayama, M.: Molecular mechanism of red cell "sickling." Science, *153*:145, 1966.

Murray, J. F., Gold, P., and Johnson, B. L., Jr.: The circulatory effects of hematocrit variations in normovolemic and hypervolemic dogs. J. Clin. Invest., *42*:1150, 1963.

Nienhuis, A. W., Barker, J. E., and Anderson, W. F.: Effect of erythropoietin on hemoglobin synthesis. *In* Fisher, J. (ed.): Kidney Hormones, Vol. 2. Academic Press, New York, in press.

Nienhuis, A. W., and Benz, E. J., Jr.: Regulation of hemoglobin synthesis during the development of the red cell. N. Engl. J. Med., *297*, 1318, 1977.

Owren, P. A.: Congenital hemolytic jaundice: The pathogenesis of the "hemolytic crisis." Blood, *3*:231, 1948.

Pape, L., Multani, J. S., Stitt, C., and Saltman, P.: In vitro reconstitution of ferritin. Biochemistry, 7:606, 1968.

Perutz, M. F.: Stero chemistry of cooperative effects in haemoglobin. Nature, *228*:726, 1970.

Pillow, R. P., Epstein, R. B., Buckner, C. D., Giblett, E. R., and Thomas, E. D.: Treatment of bone marrow failure by isogeneic marrow infusion. N. Engl. J. Med., *275*:94, 1966.

Piomelli, S., Lamola, A. A., Poh-Fitzpatrick, M. B., Seaman, C., and Harber, L. C.: Erythropoietic protoporphyria and lead intoxication: the molecular basis for difference in cutaneous photosensitivity. J. Clin. Invest., *56*:1519, 1975.

Prchal, J. F., Adamson, J. W., Murphy, S., Steinman, L., and Fialkow, P. J.: Polycythemia vera: the in vitro response of normal and abnormal stem cell lines to erythropoietin. J. Clin. Invest., 1978 (in press).

Propper, R. D., Cooper, B., Rufo, R. R., Nienhuis, A. W., Anderson, W. F., Bunn, H. F., Rosenthal, A., and Nathan, D. G.: Continuous subcutaneous administration of deferoxamine in patients with iron overload. N. Engl. J. Med., *297*, 418, 1977.

Pruzanski, W., and Shumak, K. H.: Biologic activity of cold-reacting auto-antibodies. N. Engl. J. Med., *297,* 538, 1977.

Ratto, O., Brescoe, W. A., Morton, J. W., and Comroe, J. H., Jr.: Anoxemia secondary to polycythemia and polycythemia secondary to anoxemia. Am. J. Med., *19*:958, 1955.

Reissmann, K. R.: Studies on the mechanism of erythropoietic stimulation in parabiotic rats during hypoxia. Blood, *5*:372, 1950.

Ricketts, C., Jacobs, A., Cavill, I.: Ferrokinetics and erythropoiesis in man: The measurement of effective erythropoiesis, ineffective erythropoiesis and red cell life span using ^{59}Fe. Br. J. Haematol., *31*, 65, 1975.

Rosenberg, L. E., Lilljeqvist, A-C., and Hsia, Y. E.: Methylmalonic aciduria: metabolic block localization and vitamin B_{12} dependency. Science, *162*:805, 1968.

Rosse, W. F.: Quantitative immunology of immune hemolytic anemia. II. The relationship of un-bound antibody to hemolysis and the effect of treatment. J. Clin. Invest., *50*:734, 1971.

Rosse, W. F., Dourmashkin, R., and Humphrey, J. H.: Immune lysis of normal and paroxysmal nocturnal hemoglobinuria (PNH) red blood cells. II. The membrane defects caused by complement lysis. J. Exp. Med., *123*:969, 1966.

Schmid, R.: Bilirubin metabolism in man. N. Engl. J. Med., *287*, 703, 1972.

Schroeder, W. A., Huisman, T. H. J., Shelton, R., Shelton, R. B., Kleihauer, E. F., Dozy, A. M., and Robberson, B.: Evidence for multiple structural genes for the γ chain of human fetal hemoglobin. Proc. Nat. Acad. Sci. U.S.A., *60*:537, 1968.

Shahidi, N. T., and Diamond, L. K.: Testosterone-induced remission in aplastic anemia of both acquired and congenital types. N. Engl. J. Med., *264*:953, 1961.

Shahidi, N. T.: Androgens and erythropoiesis. N. Engl. J. Med., *289*:72, 1971.

Skalak, R., and Brånemark, P. I.: Deformation of red blood cells in capillaries. Science, *164*:717, 1969.

Smith, J. R., and Landaw, S. A.: Smokers' polycythemia. N. Engl. J. Med., *298*:6, 1978.

Spaet, T. H., Bauer, S., and Melamed, S.: Hemorrhagic thrombocythemia. A blood coagulation disorder. Arch. Intern. Med., *98*:377, 1956.

Stamatoyannopoulos, G., Bellingham, A. J., Lenfant, C., and Finch, C. A.: Abnormal hemoglobins with high and low oxygen affinity. Ann. Rev. Med., *22*:221, 1971.

Stewart, W. B., Yuile, C. L., Claiborne, H. A., Snowman, R. T., and Whipple, G. H.: Radio iron absorption in anemic dogs. Fluctuations in the mucosal block and evidence for a gradient of absorption in the gastrointestinal tract. J. Exp. Med., *92*:375, 1950.

Storb, R., Prentice, R. L., and Thomas, E. D.: Treatment of aplastic anemia by marrow transfusion from HLA identified siblings. Prognostic factors associated with graft versus host disease and survival. J. Clin. Invest., *59*:625, 1977.

Streiff, R. R.: Folate deficiency and oral contraceptives. J.A.M.A., *214*:105, 1970.

Tabulation of reports compiled by the Panel on Hematology of the Registry on Adverse Reactions. Council on Drugs. American Medical Association, May, 1965, and June, 1967.

Thomas, E. D., et al.: Aplastic anemia treated by bone marrow transplantation. Lancet, *1*:284, 1972.

Thorling, E. B.: Paraneoplastic erythrocytosis and inappropriate erythropoietin production: A Review. Scand. J. Haematol., Suppl. 17, 1972.

Thorling, E. B., and Erslev, A. J.: The "tissue" tension of oxygen and its relation to hematocrit and erythropoietin. Blood, *32*:332, 1968.

Torrance, J., Jacobs, P., Restrepo, A., Eschbach, J., Lenfant, C., and Finch, C. A.: Intraerythrocytic adaptation to anemia. N. Engl. J. Med., *283*:165, 1970.

Valentine, W. N.: Hereditary hemolytic anemias associated with specific erythrocyte enzymopathies. Calif. Med., *108*:280, 1968.

Valentine, W. N., Paglia, D. E., Fink, K., and Madokoro, G.: Lead poisoning. Association with hemolytic anemia, basophilic stippling, erythrocyte pyrimidine-5'-nucleotidase deficiency, and intraerythrocytic accumulation of pyrimidines. J. Clin. Invest., *58*, 926, 1976.

Vincent, P. C., and de Gruchy, G. C.: Complications and treatment of acquired aplastic anemia. Br. J. Haematol., *13*:977, 1967.

Ward, H. P., Kurnick, J. E., and Pisarczyk, M. J.: Serum level of erythropoietin in anemias associated with chronic infection, malignancy and primary hematopoietic disease. J. Clin. Invest., *50*:332, 1971.

Waxman, S., Metz, J., and Herbert, V.: Defective DNA synthesis in human megaloblastic bone marrow: Effects of homocysteine and methionine. J. Clin. Invest., *48*:284, 1969.

Weatherall, D. J., and Clegg, J. B.: The Thalassemia Syndromes. Blackwell Scientific Publications Ltd., London, 1972.

Weed, R. I.: Hereditary spherocytosis. Arch. Int. Med., *135*, 1316, 1975.

Weed, R. I., LaCelle, P. L., and Merrill, E. W.: Metabolic dependence of red cell deformability. J. Clin. Invest., *48*:795, 1969.

Weed, R. I., and Reed, C. F.: Membrane alterations leading to red cell destruction. Am. J. Med., *41*:681, 1966.

Weintraub, L. R., Weinstein, M. B., Huser, H. J., and Rafal, S.: Absorption of hemoglobin iron: Role of heme-splitting substance in intestinal mucosa. J. Clin. Invest., *47*:531, 1968.

Wiley, J. S.: Red cell survival studies in hereditary spherocytosis. J. Clin. Invest., *49*:666, 1970.

Williams, D. M., Lynch, R. E., and Cartwright, G. E.: Drug-induced aplastic anemia. Seminars Hematol., *10*:195, 1973.

Wishner, B. C., Ward, K. B., Lattman, E. E., and Love, W. E.: Crystal structure of sickle cell deoxyhemoglobin at 5 Å resolution. J. Mol. Biol., *98*, 179, 1975.

Worwood, M.: The clinical biochemistry of iron. Seminars Hematol., *14*, 3, 1977.

Wood, W. G., Clegg, J. B., and Weatherall, D. J.: Developmental biology of human hemoglobins. Progr. Hematol., *10*, 43, 1977.

Yunis, A. A., Smith, U. S., and Restrepo, A.: Reversible bone marrow suppression from chloramphenicol. A consequence of mitochondrial injury. Arch. Intern. Med., *125*:272, 1970.

4

Phagocytes

STRUCTURE

A recent trend in dynamic morphology has been to separate the leukocytes into two major groups: the phagocytes and the immunocytes. This separation has taxonomic merits and will be followed in this book.

The phagocytes can be divided into the granulocytes and the monocyte-macrophages. Both types are bone marrow derived and it appears plausible that these cells have a common precursor, either a stem cell committed to the phagocytic cell lines or a blast cell designated as a myeloblast or a myelomonoblast. This blast cell is smaller, and both nucleus and cytoplasm are less basophilic than those of the proerythroblast. It is distinguished from the lymphoblast in that it has several visible nucleoli and a nucleus with an indistinct nuclear membrane and no perinuclear halo. The pale blue cytoplasm is scant and frequently present only as a faint outline on one side of the nucleus. The subsequent differentiation to granulocytes is heralded by the appearance of coarse granules made up of lysosomes staining blue or violet with Wright's stain. They contain large amounts of a myeloperoxidase as well as lysozymes and bactericidal cationic proteins. At this promyelocytic stage, the nucleus is still blastic with nucleoli, but at the next stage, the myelocytic stage, the nuclear chromatin becomes clumped and the capacity for mitotic division ceases. New species of lysosomal granules appear, giving the mature granulocytes their characteristic morphologic appearance. The neutrophilic granules are small and pink and contain a bactericidal lactoferrin and an alkaline phosphatase. The eosinophilic granules are large and round and contain red-staining, basic mucopolysaccharides. The basophilic granules are coarse, often concealing the nucleus, and contain histamine, heparin, and acid mucopolysaccharides. The background cytoplasm of all three cell types is pink, and the nucleus becomes lobulated with 2 to 5 distinct lobes connected by thin strands (Fig. 1–11).

The differentiation from myelomonoblast to mature monocytes is undoubtedly also a process of integrated proliferation and maturation, but distinct stages are difficult to recognize. The mature monocyte is a large cell with a diameter of about 20 to 30 microns and a prominent multi-shaped nucleus. The chromatin structure is less clumped than that of the mature granulocyte or lymphocyte and appears lace-like, with small chromatin particles tied together by fine strands. The cytoplasm is grayish-blue and contains many fine lysosomes stained pink with Wright's stain. Even on fixed smears, the cytoplasm gives an impression of being "free flowing," reflecting active ameboid motions right up to the time the cell becomes permanently fixed to the glass slide. The clear cytoplasmic vacuoles frequently observed may be artifactual and caused by the smearing technique. After the monocyte leaves the circulating blood it is transformed into a lysosome-filled macrophage. Cline and Golde have reviewed the sequence of this transformation which involves a sudden burst in metabolic activities (Fig. 4–1). Energy production is increased, synthesis of hydrolytic enzymes by the endoplasmic reticulum and their subsequent packing by the Golgi apparatus into lysosomes are enhanced, and the cell enlarges until it has taken on the appearance of the large mobile macrophage found in pulmonary alveoli, peritoneal cavities, and inflammatory exudate. These cells reach a diameter of 50μ or more and send out far-reaching cytoplasmic tentacles. The cytoplasm may contain lipid droplets and lysosomes with incompletely digested material such as carbon particles, and hemosiderin granules. The oval-shaped nucleus is off to one side, is relatively small in proportion to the cytoplasm and has an open lacy chromatin network (Fig. 4–2). Although the mobile macrophages retain common phagocytic properties, they develop characteristics of the or-

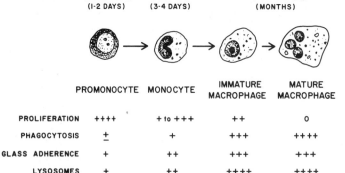

	PROMONOCYTE	MONOCYTE	IMMATURE MACROPHAGE	MATURE MACROPHAGE
PROLIFERATION	++++	+ to +++	++	0
PHAGOCYTOSIS	±	+	+++	++++
GLASS ADHERENCE	+	++	+++	+++
LYSOSOMES	+	++	++++	++++
IgG RECEPTORS	+	++	+++	+++
LYMPHOCYTE INTERACTION	?	++	++++	++++

Figure 4–1 Cellular kinetics and functional properties of the monocyte-macrophages. The mature macrophage is represented by a multinucleated epithelial giant cell, but other types include the alveolar macrophages, Kupfer cells, brain microglia, and the macrophages of the spleen, lymph nodes, marrow, and other tissues. (From Cline, M. J., and Golde, D. W.: Am. J. Med., *55*:49, 1973.)

gan to which they belong. For example, alveolar macrophages depend on oxidative phosphorylation for their energy production, whereas other macrophages depend on glycolysis. The fixed macrophage in the liver, spleen, and bone marrow appears to exist in a dynamic equilibrium with the mobile macrophage, and the characteristic foreign body giant cell or Langhans cell may represent fusion of a number of mobile macrophages. The term "reticuloendothelial system" is traditionally used to describe this large system of mobile and fixed macrophages. Since neither reticular nor endothelial cells are phagocytic, a better, but still not widely used, term is "mononuclear phagocyte system," as suggested by Meuret in 1977.

FUNCTION

Although the functions of the granulocytes and the monocyte-macrophages overlap, it seems reasonable to suggest that granulocytes function primarily as the first line of defense against microbial organisms, whereas the monocyte-macro-

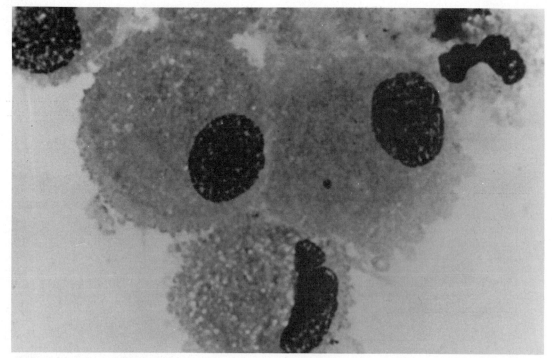

Figure 4–2 Alveolar macrophages. These macrophages live in aerobic circumstances and, in contrast to other phagocytic cells, they utilize aerobic metabolism for energy. (From Golde, D. W., Finley, T. N., and Cline, M. J.: N. Engl. J. Med., *290*:875, 1974.)

phages provide final removal of such organisms and also clear the body of its own aged and damaged cells. In order to accomplish this, the phagocytes have to (1) accumulate in sufficient numbers at the right place, (2) become attached to the foreign or nonviable material, (3) engulf, (4) dissolve, and (5) dispose of this material (Stossel, 1974).

① Granulocytes spend less than a day in the circulation before they migrate through the endothelial wall and are disposed of in various tissues. Inflammatory lesions will release specific leukotaxines which increase capillary permeability and induce local migration of the granulocytes. These leukotaxines are poorly defined but, as shown by Ward, Cochrane, and Müller-Eberhard, they may include fragments of the activated complement C3. In addition, transformed lymphocytes release both chemotactic lymphokines and a "migration inhibition factor" which acts by arresting macrophages at sites of antigen accumulation.

② The process responsible for the attachment of granulocytes to antigens depends on the opsonization of the antigenic surface by activated complement C3. Antibodies will also cause opsonization, but primarily for monocytes and macrophages which have abundant binding sites for both the Fc region of IgG and for the C3 fragment. Consequently, cells coated with non-complement binding antibodies, as found, for example, in acquired hemolytic anemia or idiopathic thrombocytopenic purpura, are primarily phagocytized by the mononuclear phagocyte system. The mechanism responsible for the attachment of phagocytes to antigens prior to antibody formation and complement activation or to devitalized cells is still obscure.

③ After the attachment, the membrane responds by engulfing the material in toto (Fig. 4–3). Inside the cytoplasm the engulfed material is enveloped by internalized surface membrane and distinct phagosomes are formed. Lysosomal granules become attached and empty their cargo of hydrolytic enzymes into the phagosomes, killing and/or dissolving their content (Fig. 4–4) and morphologically degranulating the phagocytes. The process of killing involves peroxidation of H_2O_2, which in the presence of iodide derived from tyrosine will destroy microbial membranes. Subsequent dissolution involves the integrated action of numerous hydrolytic enzymes. The ingestion of foreign or devitalized material is associated with a rapid increase in energy production and the generation of H_2O_2. Since the granulocytes contain only a few mitochondria, the major energy-producing pathway is glycolysis, and phagocytosis appears to stimulate both the Embden-Meyerhof pathway and the hexose monophosphate shunt. It has been proposed that increased demands for ATP energy cause an accumulation of NADH, which in the presence of an oxidase

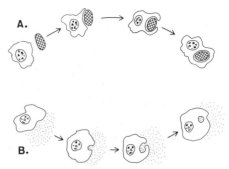

Figure 4–3 Endocytosis. The process of engulfing a portion of the cell's exterior into its interior. A. "Phagocytosis" refers to the inclusion of relatively large particles. The phagocyte membrane sends out pseudopodia to grasp the particle, utilizing a propulsive mechanism biochemically similar to that of muscle. B. "Pinocytosis" refers to the cellular interiorization of smaller particles included as a droplet of the fluid exterior into an interior membrane-lined vesicle.

generates H_2O_2. Excess H_2O_2 will in turn oxidize reduced glutathione and stimulate shunt activity (Fig. 4–5).

The final release of the degradation products tends to amplify the inflammatory response. Released lysosomal enzymes may cause injury to surrounding tissues, endogenous pyrogens cause fever, thromboplastic products may cause fibrin obstruction of vessels, and cationic proteins cause vasodilatation.

In addition to participating in the phagocytic inflammatory response to foreign antigens, the tissue macrophages play a key role in the important process of antigen-induced blast transformation of lymphocytes. This process may be dependent on a preliminary processing or digestion of the antigens by the macrophages. However, it is equally possible that the macrophage surface provides sites of attachment for both antigens and lymphocytes, permitting optimal interaction (Fig. 4–6).

The tissue macrophages are also responsible for the daily destruction of aged blood cells, denatured plasma proteins, and plasma lipids. This large and somewhat unappreciated function is accomplished through phagocytosis of whole cells and pinocytosis of small droplets containing plasma proteins and lipid microcolloids (Fig. 4–3). There still is no clear explanation of the process by which the macrophage recognizes non-viable blood cells or plasma constituents. Studies of red blood cells have revealed that aging is associated with a decreased membrane content of sialic acid resulting in a decreased negative change, but whether it be this or another subtle membrane change that is responsible for the fatal interaction with macrophages is unknown. The avidity of the tissue macrophage to slightly altered cells,

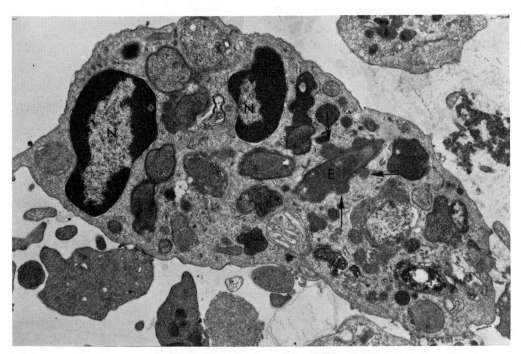

Figure 4–4 Electron microscopic picture of a human granulocyte after phagocytosis of *E. coli* (*E*). Coalescence of lysosomes with the phagocytic vacuoles is seen at arrows. *N* = nucleus. (From Zucker-Franklin, D., Elsbach, E., and Simon, P. J.: Lab. Invest., *25*:415, 1971. U.S.–Canadian Division of the International Academy of Pathology. The Williams and Wilkins Company [Agent].)

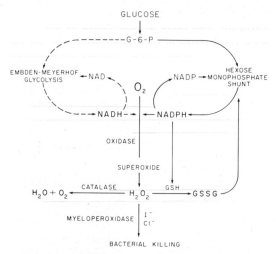

Figure 4–5 Generation of superoxide and hydrogen peroxide by an oxidase which transfers electrons from reduced pyridine nucleotides to molecular oxygen. The reduced pyridine nucleotides are primarily but not exclusively generated via the hexose monophosphate shunt. The H_2O_2 can be used for bacterial killing via a myeloperoxidase pathway utilizing the halides, iodide and chloride. Excess H_2O_2 is destroyed by catalase or by reduced glutathione (GSH), which in its oxidized state further activates the monophosphate shunt. (Adapted from Karnofsky, et al., 1970, and Stossel, 1977.)

to denatured proteins, or to macrocolloids has been used diagnostically to measure the size and blood flow of organs containing many macrophages — such as the liver, spleen, and bone marrow. The technique has been to label a cell or protein with a radioactive tracer, expose the labeled material to heat or chemicals, and use scanning techniques to determine the tissue transit or deposit of the isotopes. Similarly, certain isotopes of gold or technetium can be prepared in a colloidal form, and the clearance rate from blood and the uptake in the tissues can be used in the diagnostic evaluation of the size and function of mononuclear phagocyte organs (Fig. 4–7).

Macrophages are also placed in the mainstream of iron metabolism. A variety of tissue macrophages possess inducible heme oxidase activity, enabling them to break down red cell hemoglobin. The released iron is incorporated into ferritin and subsequently into insoluble hemosiderin. Macrophages of the liver, spleen, and bone marrow can again return iron to transferrin for transport back to the erythroid marrow. Alveolar macrophages are lacking in the ability to provide reutilization of iron, and indeed, in pulmonary hemosiderosis, abundant iron-laden alveolar macrophages are demonstrable even in the face of iron deficiency anemia and an absence of storage iron elsewhere.

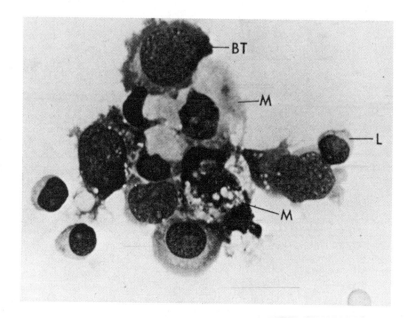

Figure 4–6 An "immunologic island" composed of central macrophages (*M*), surrounding lymphocytes undergoing blast transformation(*BT*)and untransformed lymphocytes (*L*). (From Cline, M. J.: *In* Williams et al. (Eds.): Hematology, 2nd Ed. McGraw-Hill Book Co., New York, 1977.)

Tissue macrophages presented with a phagocytic load may show a temporary decrease in efficiency, a phenomenon that Wagner and Iio called "blockade." There is a degree of specificity, however, since blockade induced by one injected material does not necessarily block the subsequent clearance of a different particle. Nevertheless, blockage produced by excessive hemolysis may cause impaired removal of foreign antigens. Fortunately, a chronic challenge to macrophage function causes "overwork hyperplasia" with an appropriate compensating increase in the mass of the mononuclear phagocyte system.

The pathophysiologic relationship of eosinophils and basophils to so-called "allergic reactions" is still unexplained. The basophils have been shown to contain sites of attachment for IgE antibody, and their degranulation is associated with the release of histamine. However, the eosinophils, which are much more closely identified

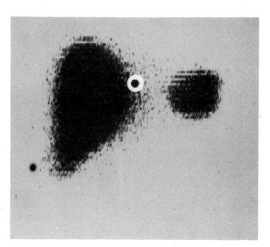

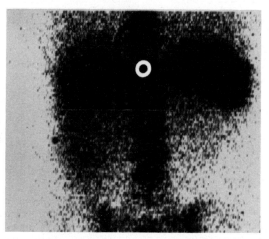

Figure 4–7 Body surface scans after intravenous injection of technetium (^{99m}Tc) sulfur colloid. Anterior views are shown. The position of the xiphoid is shown by the white circle. Left: In a normal individual 85–95% of the colloid is taken up by the macrophages of the liver because of the large hepatic blood flow, but the spleen is also well visualized. Right: In a patient with cirrhosis, hepatic uptake is reduced. The enlarged spleen is shown with increased colloid uptake, and the bone marrow macrophages now participate in the clearance, as shown by uptake over the vertebral column and pelvis. The clearance rate from the circulation is also slowed, leaving a heavy "background." (Kindly provided by Dr. M. Croll. Division of Nuclear Medicine, Lankenau Hospital, Philadelphia, PA.)

with allergy than the basophils, have not as yet been found to interact specifically with antigen-antibody complexes (Beeson and Bass, 1977).

KINETICS

Because of the relatively long tissue phase prior to and following the brief appearance of the granulocyte in the bloodstream, information about the rate and control of production and destruction has been difficult to obtain. However, reliable labeling techniques have been developed, both cohort labeling of DNA with ^{32}P or with tritiated thymidine and random labeling with radioactive diisopropyl fluorophosphate or with ^{51}Cr. Utilizing such techniques it has been possible to construct a model for granulocyte kinetics similar to models developed for erythrocytes and thrombocytes (Fig. 1–7).

In order to account for granulocyte renewal and control it is a necessity to accept the existence of a stem cell precursor pool. As described in the bone marrow section, this pool is probably divided morphologically or functionally into a multipotential stem cell pool and several unipotential stem cell pools committed to specific cell lines. The culturing of bone marrow on soft agar has disclosed the existence of a colony-forming cell, CFU-C, which, when stimulated by a colony-stimulating factor, CSF, will grow colonies containing thousands of granulocytes and monocytes. The CFU-C is believed to be the unipotential stem cell committed to the granulocyte-monocytic cell line. After blast transformation, the myeloblasts divide about three to five times and simultaneously mature into myelocytes. Warner and Athens have proposed that the number of divisions is not predetermined but actively regulated, and that skipped divisions or additional divisions may adjust the responsiveness of granulocytic production to peripheral demands. After the myelocytes have become mitotically inactive, maturing cells accumulate as a marrow granulocyte reserve. This reserve is under normal conditions made up by about five days' worth of granulocytes. Following their final release from the bone marrow, the granulocytes spend less than one day in the bloodstream, establishing two pools of about equal size — a circulating pool and a marginated pool. From the bloodstream they migrate into the tissues in which they will be destroyed either randomly in defense actions or by senescence about two to three days later (Boggs, 1967; Robinson and Mangalik, 1975).

Table 4–1 gives some approximations of the size of the various granulocytic pools. The combined size of the marrow pools is almost 1.5 times that calculated for the nucleated red blood cell pools, despite the fact that the daily production of

TABLE 4–1   GRANULOCYTIC POOLS

Cell Types	Number of Cells in 10⁹ per kg. Body Weight
Proliferating Cells	2.1
Marrow Granulocytic Reserve	5.6
Circulating Granulocytes	0.3
Marginated Granulocytes	0.2
Daily Production and Destruction	0.9

red cells is about twice the daily production of granulocytes. This, of course, is due to the fact that the marrow contains a large reserve of maturing and mature granulocytes.

In peripheral blood, the normal granulocyte count should always be considered a range rather than a value. The fluctuating equilibrium between circulating and marginated cells precludes a completely stable granulocyte count and the existence of an extensive granulocyte reserve in the bone marrow permits the granulocyte count to adjust temporarily to the demands for phagocytic cells.

The exact mechanism regulating granulocyte production is still unknown, although it undoubtedly involves a feedback between circulating granulocytes and the bone marrow. In support of the existence of a feedback mechanism is the observation that the granulocyte count in some patients with depleted bone marrow reserves exhibits an oscillatory pattern and that each period in this pattern is about 11 to 15 days, about twice the length of time it takes for myeloblasts to become mature granulocytes (Fig. 4–8). The reason for not observing such oscillations more often probably is the fact that under normal conditions the large bone marrow reserve pool will dampen or obliterate the amplitude of oscillations.

Various factors have been claimed to be responsible for maintaining the feedback adjustment between the peripheral demands for granulocytes and the bone marrow supply of granulocytes. Several granulocyte-mobilizing factors have been described, including endotoxin, etiocholanolone, Menkin's tissue leukotaxines, and a leukocyte-mobilizing factor, but, as emphasized by Craddock and co-workers, it seems unlikely that any of these are involved in the physiologic regulation of granulocyte production. Other factors released by mature circulating granulocytes have been claimed to act as inhibitors or chalones of mitotic divisions within the myelocyte pool. Recent studies, summarized by Golde and Cline in 1974, have suggested that the true granulopoietin is a glycoprotein derived from monocytes and macrophages and named colony stimulating factor or CSF. This glycoprotein, which is present in both plasma and urine, is necessary for the

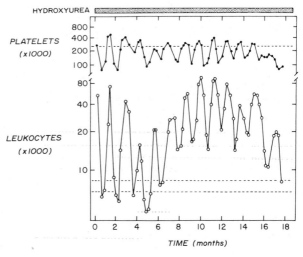

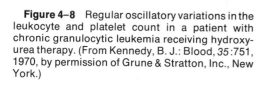

Figure 4–8 Regular oscillatory variations in the leukocyte and platelet count in a patient with chronic granulocytic leukemia receiving hydroxyurea therapy. (From Kennedy, B. J.: Blood, *35*:751, 1970, by permission of Grune & Stratton, Inc., New York.)

induction of clonal growth of granulocyte precursors in vitro (Stohlman and Quesenberry, 1972). Consequently it is tempting to construct a feedback model for the control of granulocyte production, as outlined in Fig. 4–9. This model, however, is quite hypothetical since the existence of a granulopoietin and its identification with CSF are based primarily on in-vitro data. Nevertheless, Richard and co-workers have shown that CSF is present in higher concentrations in leukopenic individuals than in normals, and Metcalf and Stanley have shown that it may increase granulocyte production when injected into mice. Furthermore, the apparently well-established existence of a circulating eosinophilopoietin (Mahmond, et al., 1977) gives support to the operation of granulocytic feedback systems based on the release and action of specific poietins.

The kinetics and regulation of the monocyte-macrophage complex are even less understood than those of the granulocyte complex (van Furth, 1970). The monocytes appear to have a shorter intramedullary life span than the granulocytic precursors, since they tend to emerge earlier than the granulocytes after a temporary bone marrow suppression. The life span of the monocyte in the circulation is probably about 36 hours or three times longer than that of the granulocyte. The extravascular life span after it has been transformed to mobile of fixed macrophages is undoubtedly long and may be counted in months if not years.

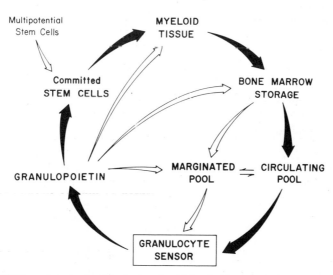

Figure 4–9 Hypothetical model of a feedback circuit which could account for the physiologic control of the granulocyte count.

PATHOPHYSIOLOGY

GRANULOCYTE DISORDERS

Classification and General Considerations

Disorders of the granulocytes are traditionally classified according to the number of circulating granulocytes into granulocytopenias and granulocytoses. However, a classification based on function and kinetics is of more contemporary importance. Using such criteria, the following classes of disorders can be recognized: quantitative abnormalities, qualitative abnormalities, and myeloproliferative disorders (Table 4–2).

The pathophysiologic effect of quantitative disorders is determined by the size of the actual and potential granulocyte pools. In granulocytopenia the lack of defense against microorganisms and other foreign invaders dominates the clinical picture, whereas in granulocytosis the problems are more subtle. Although much larger and stickier than the red cells, the viscosity of blood with a high granulocyte count is about the same as for normal blood with the same total hematocrit (white cell crit plus red cell crit), and hyperviscosity due to granulocytosis is rare unless the white blood cell count measures in the hundreds of thousands. More common is bone tenderness caused by expansion of the bone marrow and uric acid arthropathy or nephropathy caused by destruction of granulocytes. The qualitative disorders are characterized by impaired granulocyte defense despite a normal number of circulating neutrophils. Finally, the clinical manifestations of myeloproliferative disorders are related to the extent and character of cellular proliferation and cellular replacement.

TABLE 4–2 CLASSIFICATION OF
GRANULOCYTE DISORDERS

I. Quantitative Abnormalities
    Granulocytopenia
    Granulocytosis

II. Qualitative Abnormalities
    Defective delivery
    Defective phagocytic activity
    Defective bactericidal activity

III. Myeloproliferative Disorders
    Polycythemia vera
    Chronic granulocytic leukemia
    Myelofibrosis
    Thrombocythemia
    Erythroleukemia
    Acute granulocytic leukemia
    Acute myelomonocytic leukemia

Quantitative Abnormalities

Granulocytopenia. When the absolute granulocyte count is less than 3000 per cu. mm., the term granulocytopenia is used, but even at this level there are adequate numbers of granulocytes for normal defense activities. When the absolute number reaches 1000 per cu. mm., the patient becomes vulnerable to microbial attacks, but serious risk is usually first experienced at absolute counts of less than 500 per cu. mm. When playing this numbers game it is important to take into account the presence of monocytes which, although not as readily phagocytic as granulocytes, do contribute to the defense. The term *agranulocytosis* is usually reserved for the serious granulocytopenias in which both the marginated pool and the bone marrow reserve have been depleted. A depletion of the marrow reserve leaves the proliferating immature cells as the only myeloid cells present in the marrow and has given rise to the erroneous expression "maturation arrest." The immature cells are not arrested at all, but as soon as they reach maturity they are swept out of the marrow to shore up peripheral defenses.

The granulocytopenias may be caused by decreased production, ineffective production, or increased destruction. Decreased production is responsible for the granulocytopenia observed in patients with disorders causing bone marrow replacement or bone marrow aplasia. Most acutely it is seen after exposure to radiation or to radiomimetic drugs. The granulocytopenia here is part of a general suppression of cellular proliferation in the bone marrow, but because of the short granulocyte life span and the limited reserves, granulocytopenia is observed earlier than thrombocytopenia or anemia. Pisciotta has described a similar suppressive effect on the bone marrow of certain susceptible individuals by the use of phenothiazine-type drugs. These appear to have a predominant effect on the myeloid cells, with less suppression of the erythroid cells and almost complete sparing of the megakaryocytic elements. Underproduction of granulocytes has also been found to be responsible for a number of hereditary and acquired granulocytopenias. Of special interest is *cyclic neutropenia,* a disorder in which at regular intervals patients develop granulocytopenia, fever, mouth ulcerations, and infections. The pathogenesis has been linked to hormonal cycles, but recent studies indicated that the recurrent granulocytopenia may be caused by an undampened feedback between the peripheral granulocyte pool and granulocytic committed stem cells (Fig. 4–8).

Ineffective granulocytopoiesis is undoubtedly responsible for the granulocytopenia observed in *megaloblastic anemias* as well as in some of the *preleukemic syndromes.* Blume and co-workers have suggested that the granulocytopenia observed in *Chediak-Higashi's syndrome* may be caused by intramedullary autodestruction by the large abnormal lysosomes which characterize the cells in this interesting disease.

Increased peripheral destruction is caused by increased utilization, antibody-coating of the granulocytes or hypersplenism. As in patients with ineffective granulocytopoiesis the granulocytopenia is associated with a striking granulocytic hyperplasia in the bone marrow. Increased removal or destruction is an appropriate physiologic response to inflammation. An early transient granulocytopenia actually precedes the leukocytosis of bacterial infection. When the infection is particularly severe, as in septicemia, the marrow reserves of mature granulocytes may be used up, with granulocytopenia ensuing. Granulocytopenia is also commonly observed during and after viral infections, but here the mechanism is not known. Transient granulocytopenia is a feature of procedures involving exposure of large volumes of blood to foreign surfaces, such as hemodialysis coils and filtration leukopheresis columns. The surfaces presumably activate complement, which in turn causes the transient fall in granulocytes. Antibody destruction of circulating granulocytes is dramatic but rare. It is believed to involve the interaction of a drug hapten, such as aminopyrine, phenylbutazone or methyluracil, with a specific antibody and the subsequent attachment of the antigen-antibody complex to granulocytes, the so-called "innocent bystander" concept (Fig. 6–10.) These coated granulocytes are then destroyed by the macrophages particularly in the spleen. Attempts to identify autoantibodies as a cause of *chronic idiopathic neutropenia* or of the granulocytopenia of collagen vascular diseases so far have not been successful. Hypersplenism or splenic neutropenia is observed in conditions without overt antibody production but with splenomegaly. Despite many studies of the pathogenesis of the hypersplenic syndrome we still do not understand why a large spleen should destroy otherwise healthy granulocytes. It may be a question of sequestration rather than destruction similar to hypersplenic thrombocytopenia or it may involve antibodies too few to be detected by current techniques.

Granulocytosis. Granulocytosis is present when the granulocyte count exceeds 10,000 per cu. mm. When it is over 30,000 per cu. mm. the term "leukemoid reaction" is often used. Although a nonleukemic granulocytosis may reach levels of 50,000 per cu. mm. or higher, counts in excess of 100,000 per cu. mm. are extremely rare.

An acute granulocytosis of moderate degree can be caused by a mere shift of granulocytes from the marginal pool and the bone marrow reserve pool into the circulation. It is frequently observed after exposure to acute infections, trauma, emotional or physical stress or after the administration of epinephrine, adrenal steroids and endotoxin. Chronic granulocytosis is observed under conditions of sustained overproduction of granulocytes. The most common causes are bacterial infections and tissue injury. Neoplasias presumably cause granulocytosis by inducing tissue necrosis with the release of hypothetical bone marrow-stimulating substances. Eosinophilic granulocytosis is observed primarily in conditions characterized by the sustained presence of antigen-antibody complexes such as in patients with chronic parasitic invasion or with dermatologic or allergic manifestations.

Qualitative Abnormalities

A decreased resistance to infection may occur despite normal granulocyte counts if the functional competence of the granulocytes is impaired. In the so-called "lazy leukocyte syndrome" described by Miller, Oski and Harris the granulocytes do not respond appropriately to chemotaxic factors, and the granulocytes fail to accumulate and produce an inflammatory focus. Similar dysfunction of chemotaxis and migration is also present if the classic or alternate activation of C3 is impaired. Defective attachment and phagocytosis of foreign bodies are usually caused by impaired antibody production and complement function. Impaired killing of ingested microorganisms causes recurrent and chronic infections and may lead to massive granuloma formation. Despite its rarity, this so-called "chronic granulomatous disease," studied extensively by Holmes and coworkers and by Baehner and Nathan, has provided considerable insight into normal and abnormal bactericidal function. Morphologic and metabolic studies have shown that the granulocytes are capable of phagocytosis of microorganisms but incapable of their subsequent killing and disposal. The lysosomes, present in normal number, discharge their enzymatic cargo into the phagosomes, but the enzymes apparently are not bactericidal. The usual acceleration of glycolysis and hexose monophosphate shunt activity does not occur and the production of H_2O_2 is decreased. It has been proposed that in the absence of H_2O_2 the iodination of the microbial membrane cannot take place, and the organisms remain unharmed inside the phagosomes. Support for this hypothesis has been obtained from the fact that some hydrogen peroxide-producing organisms such as lactobacillus are killed by the granulocytes from patients with chronic granulomatous disease, and phagocytosis of latex particles coated with a hydrogen peroxide-producing oxidase will restore killing of simultaneously phagocytized bacteria. Chronic granulomatous disease encompasses both sex-linked and autosomal variants. Although an inherited deficiency of a NADH oxidase could explain both the lack of H_2O_2

production and hexose monophosphate shunt acceleration (Fig. 4–5), such deficiency has not been definitely established (Hohn and Lehrer, 1975).

A distinct disorder of lysosomal morphology is characteristic of the _Chediak-Higashi syndrome,_ in which giant lysosomes can be observed in granulocytes, melanocytes, fibroblasts, and other cellular elements. As suggested by White, the granulocytic lysosome may be responsible for intramedullary autodestruction, ineffective granulopoiesis, and granulocytopenia. Whether phagocytosis and lysosomal killing also are abnormal is not known, since the decreased resistance to infection exhibited by these patients could easily be accounted for by their granulocytopenia. The abnormal melanocytic lysosomes may in some way be responsible for the hypopigmentation observed in patients with Chediak-Higashi syndrome and in the closely related lysosomal disorders of the Aleutian mink and the beige mouse.

Myeloproliferative Disorders

In 1951, Dameshek, with characteristic abandon, lumped all the disorders which involve uncontrolled proliferation of bone marrow cells into one syndrome, _the myeloproliferative syndrome._ Some investigators have objected to this blatant oversimplification of a difficult problem and marshalled impressive evidence for basic differences among the diseases included. However, so far the similarities are more numerous than the differences and the unified myeloproliferative concept has been useful in our pathophysiologic and clinical approach to these diseases.

The prototype for the myeloproliferative diseases is _polycythemia vera_ (see page 35), with its uncontrolled proliferation of erythrocytic, granulocytic, and megakaryocytic elements and its frequent termination in myelofibrosis. The cellular proliferation characterizing the other members of the syndrome involves predominantly single cell lines.

Chronic Granulocytic Leukemia. This dramatic disease was undoubtedly the disorder observed by Rudolf Virchow in 1845 and reported under the catching title _"Weisses Blut"_ or, in Greek terminology, _"leukemia."_ Even today we occasionally see untreated patients in whom the white cell crit exceeds the red cell crit and the blood appears pale and the bone marrow whitish green as in Virchow's original case.

The characteristic of early chronic granulocytic leukemia is an expansion of all granulocytic pools overflowing into peripheral blood and spleen. Since the proportional sizes of the pools closely approximate those of normal bone marrow, it has been tempting to consider this disease as being caused by an impaired cellular control with autonomy of the granulocytic stem cells. However, the manifestations cannot be explained on the basis of uncontrolled normal stem cell function, but must include dysfunction of abnormal committed and multipotential stem cells.

In 1960, Nowell and Hungerford described a specific chromosomal abnormality in the myeloid cells of patients with chronic granulocytic leukemia, an abnormality which subsequently has been found to be present in about 90 per cent of cases. It consists of a deletion of part of the long arm of the number 22-G chromosome, leaving a tiny chromosome named the Philadelphia chromosome (Ph[1]) (Fig. 4–10). A simultaneous lengthening of chromosome number 9 has suggested that the alteration is not a deletion but a translocation. This fortunate discovery has been of considerable diagnostic and biologic importance. It has separated the classic Ph[1] positive patients from a small subgroup of Ph[1] negative cases with similar physical and laboratory findings but apparently with a more aggressive course and poorer prognosis. It has also established that granulocytic, erythrocytic, and megakaryocytic cells are derived from the same stem cell, since all are Ph[1] positive in chronic granulocytic leukemia. Circulating lymphocytes and bone marrow fibroblasts are Ph[1] negative, suggesting that the mutagenic event which gave rise to Ph[1] positivity must involve a step in the stem cell hierarchy distal to the points at which the stem cells for the lymphocytes and fibroblasts branch off. Although the majority of marrow metaphases show the abnormal chromosome in patients with chronic granulocytic leukemia, normal stem cell lines must also be present since intensive chemotherapy may transform a Ph[1] positive marrow to a Ph[1] negative, as reported by Smalley and co-workers.

In most patients with chronic granulocytic leukemia there is no inkling as to the character of the insult which has caused such a somatic mutation. In a few cases, however, past exposure to radiation or to drugs suggests a cause-effect relationship. For many years radiation has been recognized to be leukemogenic in certain strains of mice, but its potential for inducing leukemia in humans was not appreciated until the early 1940s. At that time statistical studies of the incidence of leukemia in physicians showed an overall incidence of 1.7 times that in the general population, and more importantly the studies by March indicated that the incidence of leukemia in radiologists was nine times that of physicians with little personal radiation exposure. This startling finding was accentuated by the finding of a high incidence of leukemia among the Japanese survivors from the atomic bomb explosions in Hiroshima and Nagasaki. Here, as summarized by Bizzozero and co-workers, the incidence of

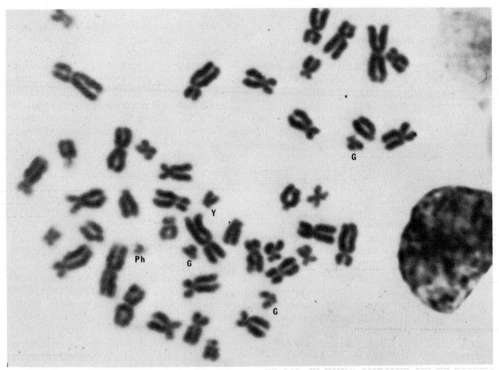

Figure 4–10 Chromosomal pattern of a male (Y chromosome) with chronic granulocytic leukemia (three normal G chromosomes and one tiny Ph¹ chromosome). (Courtesy of Dr. L. Jackson, The Thomas Jefferson University, Philadelphia.)

granulocytic leukemia, either acute or chronic, increased to about three times normal during the period from 1946 to 1955 and then slowly returned toward normal again. Studies of patients receiving therapeutic radiation have indicated that this form of radiation exposure also may be leukemogenic, but at present there are no convincing data showing that diagnostic radiation will cause leukemia. The obvious issue is whether or not the leukemogenic effect of radiation has a threshold. Some feel that any amount of radiation is potentially dangerous and should be avoided at all cost, whereas others feel that the leukemogenic risk of diagnostic radiation or radiation from natural sources or atomic bomb fallout is too small to be of public health concern.

The clinical and laboratory features of chronic granulocytic leukemia are predominantly caused by the increased body load of myeloid cells. This load may be increased up to 150 times normal and causes bone marrow expansion with sternal tenderness, anemia, splenomegaly, and granulocytosis. The nutritional demands made by the overproduction of myeloid cells may cause an increased metabolic rate, with fever and weight loss, and the final breakdown of these cells may cause uricemia, gouty arthritis, and renal stones. The red cell production is usually decreased in unrestrained cases of chronic granulocytic leukemia, probably owing to decreased "Lebensraum" in the marrow. The same may be true for platelet production. When granulocyte production has become controlled by adequate therapy the red cell and platelet mass will return to normal. The differential count of the granulocytes of peripheral blood is similar to that of the myeloid cells in normal bone marrow and is distinctly different from that of patients with leukemoid reactions in whom the cells are predominantly mature. These cells also have a normal or high content of alkaline phosphatase, whereas the cells of chronic granulocytic leukemia characteristically have a reduced content. Despite this biochemical abnormality, the phagocytic and bactericidal functions of the leukemic granulocytes appear normal. The number of basophils is usually increased and may even dominate the granulocytic picture, an unexplained but prognostically ominous sign. Serum vitamin B_{12} levels are high as is the concentration of the main B_{12} binder, transcobalamin I. The latter appears to be derived from broken-down granulocytes, but its role in the symptomatology of chronic granulocytic leukemia is unknown.

Chronic granulocytic leukemia is usually successfully managed with the use of alkylating agents such as busulfan. Unmaintained remissions may last as long as several months to a year. Incipient relapses are readily recognized by the rising granulocyte count, often accompanied by a return of splenic enlargement. Radiation therapy delivered to the spleen also successfully produces hematologic and clinical remission, but currently is considered less satisfactory than chemotherapy.

After about two to five years the disease in most patients begins to take on a more aggressive character. Myeloblasts appear in the peripheral blood, anemia becomes more severe, and thrombocytopenia develops. The spleen increases in size and the response to treatment becomes increasingly unsatisfactory. Blast cells take over the marrow and the patient eventually succumbs to the metabolic and cellular effects of an acute refractory granulocytic leukemia, the so-called "blast crisis." Some patients enter the aggressive phase by developing rapidly progressive myelofibrosis. The blast cells in this leukemia are usually Ph[1] positive, but they also display the chromosomal breaks and duplications seen frequently in acute granulocytic leukemia (Pedersen, 1973). Recent observations by Rosenthal and co-workers suggest that some of these terminal blast cell leukemias are lymphatic rather than granulocytic — observations of potential biologic and therapeutic importance. As in patients with polycythemia vera, the question has been raised as to the pathogenetic role of treatment in the final development of acute leukemia. No definite answer can be given, since in the past patients with untreated chronic granulocytic leukemia usually died from the effects of their chronic leukemia and only a few lived long enough to reach the stage in which contemporary patients develop their blast crisis.

Myelofibrosis. Bone marrow fibrosis with distortion and obliteration of marrow cavities may occur as an independent disease or as a complication of polycythemia vera or chronic granulocytic leukemia. Because of this relationship, myelofibrosis is considered a member of the myeloproliferative family. However, it seems somewhat farfetched to give the proliferation of fibroblasts the same status as the uncontrolled proliferation of blood cell precursors. In the first place, fibroblasts and other bone marrow cells do not share the same stem cell as indicated by the fact that fibroblasts of patients with chronic granulocytic leukemia are Ph[1] negative. Secondly, similar fibrotic reactions have been observed in tuberculosis, Hodgkin's disease, and carcinomatosis involving the bone marrow and are presumably reactions to tissue destruction and necrosis.

The characteristic splenomegaly of this disorder is usually believed to be caused by compensatory extramedullary hematopoiesis. However, the adult spleen appears to have lost most of its fetal capacity as a primary hematopoietic organ, and compensatory extramedullary hematopoiesis is rarely found in older people who develop an increased requirement for extra blood cell production. When foci of so-called extramedullary hematopoiesis in the spleen are found, they are probably made up of clones of bone marrow cells originating from immature cells prematurely released from the marrow and trapped in the sinusoids of the spleen. In myelofibrosis, the spleen is packed with hematopoietic tissue. Since this may occur at a time when the bone marrow is only minimally replaced by fibrous tissue and is in no need of supplementary extramedullary support, it seems more likely that the splenomegaly is caused by a pathologic myeloid metaplasia rather than by a physiologic extramedullary hematopoiesis. Foci of myeloid metaplasia are also observed in the liver but rarely elsewhere.

The most striking laboratory finding is an abnormal blood smear. The red blood cells show distorted and fragmented forms, and immature blood cells such as late erythroblasts, metamyelocytes, and myelocytes are present. It is usually assumed but has not been proved that such abnormalities are caused by cells being produced in and released from a microenvironment with less organized and regulated architecture than normal bone marrow. Progressive anemia is part of the disease, but the platelet count behaves erratically, and thrombocytosis may be as common as thrombocytopenia. It is of interest in this connection that biopsies of the fibrous marrow often reveal nests of megakaryocytes, as if these were the most hardy of the hematopoietic elements. When anemia or thrombocytopenia is severe, the question has to be raised whether the spleen destroys more cells than it produces. Erythrokinetic studies including organ scanning have been of only limited help in answering this question, and the decision to perform a splenectomy should be made only with great reluctance. The administration of androgens may cause striking improvement in the anemia in some cases (Fig. 3–29). Otherwise treatment does not appear to influence the slow but relentless progress of the disease.

Essential Thrombocythemia. Essential thrombocythemia is characterized by unrestrained proliferation of megakaryocytes. Large numbers of viable but ineffective platelets are produced causing a characteristic but unexplained mixture of bleeding and clotting problems. It is a chronic disorder, readily corrected by appropriate myelosuppressive therapy.

Chronic Erythroleukemia. Chronic erythroleukemia is a rare disorder characterized by the presence of macrocytosis, megaloblastic nucleated red cells in peripheral blood and bone marrow, ineffective erythropoiesis, and gradual progression into acute granulocytic leukemia. In the early stages it can be difficult to separate from chronic sideroblastic anemia since bone marrow examination may also disclose ringed sidero-blasts. However, granulocytopoiesis and thrombo-poiesis in erythroleukemia are almost always abnormal and ineffective.

Acute Granulocytic Leukemia. Acute granulocytic leukemia is a rapidly progressive disease characterized by the replacement of the bone marrow with immature and undifferentiated granulocytic cells. At present we relate the acute granulocytic leukemia to the myeloproliferative syndrome on the one hand and to acute lymphocytic leukemia on the other, relationships which may be spurious but nevertheless are useful in the clinical approach to this frustrating and discouraging disorder.

About 50 per cent of all leukemias are of the acute variety. There appears to be a slow but definite increase in this percentage, possibly owing to better diagnostic skills, possibly to an increased exposure to leukemogenic agents.

The acute leukemias can be divided into two major groups: the acute granulocytic and the acute lymphocytic. This subdivision of a rapidly progressive and uniformly fatal disease was initially felt to be a wasteful exercise in morphologic hair-splitting. However, at the present we recognize a fundamental difference between these two groups with regard to incidence, etiology, course, and prognosis. Acute granulocytic leukemia is a disease of adulthood, occasionally related to past exposure to radiation or chemicals, frequently with a long preleukemic phase and discourag-ingly resistant to chemotherapeutic agents. Acute lymphocytic leukemia is the predominant leukemia of childhood, rarely preceded by chemical exposure or preleukemic symptoms and highly responsive to chemotherapeutic agents. Acute granulocytic leukemia can further be subdivided into *acute granulocytic, acute promyelocytic, acute myelocytic, acute myelomonocytic,* and *acute erythroleukemia.* Acute promyelocytic leukemia is listed as a separate group because leukemias with a predominance of promyelocytes often display the characteristic syndrome of disseminated intravascular coagulation. However, owing to the high content of thromboplastic material in leukocytes, this syndrome has also been described in the other acute leukemias. The acute myelomonocytic designation is of considerable help in leukemias in which the immature cells have features of both myeloblasts and monoblasts, since it prevents the clinicians from getting into futile arguments about morphologic minutiae. The acute erythroleukemia, or so-called *Di Guglielmo's syndrome,* is a rare but dramatic acute granulocytic leukemia in which the bone marrow during the early stages is dominated by a profusion of abnormal, often multinucleated but always ineffective erythroblasts (Fig. 4–11).

The important separation of the acute leukemias into granulocytic and lymphocytic types is usually not too difficult for the experienced hematologist relying on blood and bone marrow smears stained by Wright's or Giemsa stain. Occasion-

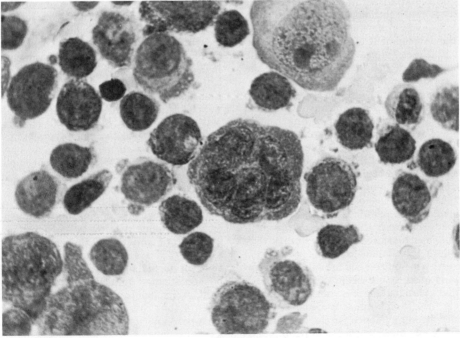

Figure 4–11 Multinucleated erythroblasts in bone marrow from patient with acute granulocytic leukemia of the Di Guglielmo variety.

ally, he is assisted by finding an eosinophilic rod in the cytoplasm of the leukemic blast cells. This so-called Auer rod is probably a giant lysosome and is never present in lymphoblasts, a useful diagnostic tidbit. Various cytochemical techniques also are being used in the differential diagnosis. The most important are the myeloperoxidase and Sudan black stains specific for the granules of acute granulocytic leukemia and tests for terminal deoxynucleotidyl transferase specific for acute lymphatic blast cells.

The etiology of acute leukemias is not known, but there is mounting evidence for the hypothesis that leukemia is caused by the action of a leukemogenic virus on stem cells rendered susceptible by genetic predisposition or chemical alteration. The presence of a genetic or chromosomal susceptibility is supported by statistical studies which indicate that the chance of developing acute leukemia is about 1 in 5 if one's identical twin has leukemia, 1 in 60 if one's nonidentical twin has leukemia, 1 in 700 if one's sibling has leukemia, and 1 in 3000 if no one else in the family has leukemia (Zuelzer and Cox, 1969). However, these data also tend to rule out an inborn mutation as the sole etiologic mechanism, since only 20 per cent of individuals with a leukemic identical twin develop the disease. Certain chromosomal defects, both congenital and acquired, appear to predispose to acute leukemia. Children with inborn chromosomal defects such as in *Down's syndrome, Fanconi's anemia,* and *Bloom's syndrome* all have an increased incidence of acute leukemia, and leukemogenic chemicals or radiation seems generally to have the capacity to cause chromosomal changes. However, the relationship between chromosomal defects and the development of acute leukemia cannot be too direct, since no single unifying chromosomal change has been found among patients with preleukemia or acute leukemia.

The potential leukemogenic effect of ionizing radiation has already been mentioned. Chemical leukemogens are playing an increasing role in the etiology of acute granulocytic leukemia. Any chemical interference with DNA replication must be considered potentially leukemogenic, and the widespread and successful use of cytotoxic and immunosuppressive agents will probably result in an increased incidence of leukemia in the future. Although these agents could cause a chromosomal mutation with the production of autonomous leukemic blast cells the possibility that they provide a latent leukemogenic virus with the opportunity for unchecked multiplication appears equally good. It has been known for about 65 years that avian leukemia is caused and transmitted by a virus, and studies by Gross 20 years ago provided strong evidence for the existence of a similar etiologic mechanism for murine leukemias. The murine leukemogenic viruses are RNA viruses and their mechanism of replication has recently been clarified by the discovery of a reverse transcriptase, an enzyme capable of incorporating the information coded in viral RNA into DNA of the host. Such an enzyme has been found in human leukemic cells but its presence there is of questionable significance, since it has also been found in human non-leukemic embryonic cells. Direct demonstration of viral particles in and around leukemic cells is difficult to achieve and, when found, their pathogenic importance is difficult to interpret (Jarrett, 1973).

Epidemiologic data suggesting direct transmission of leukemia are sparse, but strong indirect evidence for the presence of an infective agent has recently been provided by Fialkow and co-workers, who reported the course of leukemia in a girl who had received a bone marrow transplant from her brother. After some months the leukemia recurred, but this time the leukemic blast cells were cytogenetically XY cells. This unique case has generated considerable speculation and has even raised the possibility that leukemic relapses after prolonged remission are caused by reinfection rather than by the survival of a few leukemic cells, a most unorthodox view.

The orthodox view of cellular kinetics in acute leukemia is based on data obtained by Skipper and co-workers and suggests that the relapses and remissions of the disease are determined by the size of the leukemic mass. Manifest leukemia with the presence of leukemic cells in the bloodstream and with considerable leukemic bone marrow replacement is present when the leukemic mass is about 1 kg. in weight or 10^{12} cells in number. The reduction in mass to about 1 gram will cause a morphologic and symptomatic remission but will still leave about 10^9 leukemic cells at large. Further therapy will reduce the body load and prolong the remission but only total cell kill will provide a cure (Fig. 4–12). This latter assumption is derived from data in rodents in which the transplantation of a single leukemic cell into an inbred recipient will result in leukemia. However, immunologic assistance in an outbred species such as man may make it less mandatory to aim for total cell kill, a goal which probably could not be accomplished without irreparable damage to normal tissues.

By now, it has been shown convincingly that leukemic blast cells do not proliferate as actively as normal bone marrow cells (Killmann, 1968). The mitotic index and the tritiated thymidine labeling index are lower for leukemic blast cells than for normal blast cells. Even without the help of sophisticated quantitative techniques it is evident from looking at leukemic bone marrow smears that mitotic figures are relatively rare. This paradox that a rapidly growing tumor such as acute leukemia should consist of sluggishly proliferating cells has been difficult to accept.

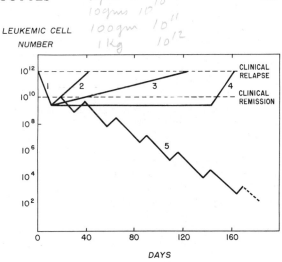

LEUKEMIC CELL NUMBER

1 gm 10^9
10 gms 10^{10}
100 gm 10^{11}
1 Kg 10^{12}

Figure 4–12 Hypothetical relationship between therapy of acute leukemia, leukemic cell number, and remission or relapse: (*1*) The effect of a successful induction therapy on cell count; (*2*) the immediate relapse which occurs after unmaintained therapy; (*3*) the slow relapse after partially effective maintenance therapy; (*4*) the prolonged remission on effective maintenance therapy; and (*5*) the hoped-for effect of repeated course of reinduction therapy on leukemic cell number. (Redrawn from Spiers, A. S. D.: Clin. Haematol., *1*:127, 1972.)

However, the therapeutic use of cytotoxic agents is based on the fact that normal bone marrow cells recover early, while there is a much more delayed recovery of leukemic blast cells; in other words, leukemic cells must have a longer generation time than normal cells. It is possible that the leukemic cell mass is made up of several cellular populations, with the majority of the cells being inert, long-lived, and slowly proliferating, while a minority have a rapid cellular turnover. It is the activity of this latter population which presumably accounts for the abrupt changes which occur in the bone marrow and peripheral blood during relapse.

In about 30 per cent of cases, the clinical and laboratory manifestations of acute granulocytic leukemia have been preceded for months or even for years by a prodromal phase which retrospectively can be designated *preleukemia.* Different degrees of neutropenia, thrombocytopenia, and anemia are present and associated with a cellular but ineffective bone marrow. Morphologic abnormalities, such as hyper- or hyposegmentation of granulocytes, megaloblastic changes, abnormal red cell morphology, ringed sideroblasts, and giant platelets, suggest defective cell development. Eventually myeloblasts appear in large enough numbers to establish a diagnosis of acute granulocytic leukemia.

The signs and symptoms of acute granulocytic leukemia usually can be attributed to mechanical or metabolic interference with the normal function of a number of organs. The leukemic cells will amass in great numbers in the bone marrow, spleen, liver, lymph nodes and blood. Bone marrow function is first and most seriously threatened, either because the finite marrow volume precludes compensatory expansion or because blast cells exert a suppressive effect on the remaining normal cells. The liver, spleen, and lymph nodes can expand considerably without functional impairment, but a liver extensively infiltrated with leukemic cells may show signs of failure, an enlarged spleen may cause sequestration and injury to normal blood cells, and lymphatic tissue with architectural displacement may be immunologically less effective. Leukostasis in the lungs with pulmonary failure, or in the brain with cerebral hemorrhage, may occur if the white cell count is exceedingly high. The effect of leukemic cells on the function of blood is less clear. Whole blood viscosity is probably not changed significantly, since an increase in the white blood cell mass usually is offset by a decrease in the red blood cell mass.

Anemia is almost invariably present at the time of diagnosis. Hypersplenic red cell destruction and ineffective erythropoiesis may contribute, but the cause is usually clear-cut — lack of space for the erythroid precursors. The anemia is best managed by judicious transfusions of packed red blood cells.

Hemorrhages and petechiae are most often the features which bring the patient to a physician. With few exceptions they are caused by thrombocytopenia and are ameliorated by transfusion of concentrated platelet preparations. The critical level of platelet count below which spontaneous bleeding occurs is hard to define, since the effect of thrombocytopenia may be aggravated by platelet dysfunction or even disseminated intravascular coagulation. In general, platelet counts below 30,000 per cu. mm. should concern, and platelet counts below 10,000 per cu. mm. are associated with spontaneous hemorrhages and petechiae.

Infections and fever are common and are most often caused by granulocytopenic impairment of host defenses. Although it has been claimed that an infection is always present when a leukemic patient develops fever, tissue necrosis and endogenous pyrogens undoubtedly contribute. Nevertheless, fever in a granulocytopenic patient in whom defenses often are reduced even further by steroids and immunosuppressive drugs should always be treated as if an infection were present. During the last decades important changes have occurred in the ecology of the infecting microorganisms. Bacteria and fungi of low virulence and high antibiotic resistance have emerged as major offenders and contribute to the chilling statistics which show that about 70 per cent of all leukemic patients die from infections. The preventive use of absorbable antibiotics has had little or no effect on infectious morbidity or mortality, but the use of careful reverse isolation techniques, laminar air flow chambers, and nonabsorbable oral antibiotics has been of some help. Complete isolation in life islands tends to isolate

patients from good nursing care and compassionate personal attention. The transfusion of normal granulocytes harvested by centrifugation or filtration leukopheresis is coming of age, and Higby and Henderson have reported on its usefulness in the management of febrile leukemic patients during their leukopenic phases.

The triad of anemia, hemorrhage, and infection will respond to effective treatment of the leukemia. Unfortunately this treatment is not specific and normal hematopoietic elements are wiped out together with the leukemic cells. If the patient survives the initial weeks of severe bone marrow failure first brought on by the disease and then temporarily aggravated by the treatment, complete remission may be achieved with the restoration of a normal bone marrow picture

TABLE 4–3 CHEMOTHERAPEUTIC AGENTS CURRENTLY USED IN TREATMENT OF LEUKEMIA

Drug	Drug Category	Mechanisms of Action
Cytosine arabinoside	Pyrimidine antagonist	Inhibition of de-novo synthesis of deoxycytidine riboside and of DNA polymerase
6-Mercaptopurine 6-Thioguanine	Purine antagonists	Inhibitions of de-novo purine synthesis
Nitrogen mustard Cyclophosphamide Chlorambucil Busulfan Melphalan	Polyfunctional alkylating agents	Cross-linkage of DNA
Methotrexate	Folic acid antagonist	Inhibition of dihydrofolate reductase. Inhibition of DNA synthesis
Daunorubicin Doxorubicin	Anti-tumor antibiotics isolated from *Streptomyces peucetius*	Inhibition of DNA and RNA synthesis
Bleomycin	Anti-tumor antibiotics isolated from *Streptomyces verticillus*	Inhibition of DNA synthesis
Prednisone	Synthetic adrenocorticosteroid	Direct lysis of lymphocytes and lymphoblasts. Inhibition of cell cycle. Inhibition of DNA synthesis and/or DNA-directed RNA synthesis.
Vincristine	Alkaloid of periwinkle plant	Metaphase arrest resulting from inhibition of mitotic spindle (microtubule) formation
L-Asparaginase	Enzyme, catalyzing the hydrolysis of L-asparaginase	Depletion of exogenous L-asparagine needed for the metabolism of malignant cells incapable of synthesizing this amino acid

and peripheral blood counts. Without treatment, survival is about 3 to 6 months. Modern multiagent treatment induces a complete remission in about 40 to 50 per cent of patients, but the median survival is still only about one year. The selection of treatment programs remains quite empiric. Some drugs shown to be quite effective in animal studies, such as hydroxyurea, are relatively inactive. Other agents known to be very effective in acute lymphatic leukemia, such as vincristine and prednisone, are far less effective in acute granulocytic leukemia. Table 4–3 lists some of the agents used currently in the treatment of leukemia, along with their presumed modes of action.

MONOCYTE-MACROPHAGE DISORDERS

Disorders of the monocyte-macrophage complex can be classified as quantitative, qualitative and malignant cellular disorders (Table 4–4).

Quantitative Abnormalities

A monocytosis with an absolute increase in circulating monocytes to more than 500 per cu. mm. is frequently a non-specific sign of some occult disease and should lead to a thorough search for a cause. Before the antibiotic era, monocytosis usually meant tuberculosis, subacute bacterial endocarditis, or some other generalized infectious disease. Now, it more often is an early "preleukemic" manifestation of a hematologic malignancy. However, it may also herald a collagen disease or a cancer.

An increase in the number of tissue macrophages may reflect an appropriate response to foreign antigens, so-called "overwork hyperplasia." It can be seen under conditions of sustained, but low-grade invasion of microorganisms, such as in *Whipple's disease, kala azar, malaria* or

TABLE 4–4   CLASSIFICATION OF MONOCYTE-MACROPHAGE DISORDERS

Quantitative Abnormalities
Reactive monocytosis
Reactive mononuclear phagocytic response

Qualitative Abnormalities
Gaucher's disease
Niemann-Pick disease

Malignant Disorders
Monocytic leukemia
Histiocytic lymphoma
Letterer-Siwe disease
Histiocytic medullary reticulosis
Hand-Schüller-Christian disease
Eosinophilic granuloma

histoplasmosis. In these conditions, the macrophage proliferation causes splenomegaly and, to a lesser extent, lymphadenopathy. Cytopenias are frequently present, and it may be difficult to distinguish between increased blood cell destruction due to hypersplenism from decreased production due to encroachment by macrophages on available bone marrow space.

Qualitative Abnormalities

The lipid storage diseases include a number of rare autosomal recessive disorders, each characterized by a deficiency in one of the catabolic enzymes involved in the breakdown of the sphingolipids (Brady, 1972). The deficiency affects all tissues, but the macrophages, by virtue of their prominent role in the catabolism of the lipid-rich membrane, are particularly prone to accumulate undegraded lipid products. This leads to the production of lipid laden and probably "blocked" foamy macrophages, stimulation of further macrophage production and eventually to a tremendous expansion of the mononuclear phagocyte system.

In *Gaucher's disease*, there is a deficiency of β-glucosidase which normally splits glucose from its parent sphingolipids, globoside and ganglioside (Fig. 4–13). The accumulation of glycosphingolipids, derived chiefly from granulocytes, gives an onion skin appearance to the pale lipid laden macrophage cytoplasm. These cells, of course, also show a positive PAS stain for carbohydrate.

SPHINGOLIPIDS

FATTY ACID – SPHINGOSIDE – SIDE CHAIN
[CERAMIDE   ]

GLOBOSIDE
CERAMIDE – GLUCOSE – GALACTOSE – GALACTOSE-N ACETYLGALACTOSAMINE
(1)   (3)

GANGLIOSIDE
CERAMIDE – GLUCOSE – GALACTOSE-N ACETYLGALACTOSAMINE – GALACTOSE
(1)   (4)   (5)

SPHINGOMYELIN
CERAMIDE – PHOSPHORYL CHOLINE
(2)

Figure 4–13   In the lysosomal degradation of glycolipid constituents of senescent cells, the carbohydrates or the phosphorylcholine constituents have to be removed sequentially before final hydrolysis of ceramide, the sphingosine-fatty acid complex. Absence of the following specific enzymes will lead to accumulation of their substrate in the macrophages.

1. β-Glucosidase deficiency: Gaucher's disease
2. Sphingomyelinase
     deficiency: Niemann-Pick
3. α-Galactosidase deficiency: Fabry's disease
4. Hexosaminidase deficiency: Tay-Sachs disease
5. β-Galactosidase deficiency: Gangliosidosis

In its typical form, Gaucher's disease is a slowly progressive disease in which the accumulation of Gaucher's cells causes massive splenomegaly and hepatomegaly, bone marrow expansion, and pulmonary infiltration. In *Niemann-Pick disease,* the deficiency is in an enzyme that normally cleaves phosphoryl choline from its parent sphingolipid, sphingomyelin. The macrophages in this condition have the appearance of typical "foam cells" and do not stain with PAS. They cause a rapidly progressive hyperplasia of the mononuclear phagocyte system and the accumulation of undegraded sphingomyelin leads to neuronal degeneration and death within a few years of life.

Cells resembling Gaucher's cells and "foam cells" can also be seen in the marrow of patients with chronic granulocytic leukemia. Here the cause lies not in a deficiency of a catabolic enzyme, but, rather, in an increased lipid load from the sphingolipid-rich granulocyte membrane. "Foam cells" are also seen in the hyperlipidemias demonstrating that the plasma may be a source of lipid in the macrophage cytoplasm (Ferrans, et al., 1971).

Malignant Disorders

The acute monocytic or myelomonocytic leukemia is for diagnostic and therapeutic convenience treated as a myeloproliferative disorder closely related to acute myelogenous leukemia. *Chronic monocytic leukemia,* however, is logically a disorder of the monocyte-macrophage system. Chronic monocytic leukemia is a rare, often slowly progressive condition with minimal lymphadenopathy and moderate splenomegaly. The blood smear shows numerous promonocytes and mature monocytes, but the morphologic identification of the cells can be quite taxing.

A number of variations have been described under designations such as *histiocytic leukemia,* *leukemic reticuloendotheliosis, hairy cell leukemia,* or *reticulum cell leukemia.* These conditions have traditionally been assigned to the monocyte-macrophage system although basic phagocytic properties of the involved cells have not always been clearly demonstrated (Katayama and Finkel, 1974). Recent attempts to identify cellular surface markers have raised the possibility that some or all of the involved cells synthesize immunoglobulins and that these conditions actually belong to the lymphoproliferative system. Such taxonomic questions may appear clinically unimportant today. However, our progress in designing chemotherapeutic agents tailored to the metabolic functions of malignant cells is so rapid that we can anticipate to have future treatments for conditions belonging to the phagocytic system that are very different from treatments for conditions belonging to the immunocytic system.

Malignant proliferative disorders of the more differentiated macrophages may result in *histiocytic medullary reticulosis.* This is a rapidly progressive and fatal febrile disorder of adults with lymphadenopathy, hepatosplenomegaly, hemolytic anemia, thrombocytopenia and leukopenia. Its hallmark is erythrophagocytosis, and red cell laden macrophages are readily demonstrable in the pleomorphic cellular infiltrate. The childhood counterpart is termed *"Letterer-Siwe" disease,* but the phagocytic cells here are less erythrophagocytic and hemolytic anemia is not a prominent factor. Chronic unrestrained proliferation of completely differentiated macrophages are found locally as *eosinophilic granuloma* or more diffusely as *Hand-Schüller-Christian disease.* These diseases have been lumped together under the term *"histiocytosis X,"* but a thorough clinical and pathologic evaluation should provide a specific diagnosis and especially should separate these probably malignant disorders from benign reactive hyperplasia of the mononuclear phagocyte system.

REFERENCES

Baehner, R. L., and Nathan, D. G.: Quantitative nitroblue tetrazolium test in chronic granulomatous disease. N. Engl. J. Med., *278*:971, 1968.

Beeson, P. B., and Bass, D. A.: The Eosinophil. W. B. Saunders Co., Philadelphia, 1977.

Bizzozero, O. J., Johnson, K. G., and Ciocco, A.: Radiation-related leukemia in Hiroshima and Nagasaki, 1946–1964. N. Engl. J. Med., *274*:1095, 1966.

Blume, R. S., Bennett, J. M., Yankee, R. A., and Wolff, S. M.: Defective granulocyte regulation in the Chediak-Higashi syndrome. N. Engl. J. Med., *279*:1009, 1968.

Boggs, D. R.: The kinetics of neutrophilic leukocytes in health and disease. Seminars Hematol., *4*:359, 1967.

Brady, R. O.: Biochemical and metabolic basis of familial sphingolipidosis. Seminars Hematol., *9*:273, 1972.

Cline, M. J.: Biochemistry and function of monocytes and macrophages. *In* Williams, W. J., et al. (Eds.): Hematology, 2nd Ed. McGraw-Hill Book Co., New York, 1977, p. 861.

Cline, M. J., and Golde, D. W.: A review and reevaluation of histiocytic disorders. Am. J. Med., *55*:49, 1973.

Craddock, C. G., Perry, S., Lawrence, J. S., Buxbaum, L., and Pieper, G.: Production and distribution of granulocytes and the control of granulocyte release. *In* Wolstenholme, G. E. W., and O'Connor, M. (Eds.): Ciba Foundation Symposium on Haemopoiesis. Churchill, London, 1960, p. 237.

Dameshek, W.: Some speculations on the myeloproliferative syndromes. Blood, *6*:392, 1951.

Ferrans, V. J., Buja, M., Roberts, W. C., and Frederickson, D. S.: The spleen in Type I hyperlipoproteinemia. Am. J. Pathol., *64*:67, 1971.

Fialkow, P. J., Thomas, E. D., Bryant, J. J., and Neiman, P. E.: Leukaemic transformation of engrafted human marrow cells in vivo. Lancet, *1*:251, 1971.

Golde, D. W., and Cline, M. J.: Regulation of granulopoiesis. N. Engl. J. Med., *291*:1388, 1974.

Golde, D. W., Finley, T. N. and Cline, M. J.: The pulmonary

macrophages in acute leukemia. N. Engl. J. Med., *290*:875, 1974.

Gralnick, H. R.: Classification of acute leukemia. Ann Int. Med., *87*:740, 1977.

Gross, L.: Viral etiology of leukemia and lymphomas. Blood, *25*:377, 1965.

Higby, D. J., and Henderson, E. S.: Granulocyte transfusion therapy. Ann. Rev. Med., *26*:289, 1975.

Hohn, D. C., and Lehrer, R. I.: NADPH oxidase deficiency in X-linked chronic granulomatous disease. J. Clin. Invest., *55*:707, 1975.

Holmes, B., Quie, P. G., Windhorst, D. B., and Good, R. A.: Fatal granulomatous disease of childhood: An inborn abnormality of phagocytic function. Lancet, *1*:1225, 1966.

Jarrett, W. F. H.: Viruses and leukemia. Br. J. Haematol., *25*:287, 1973.

Karnofsky, M. L., Noseworthy, J., Simmons, S., and Glass, E. A.: Metabolic patterns that control the functions of leukocytes. *In* Greenwalt, T. J., and Jamieson, G. A. (Eds.): Formation and Destruction of Blood Cells. J. B. Lippincott Co., Philadelphia, 1970, p. 207.

Katayama, T., and Finkel, H. E.: Leukemic reticuloendotheliosis. A clinicopathologic study with review of the literature. Am. J. Med., *57*:115, 1974.

Kennedy, B. J.: Cyclic leukocyte oscillations in chronic myelogenous leukemia during hydroxyurea therapy. Blood, *35*:751, 1970.

Killmann, S. A.: Acute leukemia: the kinetics of leukemic blast cells in man. An analytical review. Series Haematol., *1(3)*:38, 1968.

Mahmoud, A. A. F., Stone, M. K., and Kellermeyer, R. W.: Eosinophilopoietin: a low molecular weight peptide stimulating eosinophil production in mice. Clin. Res., *25*:519a, 1977.

March, H. C.: Leukemia in radiologists, ten years later. Am. J. Med. Sci., *242*:137, 1961.

Metcalf, D., and Stanley, E. R.: Haematological effects in mice of partially purified colony stimulating factor (CSF) prepared from human urine. Br. J. Haematol., *21*:481, 1971.

Meuret, G.: Disorders of the mononuclear phagocyte system. An analytical review. Blut, *34*:317, 1977.

Miller, M. E., Oski, F. A., and Harris, M. B.: Lazy leucocyte syndrome. Lancet, *1*:665, 1971.

Nowell, P. C., and Hungerford, D. A.: A minute chromosome in human chronic granulocytic leukemia. Science, *132*:1497, 1960.

O'Riordan, M. L., Robinson, J. A., Buckton, K. E., and Evans, H. J.: Distinguishing between the chromosome involved in Down's syndrome (trisomy 21) and chronic myeloid leukemia (Ph¹) by fluorescence. Nature, *230*:167, 1971.

Pederson, B.: The blast crisis of chronic myeloid leukemia. Acute transformation of a preleukemic condition? Br. J. Haematol., *25*:141, 1973.

Pisciotta, A. V.: Studies on agranulocytosis X. A biochemical defect in chlorpromazine-sensitive marrow cells. J. Lab. Clin. Med., *78*:435, 1971.

Pisciotta, A. V.: Immune and toxic mechanisms in drug-induced agranulocytosis. Seminars Hematol., *10*:279, 1973.

Richard, K. A., Morley, A., Howard, D., and Stohlman, F., Jr.: The in vitro colony-forming cell and the response to neutropenia. Blood, *37*:6, 1971.

Robinson, W. A., and Mangalik, A.: The kinetics and regulation of granulopoiesis. Seminars Hematol., *12*:7, 1975.

Rosenthal, S., Canellos, G. P., DeVita, V., Jr., and Gralnick, H.R.: Characteristics of blast crisis in chronic granulocytic leukemia. Blood, *49*:705, 1977.

Skipper, H. E.: Cellular kinetics associated with "curability" of experimental leukemia. *In* Dameshek, W., and Dutcher, R. M. (Eds.): Perspectives in Leukemia. Grune and Stratton, New York, 1968, p. 187.

Smalley, R. V., Vogel, J., Huguley, C. M., Jr., and Miller, D.: Chronic granulocytic leukemia: cytogenetic conversion of the bone marrow with cycle-specific chemotherapy. Blood, *50*:107, 1977.

Spiers, A. S. D.: Chemotherapy of acute leukaemia. Clin. Haematol., *1*:127, 1972.

Stohlman, F., Jr., and Quesenberry, P. J.: Colony-stimulating factor and myelopoiesis. Blood, *39*:727, 1972.

Stossel, T. P.: Phagocytosis, N. Engl. J. Med., *290*:717, 774, 833, 1974.

van Furth, R.: Origin and kinetics of monocytes and macrophages. Seminars Hematol., *7*:125, 1970.

Wagner, H. N., Jr., and Iio, M.: Studies of the reticuloendothelial system (RES). III Blockade of the RES in man. J. Clin. Invest., *43*:1525, 1964.

Ward, P. A.: Insubstantial leukotaxis. J. Lab. Clin. Med., *79*:873, 1972.

Ward, P. A., Cochrane, C. G., and Müller-Eberhard, H. G.: Further studies of the chemotactic factor of complement and its formation in vivo. Immunology, *11*:141, 1966.

Warner, H. R., and Athens, J. W.: An analysis of granulocyte kinetics in blood and bone marrow, in leukopoiesis in health and disease. Ann. N.Y. Acad. Sci., *113*:523, 1964.

White, J. G.: The Chediak-Higashi syndrome: A possible lysosomal disease. Blood, *28*:143, 1966.

Zucker-Franklin, D., Elsbach, P., and Simon, E. J.: The effect of the morphine analog levorphanol on phagocytosing leukocytes. Lab. Invest., *25*:415, 1971.

Zuelzer, W. W., and Cox, D. E.: Genetic aspects of leukemia. Seminars Hematol., *6*:228,1969.

5

Immunocytes

STRUCTURE

The immunocytes work together with the phagocytes to maintain the integrity of the whole organism against foreign invaders. With functional responsibilities in such close accord, it is natural that these two families of cells should share many common anatomic sites in the lym-

phoreticular system of the body. Lymphatic tissue is found throughout the body and, on cytogenetic grounds, is classified into primary and secondary types. Lymphocytes are first differentiated in the primary lymphatic tissue. They are then sent out to populate the secondary lymphatic tissue, where they function in specific immune responses. The primary lymphoid organs in mammals are the

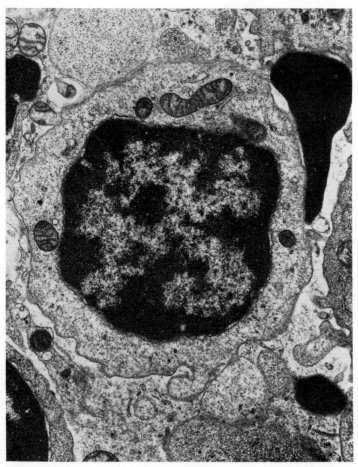

Figure 5–1 Electron microscope picture of a small mature human lymphocyte. Cytoplasm is scanty and contains mitochondria and ribosomes. Chromatin is densely packed into masses in a centrally placed nucleus. (Courtesy of Dr. A. Abraham, Divisions of Pathology and Research, Lankenau Hospital, Philadelphia, PA.)

bone marrow and the thymus. The secondary lymphatic organs, consisting of the spleen and the lymph nodes along with subepithelial lymphoid tissue in the gastrointestinal tract, are characterized by a basic arrangement of lymphocytes into follicles with germinal centers. In the marrow the lymphocytes typically are scattered among the other cellular elements; germinal follicles are not seen in either thymus or marrow. A primary lymphoid organ equivalent to the "bursa of Fabricius" in the fowl has been postulated to exist in mammalian species, but whether such a "bursa equivalent" truly exists remains an open question. A circulating pool of lymphocytes is found in the blood, mixed with other cell types, as well as in lymph, which contains few cellular elements other than lymphocytes.

Immunocytes are subclassified morphologically as lymphocytes and plasma cells. The small lymphocyte, a nondividing cell (which therefore does not take up tritiated thymidine), is about 9 μ in diameter on fixed and stained peripheral blood films. It has a skimpy rim of pale blue homogeneous cytoplasm which may contain a few azurophil-

ic granules. Its nucleus has a chromatin pattern tightly arranged in bluish-purple blocks, often with a small notch or indentation in the nuclear membrane (Fig. 5–1). The large lymphocyte has a more generous rim of cytoplasm which stains a deeper blue. Its nucleus is also larger, with nuclear chromatin blocks spaced somewhat further apart, giving the nucleus a more "loose" appearance. Nucleoli may be seen. Large lymphocytes are proliferating and take up tritiated thymidine into their nuclei. The lymphoblast has a nuclear chromatin pattern which no longer exhibits a blocklike pattern but instead is finely divided, with a "grainy" texture in the midst of which one or two nucleoli are seen. Plasma cells (or "plasmacytes") are recognized in Wright-Giemsa stains by the eccentrically placed nucleus, with densely stained chromatin blocks close together, and a deep blue-green cytoplasm, with a clear zone containing the Golgi apparatus adjacent to one side of the nucleus (Fig. 5–2). The high level of secretory activity of plasma cells is reflected not only by the intense cytoplasmic basophilia but by the frequency of cytoplasmic inclu-

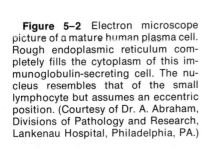

Figure 5–2 Electron microscope picture of a mature human plasma cell. Rough endoplasmic reticulum completely fills the cytoplasm of this immunoglobulin-secreting cell. The nucleus resembles that of the small lymphocyte but assumes an eccentric position. (Courtesy of Dr. A. Abraham, Divisions of Pathology and Research, Lankenau Hospital, Philadelphia, PA.)

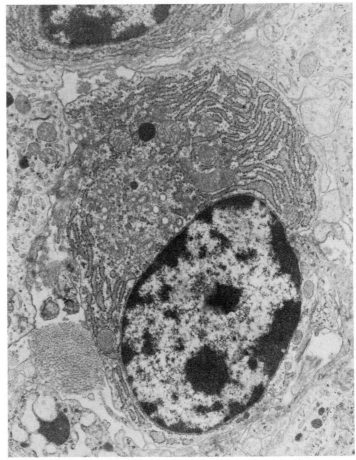

sions (such as grapelike vacuoles or crystalloidal structures). "Proplasmacytes" and "plasmablasts" show increasing looseness of nuclear chromatin and prominence of nucleoli.

FUNCTION

The immunocytes are an intelligence corps which gives *specificity* to the attack of the warrior phagocytes upon foreign antigenic foes. *Memory* of such specificity is another responsibility of the immunocytes, so that future defenses against a known antigenic opponent are more easily mustered. To a limited degree immunocytes may themselves participate directly in the attack.

Immune responses are of two types — one is cell-borne and mediated by "T" (for thymus-derived) lymphocytes, the other is humoral and mediated by "B" (for "bursa-equivalent" or "bone marrow"-derived) lymphocytes. This functional division of the immunocytes is paralleled by separate developmental lines as well as by separate (although closely intermingled) anatomic sites of distribution.

As T and B lymphocytes follow their separate pathways of maturation and development, distinctive features appear on the cell surfaces which facilitate laboratory identification (Fig. 5–3).

T cells form "E rosettes" with normal sheep erythrocytes, develop specific surface antigens, and express on their surfaces genetically controlled factors that govern a variety of immune responses.

B cells synthesize intrinsic surface immunoglobulins and in addition they also develop surface receptors for the Fc region of immunoglobu-

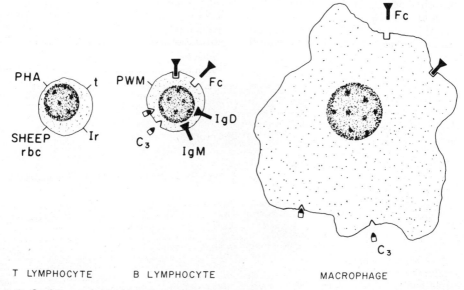

T LYMPHOCYTE   B LYMPHOCYTE   MACROPHAGE

Figure 5–3 Surface markers of lymphocytes and macrophages.

T lymphocytes are identified primarily by their tendency to form spontaneous sheep cell "E rosettes," presumably mediated by a surface receptor for sheep erythrocytes (sheep rbc). T lymphocyte specific surface antigens (t) can be identified by immunologic techniques. Indeed, antigenic differences in surface membrane may permit identification of T lymphocyte subpopulations (i.e., helper, suppressor, effector cells) in some species. Phytohemagglutinin (PHA) causes T lymphocytes to enter mitosis. Genetic factors, closely linked on the chromosome to the major histocompatibility complex, find expression on the T cell surface (Fudenberg, et al., 1978). One of these, the "immune response" (Ir) gene, controls cellular and humoral responses to many antigens. Another is responsible for cytotoxic and blastogenic reactions to lymphocytes of different histocompatibility type (graft versus host reaction, mixed lymphocyte culture).

B lymphocytes carry surface immunoglobulin IgM and IgD as intrinsic components of their membranes, identifiable by immunofluorescent methods. Other immunoglobulins present on the B cell surface may originate from the plasma through binding of their Fc regions to Fc receptor sites on the B cell membrane. (Intrinsic membrane immunoglobulin can be distinguished from bound immunoglobulin by in-vitro incubation techniques.) Attachment of aggregated IgG or of IgG coated erythrocytes or other immune complexes identify B lymphocytes via their Fc receptor sites. Complement coated erythrocytes attach at the complement (C_3) binding site to form "EAC rosettes." Pokeweed mitogen (PWM) induces blastogenesis of B lymphocytes. B lymphocytes also carry specific surface antigens.

Macrophages and monocytes have Fc and C_3 receptors and thus may be confused with B lymphocytes. However, they lack intrinsic surface immunoglobulin.

lins and for complement components (Fig. 5–4). B cells differ from T cells in their response to mitogens (Uhr, 1975).

The dividing line between T and B cells as identified by these surface markers is not as sharp as we would like. Complement and Fc receptors, for example, may be found on some subpopulations of T cells. Some T lymphocytes may carry a low-density coating of surface immunoglobulin. The fact that neutrophils and monocytes bear surface receptors for complement and the Fc fragment adds to the confusion of accurate identification. Changes in the specific antigenic composition of the surface membrane occur during normal immunocyte differentiation. Thus identification of differences in surface antigens among immunocytes by immunologic techniques may at times be more reflective of developmental stage than of any particular subpopulation. Finally, differences in surface appearance among lymphocytes have been shown by scanning electron microscopy, but the significance of this observation is still open to question (Fig. 5–5).

Cell-mediated immunity is responsible for delayed hypersensitivity, homograft rejection, graft-versus-host reaction, defense against viral, fungal, and certain bacterial infections, such as tuberculosis, and possibly even defense against the growth of neoplastic cells in the body. The T lymphocytes regulate humoral immunity but do not have the capacity to secrete circulating antibody. Their anatomic sites of distribution in the lymph nodes are in the deep cortical regions and in the periphery of the germinal follicles (Fig. 5–6). In the spleen they are found in the periarteriolar lymphatic tissue. They also constitute the majority of lymphocytes in the circulating pool of blood and lymph. The population of these specific anatomic sites with T lymphocytes is dependent upon the thymus gland, which in turn is dependent upon the marrow as the source of its stem cells. The thymus may directly "condition" a lymphocytic stem cell derived from the marrow or it may secrete a hormonal substance which conditions marrow lymphocytes at some distance from the thymus to function as T lymphocytes or both mechanisms may prevail.

The cell-mediated immune response differs from the humoral response in several important respects. After initial recognition and processing of specific antigen by phagocytes, T lymphocytes are programmed in a still unknown manner and become specifically "activated" (Fig. 5–7). This activation causes DNA synthesis, blast transformation, and subsequent cellular proliferation. It also causes the production of nonimmunoglobulin humoral factors called lymphokines which further amplify the immune response by recruiting other non-committed T lymphocytes to become specifically activated and to proliferate (David, 1973). Migration inhibition factor prevents macrophages from leaving the area, presumably

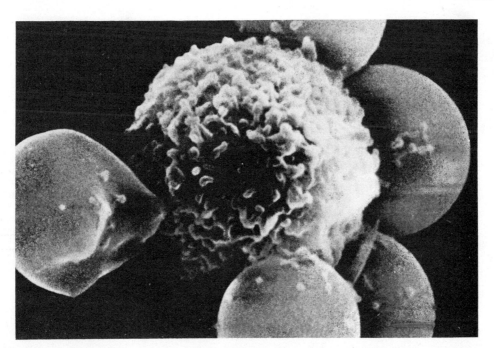

Figure 5–4 Complement coated erythrocytes adhere to a B lymphocyte to form an "EAC rosette." "E rosettes" have the same appearance but are formed by the adherence of normal uncoated sheep erythrocytes to T cells. (From Tsukada, M., et al.: Acta. Haematol. Jap., *39*, 43, 1976.)

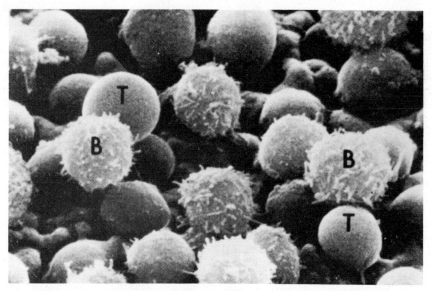

Figure 5–5 Scanning electron microscopic picture of lymphocytes, some showing roughened surfaces studded with microvilli (B) and others with smooth membrane surfaces (T). The significance of this difference in surface is uncertain, although it originally was thought to distinguish B from T lymphocytes. (From Polliack, A., et al.: J. Exp. Med., *138*:607, 1973.)

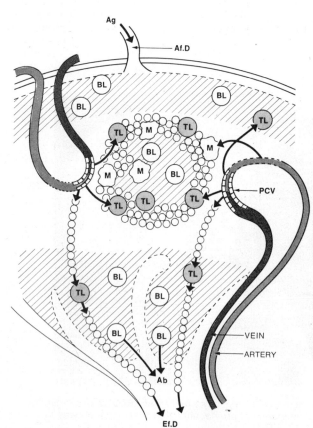

Figure 5–6 Diagram of lymph node. *TL* = T lymphocyte; *BL* = B lymphocyte; *M* = macrophage; *Ag* = antigen; *Ab* = antibody; *Af. D* = afferent lymphatic duct; *Ef. D* = efferent lymphatic duct; *PCV* = post-capillary venule. The cross-hatched zones represent areas populated by B lymphocytes (superficial cortical zone, germinal centers, and medullary cords). Areas containing open circles represent T lymphocyte regions (deep cortical zone, follicle periphery). T lymphocytes circulate in close proximity to macrophages, allowing interaction between these cells and specific antigen. (From Craddock, C. G., et al.: N. Engl. J. Med., *285*:380, 1971. Reprinted by permission.)

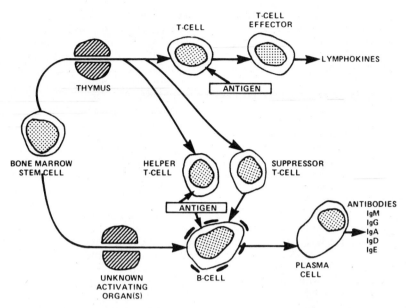

Figure 5–7   The cellular (T) and humoral (B) immune systems. The participation of macrophages is important both for antigen processing as well as for the afferent effector arm of the immune response. Lymphokines are non-immunoglobulin substances secreted by T lymphocytes. They include macrophage migration inhibition factor, transfer factor, and other active principles. (From Waldman, T. A.: Ann. Allergy, *39*:79, 1977, with permission.)

serving the cause of antigen localization and destruction. Most of the activated T lymphocytes serve as "effector" cells by exerting a cytotoxic effect, by complement activation, and by attracting macrophages. Some cytotoxic ("killer") lymphocytes directly attack cellular antigens. Others require antibody combined with antigen on the foreign cell surface in order to seek out the cell for destruction (Podleski, 1976). Some of the activated T cells produce a population of small nondividing lymphocytes which bear a "memory" of the event. These "memory cells" remain for very long periods of time, possibly even a lifetime, in a resting and nondividing state, ready to resume immediate proliferation upon re-exposure to the specific antigen. Subpopulations of T lymphocytes called helper and suppressor cells regulate the humoral immune response, as described below. Individuals may differ in their immune responsiveness to specific antigens because of inherited differences in the "immune response" gene, which is closely related on the chromosome to the major histocompatibility locus and plays an important role in regulating the T cell response (Paul and Benacerraf, 1977).

B immunocytes occupy the superficial cortical regions, the medullary cords, and the germinal centers of the follicles of the lymph nodes, spleen, gastrointestinal tract, and other tissues (Fig. 5–6). The B immunocytes form an immobile pool; the majority do not circulate. They are also derived from a bone marrow stem cell but their

further development is not dependent upon the thymus. B lymphocytes must also be programmed with information about a specific antibody, and for many antigens they cooperate with T lymphocytes in this programming process (Fig. 5–7). Possibly the relatively immobile B lymphocytes require the cooperation of the freely circulating T cells to achieve rapid widespread activation throughout the body. Surface membrane immunoglobulins on B lymphocytes are exclusively of the IgM and IgD types and act as receptors for specific antigens. The formation of antigen-antibody complexes on the B lymphocytes causes them to proliferate and mature into antibody-secreting plasma cells. As B cells differentiate into plasma cells they lose their intrinsic membrane immunoglobulin. The plasma cell represents the most mature form of the activated B lymphocyte and no longer has the capacity to divide. The antibodies produced effect the immune response by virtue of their properties as agglutinins, lysins, and opsonins. Like T lymphocytes, some B lymphocytes have the capacity to develop into long-lived memory cells.

The secretion of antibodies of great diversity into plasma and extravascular fluids is the special prerogative enjoyed by the B cells. An understanding of the molecular structure of antibodies is necessary to appreciate how precise specificity yet wide diversity are combined in one family of closely related proteins. The immunoglobulins fall into five families of proteins. IgG immunoglobulins, of molecular weight 160,000 and sedimentation constant 7S, are normally present in serum at a concentration of about 1250 mg. per 100 ml., constituting by far the major type. Their relatively small molecular size permits transport across the placenta. IgA immunoglobulins (normal serum concentration 250 mg. per 100 ml.) are the major type found in body secretions (saliva, tears, colostrum, and gastrointestinal, respiratory, and urinary tract fluids). They form polymers of 9S, 11S, and 13S from the basic unit of 7S. IgM immunoglobulins (normal serum concentration 120 mg. per 100 ml.) are large 18S molecules, also an association of 7S units, especially well suited for agglutination and complement fixation. The IgM synthesized in the B cell membrane is monomeric, however. The other two families of immunoglobulins, IgD and IgE, are present in much lower concentrations, 3 mg. per 100 ml. and 0.03 mg. per 100 ml., respectively. IgD functions almost exclusively as a membrane-bound immunoglobulin; very little is secreted into the plasma. IgE exists primarily in complex formation with mast cells, where it awaits combination with antigen, triggering mast cell release of histamine and other active products. IgE is important in allergic reactions involving the skin, the lungs, and other tissues (Table 5–1).

All the immunoglobulin families have a basic structure in common (Fig. 5–8). This unit consists of two light (or "L") and two heavy (or "H") chains, so termed because of their difference in molecular weight (22,000 as opposed to 52,000). Disulfide bridges bind the H chains to each other and to the L chains. Hydrogen bonding also helps hold the molecular pieces together. The N-terminal ends of an L and H chain together form the antigen binding site. Since there are two such regions on the molecular surface, the immunoglobulin unit is divalent; i.e., it can combine with two antigen molecules. Univalent antibody can be artificially produced by cleavage of the molecule with papain. Such treatment produces one Fc fragment, which carries the C-terminal ends of both H

chains, and two Fab fragments, each of which carries the N terminal of one H and one L chain. The Fab fragments function as univalent antibodies. The Fc portion of the molecule is of particular importance in bringing about complex formation with phagocyte and lymphocyte Fc receptors. The molecule contains a variable amount of carbohydrate attached to the H chain.

The amino acid sequence of the H and L chains is governed by the same kinds of genetic controls that govern the structure of other body proteins. The H chains each contain about 450 amino acid residues, and the L chains about 214. About three fourths of the H chain and one half of the L chain are invariant in their amino acid structure. Specificity, however, lies in the remaining one fourth of the H chain and one half of the L chain where regions of the molecule show great variation in amino acid structure which determines their specificity for antigen. These two structural regions of H and L chains have been called "C" (for common) and "V" (for variant).

There are only two different types of L chains — κ and λ. Only one type is present in any given molecule, but both types are represented in all immunoglobulin families. Class specificity lies in the type of H chain.

There are four subclasses of IgG H chains (γ1, γ2, γ3, γ4). IgA has α heavy chains and is a polymer of two, three, or four 7S units plus a "secretory component" which facilitates transport into body secretions (Walker and Isselbacher, 1977). IgM, a pentamer of 7S units, has μ heavy chains (Fig. 5–9). Subclasses of α and μ heavy chains have also been described. IgA and IgM contain considerably more carbohydrate than IgG.

In basic respects the genetic control of immunoglobulin synthesis resembles that of hemoglobin. The major subunits of the molecule — L and H chains of immunoglobulin and α and β chains of hemoglobin — are under the control of gene regions which are separate and independent and

TABLE 5–1 COMPARISON OF IMMUNOGLOBULIN CLASSES

	IgG	IgA	IgM	IgD	IgE
Serum concentration (mg. per 100 ml.)	1250	250	120	3	0.03
Sedimentation constant S_{20}	6.6S	7S, 9S, 11S, 13S	18S	6.5S	7.9S
Carbohydrate (total %)	2.9	5–10	11.8	10–12	11
Heavy chains	γ	α	μ	σ	ϵ
Light-chain frequency kappa:lambda ratio	2:1	1:1	3:1	1:4	

IgD functions almost exclusively as a B lymphocyte surface immunoglobulin and IgG and IgA as plasma immunoglobulins. IgM serves both as a surface immunoglobulin and is secreted into the plasma in significant quantities. IgE is secreted by plasma cells but is mostly bound to mast cells, where it awaits complex formation with antigen.

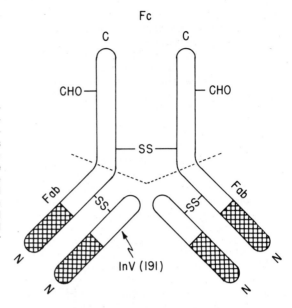

Figure 5–8 Diagram of the structure of the 7S immunoglobulin. C and N represent C-terminal and N-terminal amino acids, respectively. *CHO* = carbohydrate. Disulfide bonds connect the smaller L chains with the larger H chains, and the latter with each other. The interrupted line represents papain cleavage into Fc and Fab fragments. The Fc region may combine with Fc receptors on the surfaces of B lymphocytes and macrophages. The Fab fragments contain the antigen binding sites. The InV locus at the 191st amino acid residue of the L chain is shown. The crosshatched areas represent the variable regions, and the clear areas the common regions.

yet which must coordinate their efforts in order to produce balanced synthesis of the subunits, thus avoiding shortages or surpluses of unpaired polypeptide chains. The extraordinary molecular diversity of the immunoglobulins, however, is a major point at which genetic control of this system of body proteins differs from all others. The synthesis of specific immunoglobulin, including the common and variable region for each H and L chain, is under the control of one clone of B immunocytes. The body contains numerous such clones, leading to heterogeneous production of almost countless different immunoglobulin molecules. Both lymphocytes and plasma cells synthe-

size immunoglobulin, plasma cells producing about two thirds of the IgG. On the other hand, about 90 per cent of IgM is produced by lymphocytes. The gene regions controlling the common structural regions of L and H chains are inherited. Inherited amino acid substitutions may affect these common regions. Thus, INV-1 and INV-3 are genetic alleles affecting the κ chain at the 191st amino acid site, where either leucine or valine, respectively, is placed. Precisely how B immunocytes develop gene regions in different clones to control the variant regions of the L and H chains remains a mystery. A somatic theory postulates that the antigen, after being processed

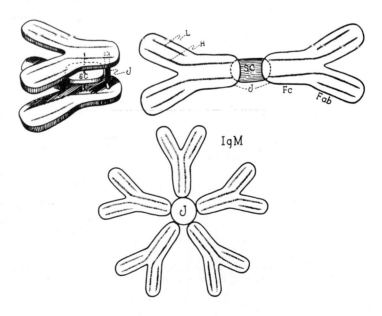

Figure 5–9 Assembly of 7S units in higher molecular weight immunoglobulins, IgA (*above*) and IgM, showing "secretory component" (*SC*) and "joining piece" (*J*). Joining piece is necessary to form polymers. Secretory component is produced by mucosal epithelial cells and is necessary for the transport of dimeric IgA into body secretions, It appears to protect IgA from the action of digestive enzymes. (Reprinted, by permission, from Tomasi, T. B.: The New England Journal of Medicine, *287*:501, 1972.)

by a macrophage, somehow produces a "reverse flow" of information which thus establishes itself as a permanent record in the programmed genome of a given clone of B cells. The germ line theory postulates that all genetic information, common as well as variant, is obtained through inheritance.

KINETICS

The differentiation, proliferation, and fate of the body's lymphocytes contrast sharply with those of the other cellular elements of the blood. The maturation and proliferation processes which give rise to a specialized peripheral lymphatic tissue are not accompanied by significant morphologic changes other than that change which sets apart the large proliferating cells from the small non-proliferating cells. The marrow serves as the ultimate source of all lymphocytes and together with the thymus is considered a primary lymphatic structure concerned with the differentiation and proliferation of a peripheral population of mature, specialized lymphocytes in

the blood, lymphatics, lymphatic tissue, and spleen. The fully developed red cells, granulocytes, and platelets have a finite life span at the end of which the cell disintegrates. In the case of the peripheral lymphatic tissue, the cells retain the ability to undergo cell division once again by a process of "blastogenesis." The peripheral lymphatic system is also charged with the task of maintaining immunologic memory, which it does by means of a small population of exceedingly long-lived cells which may survive for many years and then once again re-enter cell division upon specific stimulation by antigen. Thus, the cell life span of lymphocytes varies tremendously.

The information which has been obtained about lymphocyte kinetics has relied heavily upon cytologic techniques of DNA labeling by tritiated thymidine. Lymphocytes identified by chromosomal markers have also been used.

The lymphocytes in the primary lymphatic tissue — the marrow and the thymus — undergo relatively rapid and continuous proliferation quite independently of specific antigenic stimulation (Fig. 5–10). For decades evidence has been

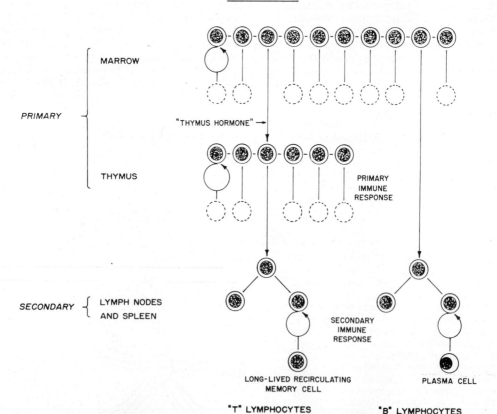

LYMPHOPOIESIS

MARROW

PRIMARY

"THYMUS HORMONE" →

THYMUS

PRIMARY IMMUNE RESPONSE

SECONDARY { LYMPH NODES AND SPLEEN

SECONDARY IMMUNE RESPONSE

LONG-LIVED RECIRCULATING MEMORY CELL

PLASMA CELL

"T" LYMPHOCYTES   "B" LYMPHOCYTES

Figure 5–10 Diagram of lymphopoiesis. Interrupted circles represent effete cells in marrow and thymus which do not achieve perpetuity in the secondary lymphatic tissue. Proliferation takes place in both the primary and secondary tissues, in the latter as a result of specific immune response.

presented for and against the theory that the marrow lymphocytic stem cell is pluripotential and also gives rise to the diverse cells of the myeloid series. Indeed the recent observation that an acute lymphoblastic crisis may complicate the course of chronic myelogenous leukemia argues in favor of a common ancestral stem cell for the lymphoid and myeloid cell lines.

Marrow and thymic lymphopoiesis appears to be more active than a fully developed adult's peripheral lymphatic tissue would require for replenishment, and therefore it is reasonable to assume that the bulk of lymphopoiesis in these organs is wasteful, most of the proliferated cells undergoing destruction in order to prevent massive accumulation of unwanted numbers. Relatively few are directed to assume positions in peripheral secondary lymphatic tissue. Under normal conditions, the secondary lymphatic tissue is not actively proliferating, but upon exposure to antigen, specifically stimulated cells undergo rapid division, with germinal centers showing the greatest level of activity.

The bulk of the T lymphocytes of the peripheral lymphatic tissue recirculate. They follow a path from blood to lymph node and spleen through lymphatic channels back to blood. Egress from the blood into the lymphatic tissue occurs through the wall of the postcapillary venule, where the T cells percolate through the periphery of follicles and the deep cortical areas eventually to be collected into the efferent lymphatic (Fig. 5–6).

Approximately 10 hours are required for lymphocytes to leave the blood and appear in the thoracic duct. The T cells do not recirculate through the marrow or thymus to any significant degree. The T cell system can be lymphocyte-depleted by means of thoracic duct drainage or extracorporeal irradiation, leaving the T areas of the lymphatic tissue empty. The recirculating population consists of "short-lived" and "long-lived" cells. This conclusion is based on experiments in animals given continuous injections of tritiated thymidine over a period of many months. In rats, about 40 to 45 per cent of small lymphocytes take up label in 5 to 10 days. The labeling index continues to increase thereafter, but even after nine months, about 5 to 10 per cent of the small lymphocytes remain unlabeled. They are considered to be the long-lived memory cells. All large lymphocytes label within three days. The gradual slope of decline of the DNA labeled cells shows a slow replacement rate and a long survival time of most small lymphocytes.

The B cells are largely noncirculating. They maintain a fixed position in the germinal centers, medullary cords, and superficial cortical zones of the secondary lymphatic tissue. Apparently the majority of cells produced are short-lived. Mature plasma cells probably do not survive longer than two or three days. A small proportion of B cells mature in the marrow because a few plasma cells are normally seen there.

PATHOPHYSIOLOGY

Classification and General Considerations

The system of fixed and circulating immunocytes which constitute the secondary lymphatic tissue provides a vital defensive function. Thus, the most common alterations occur in reactive response to the presence of foreign antigens, such as local or systemic infections. The reaction may consist of focal or generalized adenopathy, splenomegaly, the presence of large "young" lymphocytes or plasmacytoid cells in the circulation, or an elevation of the absolute lymphocyte count. Another common reactive change is a generalized increase in all immunoglobulin types.

Neoplastic alterations of the immunocytes represent inappropriate proliferative responses which produce an increase in the number of immunocytes and may be associated with either an increase or a decrease in the concentration of immunoglobulins. These conditions are often associated with functional impairment of cellular or humoral immune mechanisms which, in turn, leads to an abnormal susceptibility to a variety of infections which are often quite different from those commonly observed in patients with an intact immune system (Levine and associates, 1972). Autoimmune phenomena, such as hemolytic anemia or thrombocytopenia, are also observed in patients with lymphoproliferative disorders. In clinical practice the problem of distinguishing neoplastic from reactive conditions affecting the immune system may be difficult, and judgments must be made with great care because of the vast differences in prognosis and treatment between the two states.

An over-all classification of disorders of the immunocytes is summarized in Table 5–2.

Quantitative Disorders

Lymphocytopenia and Hypogammaglobulinemia. A reduction in the number of circulating lymphocytes below the normal level of 1000 to 1500 per cu. mm. comes about through either increased loss or decreased production. The alteration represents primarily a change in the T cells, which constitute the majority of circulating lymphocytes. Mechanical loss of lymphocytes can be produced by tapping the circulating stream at the thoracic duct and draining off the lymph. A similar mechanism may explain the lymphocytopenia of intestinal lymphangiectasia and other disorders associated with leakage of lymph into the gastrointestinal tract. Lymphocytes are extraordinarily radiosensitive and a fall in the lym-

TABLE 5–2 CLASSIFICATION OF
IMMUNOCYTE DISORDERS

I. *Quantitative Disorders*
   Lymphocytopenia and hypogammaglobulinemia
      Primary
         Congenital
         Acquired
      Secondary
   Lymphocytosis and hypergammaglobulinemia
      Reactive
      Immunoproliferative

II. *Qualitative Disorders*

III. *Immunoproliferative Disorders*
   Leukemia
      Chronic lymphatic
      Acute lymphatic
   Lymphoma
      Hodgkin's
      Non-Hodgkin's
   M-component disorders
      Plasma cell myeloma
      Macroglobulinemia
      Benign monoclonal gammopathy
   Other variants
      Leukemic reticuloendotheliosis
      Mycosis fungoides
      Sézary syndrome

phocyte count of the peripheral blood precedes the decrease in either granulocytes or platelets caused by radiation. Lymphocytopenia is often present in patients during acute stress or therapy with corticoids. The studies of Fauci and Dale have demonstrated that glucocorticoids produce lymphocytopenia by shifting the distribution of lymphocytes from the intravascular to the extravascular space. The effect is transitory. In patients with certain lymphoproliferative disorders, however, glucocorticoids may produce the opposite effect and temporarily raise the blood lymphocyte count by means of altering the body distribution from extra- to intravascular sites. Adrenal steroids also cause cell lysis and inhibit cell proliferation, but these actions are limited to certain sensitive lymphocyte subpopulations. Steroid sensitivity is highly species-dependent.

The secondary lymphatic tissue is the immediate source of the circulating lymphocytes. Ablation of this source by malignant replacement, as in the case of advanced Hodgkin's disease or widespread metastatic carcinoma, or its destruction by irradiation of the lymph node-bearing regions of the body, leads to an inability of these regions to return adequate numbers of lymphocytes into the blood through the lymphatics. Chemotherapeutic alkylating agents will also affect

lymphocyte replacement by interfering with the proliferating and the short-lived small lymphocyte pools.

Hypogammaglobulinemia occurs as an acquired or congenital syndrome, but it is not necessarily associated with lymphocytopenia, since the source of immunoglobulins is not T lymphocytes but rather the non-circulating B cells. In infants or children, hypogammaglobulinemia usually represents a congenital immune deficiency. In adults, the condition is acquired either by increased loss in the urine or the gastrointestinal tract as a complication of nephrotic syndromes or protein-losing enteropathy, or by decreased production, usually secondary to a lymphoproliferative disorder.

Primary acquired late onset hypogammaglobulinemia ("common variable") varies greatly in severity and in the pattern of immune deficiency (Geha and associates, 1974). Recurrent sinopulmonary infections and malabsorption are among the more common of the clinical complications. At least one variety is thought to be the result of increased activity of a subpopulation of suppressor T lymphocytes acting to inhibit the normal development of B cells into mature secretory plasma cells.

The *congenital immune deficiency syndromes* of childhood form an array of rare but intriguing conditions upon which much of our understanding of the normal immune mechanism is based. The *Bruton type of agammaglobulinemia* is a sex-linked developmental defect of the B system of lymphocytes and plasma cells. Those regions of the secondary lymphatic tissue populated by these cells are empty, whereas the thymic-dependent areas remain intact. Circulating lymphocytes are present in normal numbers, but the concentration of immunoglobulins in the plasma is very low. The numerous infections which occur, usually in the sinopulmonary tract, can be prevented by the therapeutic use of gamma globulin injections. The *DiGeorge syndrome* is a severe developmental defect of the third and fourth pharyngeal pouches with consequent thymic aplasia and a profound lack of the thymic-dependent system of T cells. The corresponding regions of the T system are depleted of lymphocytes, and this is associated with lymphocytopenia but normal plasma immunoglobulin concentrations. *Swiss type lymphocytopenic agammaglobulinemia* ("combined immunodeficiency") affects both systems of immunocytes and thus would appear to trace its origins back to the common stem cell of origin in the bone marrow. A number of cases of severe combined immunodeficiency have been associated with deficiency of the enzyme adenosine deaminase (Parkman and co-workers, 1975). The adenosine which accumulates is toxic to lymphoid cells. Combined immunodeficiency may be corrected by bone marrow transplantation, whereas thymic transplantation should suffice in the DiGeorge syndrome (Bortin and Rimm, 1977).

Other congenital immune deficiency syndromes have been described, some resembling the Swiss type, others of a more mixed nature, such as *Wiskott-Aldrich syndrome* and *hereditary ataxia telangiectasia*. The features of Wiskott-Aldrich syndrome include sex-linked inheritance, thrombocytopenia, eczema, and susceptibility to infection associated with impaired ability to form antibody in response to polysaccharide antigens. The level of IgM is low, but IgG is normal and concentrations of IgA are often very high. Death in childhood is the result, owing either to severe infection or to the development of malignant disease, often of a lymphoma-like character. Successful therapy with transfer factor has been reported. In ataxia telangiectasia, the immune deficiency affects IgA and IgE along with qualitative deficiency in cell-mediated response.

The physiologic hypogammaglobulinemia of infancy must be distinguished from the congenital immune deficiency syndromes. Following the gradual disappearance from the infant's circulation of maternal IgG, endogenous synthesis takes over, raising IgG and IgM levels to about three fourths the adult level by one year of age. IgA levels increase more slowly, reaching adult levels by about two years.

Lymphocytosis and Hypergammaglobulinemia. Lymphocytosis is defined as an increase in the absolute lymphocyte count above 4000 per cu. mm. in adults, above 7000 cu. mm. in young children, and above 9000 per cu. mm. in infants. In "relative" lymphocytosis, the proportion of lymphocytes in the peripheral blood is increased because of concomitant granulocytopenia, but the absolute number is not above the normal range.

The leukocyte response evoked by a particular infection varies with the particular organism and also with the stage of the infection. Some infections, mostly viral but including some bacterial, are noted for their ability to evoke a lymphocytic response. Pertussis and acute infectious lymphocytosis are two childhood illnesses with a particularly striking tendency to raise the blood lymphocyte count — predominantly small mature forms — to very high levels in the range of 15,000 to 50,000 per cu. mm., but occasionally to as high as 100,000 per cu. mm.

Infectious mononucleosis is associated with a more modest lymphocytosis, usually not in excess of 20,000 per cu. mm., but there is a greater proportion (usually about 20 per cent of the total) of young and "atypical" forms (Lai, 1977). These are as large as 15 to 25 μ in diameter, with a generous rim of cytoplasm, often deep blue, foamy, and containing vacuoles, with an irregular outline which tends to cling to adjacent red cells. The nucleus is also larger, its chromatin

clumps are somewhat more widely spaced, and its outline is often indented, irregular, or lobulated into "monocytoid" forms. One or two nucleoli per nucleus are occasionally seen.

Infectious mononucleosis is caused by the Epstein-Barr virus (EBV). B lymphocytes become infected with EBV. T lymphocytes then undergo a reactive proliferative response, giving rise to the atypical lymphocytes in the peripheral blood. EBV antigen can be identified on B cell membranes but is absent from the T cells. The humoral response is also of use in establishing the diagnosis by means of a significantly positive heterophile antibody titer.

During this period of T cell response in infectious mononucleosis, as in other viral infections, there is a temporary period of anergy associated with loss of the delayed hypersensitivity response. The explanation for this transient decrease in immune reactivity is unknown.

The EBV also appears to be of importance in the causation of the African type of *Burkitt's lymphoma* and of nasopharyngeal carcinoma (Klein, 1975). It is constantly associated with both these neoplasias. Why certain individuals respond to EBV infection with a benign self-limited disorder and others are stricken with malignancy is a mystery. Presumably the immunologic T cell response differs in the two circumstances; its failure to contain the infection under certain circumstances leads to a neoplastic transformation. EBV is also associated with Hodgkin's disease, but its importance in the genesis of this neoplasia is questionable.

The heterophile antibody test is positive in the great majority of cases, distinguishing infectious mononucleosis from a large number of other infections which may give rise to a similar blood picture, although usually with fewer atypical lymphocytes. These infections include measles, mumps, adenovirus, viral hepatitis, cytomegalovirus, toxoplasmosis, brucellosis, typhoid fever, *Listeria monocytogenes,* and even tuberculosis. These infections sometimes cause only a relative lymphocytosis, the most prominent change being a reduction in circulating granulocytes. Relative lymphocytosis is also a feature of the very early (usually preclinical) stages of bacterial infection, as granulocytes begin to leave the circulation to go into the infected tissues, or the very late stages of severe and overwhelming bacterial infection after exhaustion of granulocyte reserves. In the latter circumstance, the relative lymphocytosis is an ominous prognostic indicator. As one would predict from the effect of adrenal steroids on lymphocytes, adrenal insufficiency may cause a rise in the blood lymphocytes.

An inappropriate increase in the absolute lymphocyte count, not explainable on the basis of either immunoreactive states or endocrine disease, is indicative of a lymphoproliferative disorder, usually lymphatic leukemia. Small mature lymphocytes predominate in chronic lymphatic leukemia. In the early stages of this disorder the elevation may be slight, but counts are usually in the range of 50,000 to 250,000 per cu. mm. when the diagnosis is first made. A rare patient may reach values as high as 1,000,000 per cu. mm. The leukocytosis of acute lymphatic leukemia is usually lesser in degree. Instead of the small mature lymphocyte, it features immature lymphoblasts.

One of the most important problems in clinical hematologic diagnosis is the distinction between leukemia and "leukemoid" reactions. The clinical course, whether benign and self-limited or persistent or progressive, is one obvious point of difference. The ability to distinguish the morphologic features of leukemic lymphoblasts from the young and atypical lymphocytes found in infectious states is another. The association of anemia, thrombocytopenia, and/or granulocytopenia suggests leukemia, but these findings singly or in combination are sometimes seen in infections. Perhaps the most salient pathophysiologic point of distinction lies in the fact that replacement of the primary lymphatic organ, the bone marrow, is a prominent feature of leukemia. Reactive states cause proliferation mostly in the secondary lymphatic tissue; the reactive young and "atypical" lymphocytes which characterize infectious

mononucleosis and other infections therefore do not replace the normal marrow cells to any significant degree. Lymphocytes and plasma cells may increase in the marrow as a reactive change, but they usually are in the range of 5 to 15 per cent of the total marrow cells, hardly ever above 30 per cent, and never replace the marrow tissue as leukemic proliferation usually does.

An increase in plasma immunoglobulin concentration above the normal range is a common response not only in many infectious diseases but also in other conditions, such as liver cirrhosis, carcinoma, sarcoidosis, and lupus erythematosus, to name a few. Such responses are polyclonal and affect a variety of immunoglobulins. This is reflected in the serum electrophoretic pattern by a diffuse increase, or "broad-band" hypergammaglobulinemia. Immunoelectrophoretic analysis shows increases in all immunoglobulin families, IgG, IgA, and IgM. In an acute immune response, the increase in IgM occurs first. The finding in a serum electrophoretic pattern of hypergammaglobulinemia due to a narrow dense band in the broad region where the gamma globulins are normally found has a different significance. It is the secretory product of a monoclonal line of B cells producing only one type of immunoglobulin. This narrow band is often referred to as a "spike," but the term "M-component," for monoclonal component, is more appropriate (Fig. 5–11). The pres-

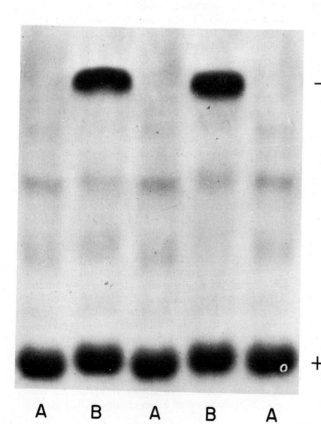

Figure 5–11 Electrophoretic separation of serum proteins on cellulose acetate. A is normal serum. B is abnormal serum containing an M-component located near the cathodal end of the strip in the gamma zone. (The cathodal end is at the top and the anodal at the bottom of the picture.)

A B A B A

ence of an M-component in the serum or urine requires investigation of the patient for a malignant proliferative disorder of the B cells, i.e., myeloma or primary macroglobulinemia. On the other hand, the mere presence of such a component does not by itself establish such a diagnosis.

Qualitative Disorders

There are several points in the immune response at which qualitative defects in lymphocyte function may be the primary factors responsible for a poor immune response. In contrast to the granulocytic series, however, it is difficult to separate functional defects of the lymphocyte from numerical deficiency, since the process of specific activation (with the assistance of modifying factors) sets off a series of cell proliferations of the specifically activated clone. Thus, a qualitative defect at the afferent level of the immune response will be reflected in deficient numbers at the efferent limb.

Malignant transformation of cells in the body is increasingly being viewed as a qualitative breakdown in the function of "surveillance" lymphocytes whose function it is to recognize specific "tumor" antigens on the surface of such cells and to bring about their destruction. The association of defective lymphocyte function with malignant transformation in the congenital immune deficiency states is indeed a striking example of a lack of surveillance. In a similar fashion, individuals who are under prolonged immunosuppressive therapy also show an increased tendency to develop malignant disease, often a lymphoma. Immune deficiency is a common feature of most of the lymphoproliferative disorders, but whether it precedes the development of the neoplasia or comes as a consequence of it — or both — remains a controversial subject.

Immunoproliferative Disorders

The neoplastic alterations of the lymphoid tissue produce an array of conditions quite distinct from but equally as rich in diversity as the myeloproliferative group of hematologic syndromes. The rapid expansion of basic knowledge about lymphocytes has produced a flurry of new concepts of lymphoproliferative disorders which rely on cell markers as well as traditional histopathology (Jaffe and co-workers, 1977). The rapidly emerging concepts are forcing reappraisal of old ideas.

The lymphatic leukemias primarily invade the bone marrow, with a prominent tendency to infiltrate the circulating bloodstream. The condition spreads to involve lymph nodes, spleen, and in-deed many other tissues in the body. The lymphomas are a group of related conditions which affect the secondary lymphatic tissue first with tumor formation which subsequently spreads to the other tissues including the marrow, without much tendency in most cases to release significant numbers of malignant cells into the circulation. The third major group of immunoproliferative conditions, plasma cell myeloma and primary macroglobulinemia, cause extensive marrow replacement but show little tendency to infiltrate the blood. They do give rise to a high frequency of aberrations of immunoglobulin synthesis.

Lymphoproliferative disorders may be classified according to their origins from a T or B cell line and also with respect to the functional stage of cell differentiation from which the monoclonal neoplasia springs. The T cell neoplasias include acute lymphatic leukemia, lymphoblastic lymphoma, mycosis fungoides, and Sézary syndrome. The B cell disorders include the M-component disorders, chronic lymphatic leukemia, and most of the non-Hodgkin's lymphomas. Hodgkin's disease continues to elude a niche in this schema (Table 5–3).

Chronic Lymphatic Leukemia (CLL). This disease increases in frequency with advancing age, whereas acute lymphatic leukemia is mostly a disease of childhood. The terms "chronic" and "acute" were originally descriptive of the clinical courses, but therapeutic advances in the management of the acute variety have narrowed the gap in life expectancy between the two. As a result, the terms are now more indicative of the morphology of the leukemic cell than of the prognosis. The small mature lymphocyte is the hallmark of chronic lymphatic leukemia; the lymphoblast is the sign of the acute variety.

CLL is rare in childhood but not uncommon in mature and older adults; two thirds of patients are over the age of 60. There is a 2:1 sex predominance in favor of males. The diagnosis is usually easily made by the observation that large numbers of small mature lymphocytes have accumulated in the blood and bone marrow. In comparison with the normal these lymphocytes are often more friable, have deeper nuclear clefts, and sometimes have more cytoplasm. Immature lymphoid cells are less than 5 per cent of the total. The absolute lymphocyte count in the blood is usually elevated to 10,000 to 150,000 per cu. mm. or even higher at the time of initial diagnosis, although a "subleukemic" (or "aleukemic") variety may be seen in which the cellular infiltration is confined to the marrow. Generalized lymphadenopathy and splenomegaly are common. Lymphocytic infiltration of the liver and of other body tissues increases as the disease progresses. The median life expectancy is about five years, but the clinical course is variable. One fifth of the patients, often

TABLE 5–3 CLASSIFICATION OF IMMUNOPROLIFERATIVE DISORDERS
ACCORDING TO FUNCTIONAL STAGE OF DIFFERENTIATION
(EARLY, INTERMEDIATE, OR LATE)

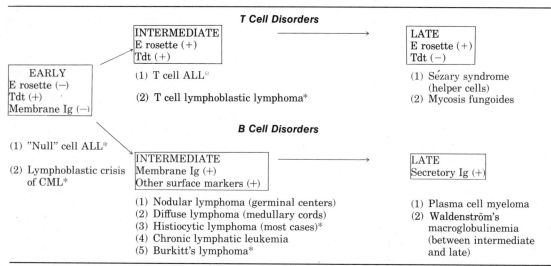

*Neoplastic cells predominantly transformed into large cells or "blasts."
Abbreviations: ALL = acute lymphatic leukemia   CML = chronic myelogenous leukemia
              Tdt = terminal deoxynucleotidyl transferase   Ig = immunoglobulin
NOTE: "Null" cell ALL and lymphoblastic crisis of CML may originate from an undifferentiated marrow lym-
         phoid cell line or from early cell lines with incompletely developed T or B cell characteristics (Gralnick
         and associates, 1977). Hodgkin's disease is not included in this schema.

those in the somewhat younger age group, are resistant to therapy and die within a year. At the other extreme, one third of patients are still alive after 10 years.

From the pathophysiologic point of view this disorder is better described as an abnormality of cell accumulation rather than one of cell proliferation. The leukemic cell population is predominantly non-dividing and inert. Immunoglobulins of the IgM type and sometimes also of the IgD type are present on the lymphocyte membrane. They are monoclonal and indicate the origin of CLL from a single line of B lymphocytes. Etiology is obscure, but the rarity of CLL among individuals of Oriental extraction along with a significant occurrence of multiple cases within the families of affected patients suggests that genetic factors are important.

Although years may pass without the occurrence of significant symptoms, many patients have anorexia, fatigue, weight loss, and sweats. Growth of lymphatic tumors may cause mechanical symptoms. Anemia, thrombocytopenia, and granulocytopenia are unfavorable signs and usually indicate impending trouble in any one or a combination of the functions these respective cellular elements fulfill. The most important cause of this cytopenia is the crowding out from the marrow of the normal precursor cells by the closely packed lymphocytes. Massive splenic enlargement may add to the severity of the cytopenia by trapping and sequestering or destroying any one or a combination of the blood cells. About 5 to 10 per cent of patients have an associated Coombs'-positive autoimmune hemolytic anemia, with spherocytosis, reticulocytosis, and erythroid hyperplasia in an otherwise lymphocytic marrow, along with the other usual signs of hemolysis. Death as a result of infectious complications runs high, since the disease fundamentally represents a breakdown in the normal defense mechanism. The susceptibility to infection may stem either from severe neutropenia or from the impediment to the production of circulating antibody. About half the cases show decreased serum immunoglobulin concentrations and about 5 per cent show an M-component in the serum electrophoretic pattern. The abnormal lymphocytes are poorly responsive to mitogenic stimulation with phytohemagglutinin, as would be expected of B lymphocytes.

The goal of therapy is to relieve symptoms and to improve anemia, thrombocytopenia, or granulocytopenia by reducing the size of the lymphocyte mass. Since cell proliferation is not a prominent feature, chemotherapeutic agents which depend on the DNA synthetic or mitotic phases of cycling cells are not useful. Chemotherapeutic destruction of the lymphocyte mass by alkylating agents (chlorambucil or cyclophosphamide) and adrenal glucocorticoids used singly or in combination are the mainstay of treatment.

Therapy has no doubt decreased morbidity and improved quality of life in CLL, but it seems likely that it has not dramatically increased life expectancy. Although peripheral blood counts improve, hypogammaglobulinemia is often not affected by treatment. The goal is to achieve "control" of the disease rather than "complete remission," as in the acute leukemias, since there is no evidence that added clinical benefit would accrue from the additional therapy that would be necessary. If properly managed, many patients may live out their normal life span with this disease. It rarely changes character, and the danger lies almost entirely in the immune deficiency and in bone marrow and organ impairment from lymphocyte encroachment.

Acute Lymphatic Leukemia (ALL). Primarily a disease of childhood with peak incidence at the age of four, ALL affects 20- to 30-year-old adults with a frequency about equal to that of acute granulocytic leukemia. Above that age, 90 per cent or more of the acute leukemias are granulocytic. The onset is relatively sudden, with symptoms of anemia, bleeding, or fever. Preleukemic manifestations are absent. Bone pain is not uncommon. The white blood cell count is usually increased, occasionally to values of 100,000 per cu. mm. or higher, with infiltration of the blood with lymphoblasts, but about one third of the cases present with a normal or low white cell count. Anemia and thrombocytopenia are the rule, but immunologic abnormalities are not observed, except inasmuch as they may come later as a result of the immunosuppressive effects of therapy. Intracranial hemorrhage is a life-threatening event, the likelihood of which is increased if severe thrombocytopenia occurs together with extreme elevations of the white cell count. Serum uric acid concentrations often are high, and precautions are necessary to avoid urate nephropathy. Neurologic manifestations due to infiltration of the central nervous system or of peripheral nerves are not uncommon. A slight to moderate degree of lymphadenopathy and hepatosplenomegaly are often present. Many other body tissues also become infiltrated with leukemic cells. Slow but unrestrained proliferation of the lymphoblasts crowds out normal blood precursor cells and produces death within a few months from hemorrhage or infection if the condition is not treated. Successful treatment eradicates all visible evidence of malignant tissue and allows the normal marrow cells to repopulate the marrow and to restore peripheral blood counts to normal, a state called "complete remission."

About a quarter of the cases of acute lymphatic leukemia (ALL) are positive for T cell membrane markers (Belpomme and associates, 1977). These tend to have a greater frequency of thymic and subcutaneous tumor formation, higher white cell count, greater likelihood of central nervous system involvement, and a generally less favorable outcome. Almost three quarters do not show any of the usual surface markers, and have therefore been called "null," or "non-T non-B" cell ALL. However, almost all ALL cells are positive for the marker enzyme "terminal transferase" (terminal deoxynucleotidyl transferase) (Greenwood and associates, 1977). This enzyme is highly characteristic of thymocytes and is also present in marrow, but it is absent from fully mature T cells. Its presence in almost all cases of ALL suggests that "null" cell ALL is in fact a neoplasia of an undifferentiated T cell line which has not yet developed the characteristic T cell surface markers. About one third of cases of acute blastic transformation of chronic myelogenous leukemia are also positive for terminal transferase. This finding indicates a lymphoblastic rather than a myeloblastic origin. Indeed, the morphologic appearance of these cells and their responsiveness to vincristine and prednisone treatment also support the concept of their lymphoid origin.

By means of experiments using tritiated thymidine, Mauer and his co-workers have found that the leukemic cells in patients with ALL do not proliferate in a uniform fashion. There appear to be two pools, one consisting of larger blasts which take up tritiated thymidine and are thus proliferating, while the other is made up of smaller blast cells which do not take up the DNA label and thus are not in a state of proliferation (Fig. 5–12). The cell cycle times of the proliferating leukemic cells generally vary in the range from three to ten days, although some apparently do not divide more often than once every 20 days. The large proliferating blasts predominate in the bone marrow; the small non-proliferating blasts are relatively more frequent in the circulating blood, where they have a relatively short life span with $T^{1/2}$ of about 25 hours. The importance of the non-proliferating pool of leukemic cells lies in its resistance to modalities of therapy which depend on cells being in a state of cycle, i.e., entering phases of DNA synthesis and/or mitosis. These non-dividing cells have the capacity to re-enter a proliferative phase after some period of dormancy, suggesting that they may be the bearers of the seeds of relapse, which is such a constant feature of the disease.

Chromosomal abnormalities, usually aneuploidy, are inconstantly present in ALL. They vary from case to case, but seem to remain constant in any given patient throughout the course of the disease. Their relationship to pathogenesis is unknown. Other aspects of cytogenetics and etiology of acute leukemia are discussed in the section on acute granulocytic leukemia.

The following concepts of chemotherapeutic strategy have been developed for the treatment of acute leukemia:

Induction — the initial stage of chemotherapy

% LABELED
BLAST CELLS

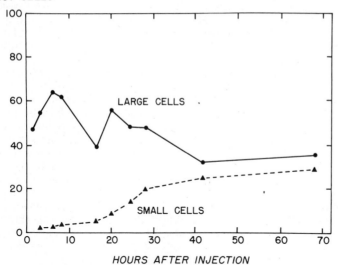

HOURS AFTER INJECTION

Figure 5–12 The labeling of large and small blast cells in a patient with acute leukemia after an injection of tritiated thymidine. The large cells are proliferating and therefore immediately take up the label. Initially, small cells take up no label because they are not dividing. Large blasts, however, become small non-dividing blasts, causing a belated appearance of the label in these cells. (Redrawn from Mauer, A. M., et al.: Human Tumor Cell Kinetics. National Cancer Institute Monograph No. 30, p. 71.)

designed to bring about complete remission in leukemia, i.e., alleviation of the symptoms, restoration of normal blood counts, and a return to a normal bone marrow in which less than 5 per cent of the cells are blasts. In ALL, vincristine and prednisone given together produce complete remission in about 90 per cent of new cases. The two agents act on different phases of the cell cycle, vincristine on the M (mitotic) phase and prednisone chiefly on the G_1 (intermitotic) phase. This example illustrates an important principle which has proved itself in certain other oncologic circumstances, namely, that combinations of agents are more effective and have no more toxicity than when each of the agents is used singly. Meticulous supportive care during induction with such measures as platelet transfusion, protective isolation, and the judicious use of antibiotics is important to the attainment of a successful outcome, especially in acute granulocytic leukemia, in which remission is so much more difficult to achieve than in ALL.

Consolidation and Intensification—a relatively intensive phase of chemotherapy which may be administered for an arbitrary period of time after the induction of complete remission. The object is to further reduce the number of leukemic cells, already so few that they are clinically inapparent, and thus delay clinical relapse by increasing the number of cell doublings necessary to grow enough leukemic tissue to produce clinical signs and symptoms. During this phase the improved bone marrow function brought about by the remission induction markedly increases the patient's hematologic tolerance to the cytotoxic effects of the chemotherapy.

Maintenance — a prolonged therapeutic effort to maintain the patient in a continuous state of complete remission for as long a time as possible. Without such treatment the remission in ALL lasts only one to four months. Those patients who relapse sooner after unmaintained remission probably have a shorter leukemic cell cycle time than those who stay in remission longer. Single or multiple agents, given alone or together, continuously, sequentially, or in cycles, have been used. Methotrexate, 6-mercaptopurine, and cyclophosphamide have been particularly useful. Nonspecific immune stimulation with such agents as BCG vaccine also appears to be active in maintaining remission.

Reinforcement — the application during the period of maintenance therapy of treatments of the type with which remission was first induced. For example, in ALL, vincristine and prednisone given from time to time during maintenance therapy appear to lengthen remission duration significantly.

Total Therapy — the effort, in addition to all the above stratagems, to eradicate hidden nests of leukemic cells which otherwise escape the chemotherapeutic onslaught. The central nervous system is a favorite hideout for such nests, a fact amply documented by the 30 to 50 per cent incidence of meningeal leukemia in ALL, a complication which almost always arises when the patient is in bone marrow remission. Meningeal leukemia causes symptoms and signs of increased intracranial pressure — headache, nausea and vomiting, and papilledema. Leukemic cells are found in the cerebrospinal fluid along with an elevated pressure, a decreased glucose concentration, and often some elevation of the protein concentration. With the exception of prednisone and the nitrosourea derivatives, chemotherapeutic agents do not readily cross the blood-brain barrier. The response to intrathecal therapy with methotrexate or to irradiation of the craniospinal axis is prompt. Based on the frequency of this complication and on the efficacious nature of the therapy, the most recent addition to the therapeutic strategy in ALL is the prophylactic treatment of this body site, in the hope of eliminating secluded nests of leukemic cells, with either intrathecal chemotherapy or radiation therapy or both. Simone has recently summarized the experience with "total therapy" at St. Jude's Hospital in Memphis.

The development of therapeutic strategy over the years has been paralleled by a progressive increase in life expectancy in children with ALL (Fig. 5–13). Hope is turning to expectation that many children with ALL will be cured as a result of "total therapy." In adults with ALL, the results of treatment have not been as good, with the increase in life expectancy having been lengthened from a median of four to six months to about 18 months.

Malignant Lymphoma, Hodgkin's Type. Noted for its predilection for young adults, Hodgkin's lymphoma makes up about one third of all cases of lymphoma (Moran and Ultman, 1974). All age groups are affected, a low frequency in childhood rising to about 2.5 cases per 100,000 population in adolescents and young adults. After the age of 50, the frequency increases along with that of

other malignant disease. Males predominate 3:2, and females appear to have a better prognosis. In contrast to the other lymphomas, Hodgkin's is more likely to start in the low cervical or supraclavicular lymph nodes and to cause high fever and intense itching. A small percentage of cases arise outside of the lymphatic system. Sometimes it is the cause of fever of unknown origin, even in the absence of apparent external lymphadenopathy.

Often the peripheral blood is entirely normal, but a variety of different changes can be seen. Increases in the granulocyte and platelet counts are not uncommon. Monocytosis and eosinophilia are less frequent. Coombs'-positive acquired hemolytic anemia occurs in occasional patients, but anemia, when it is present, is usually the variety seen with chronic disease. Pancytopenia may be caused by any combination of the factors of bone marrow invasion, hypersplenism, and bone marrow suppression from treatment. Absolute lymphocytopenia is a sign of rather advanced involvement of the lymphatic system significantly associated with an impairment of delayed hypersensitivity and other cellular immune responses. T cell function is impaired while the ability to form specific antibody is usually preserved. The cellular immune defect leads to the occurrence of complicating infections which are often of an unusual nature, such as aspergillosis, moniliasis, and other fungal diseases; *Pneumocystis carinii* infection; and localized or generalized herpes zoster. Rare "epidemics" have suggested that it may be spread as an infectious disease with a low

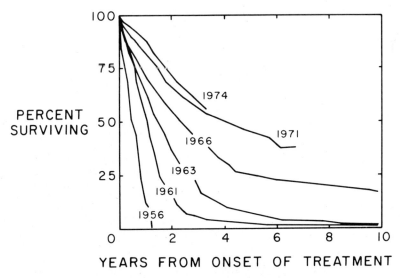

Figure 5–13 Improved survival in acute lymphatic leukemia between 1956 and 1977 in patients under age 20 at time of diagnosis. The years indicated are the start of treatment. A series of modifications in the treatment protocols over the years has been associated with progressive improvement in survival, with a significant proportion of long-term survivors off all treatment for several years. (Redrawn from data of Cancer and Leukemia Group B, by permission of Dr. James F. Holland)

order of contagion, but there is no proof that Hodgkin's disease is caused by an oncogenic infectious agent.

In contrast to the other lymphomas, Hodgkin's tends to begin in one site and to spread locally from one involved lymph node region to the next nearest group of lymph nodes, accounting for the high cure rate after local treatment and for the better results obtained by "extended field" as compared to "limited field" radiotherapy (Fig. 5–14). The other lymphomas are more likely to be "polycentric" rather than "unicentric" at the time of their origin. With the passage of time, however, the tendency is strong for relentless progression of lymphoma of any type, first within the lymphatic system, and then finally to extralymphatic structures such as liver, bone, lungs, and other organs. The course in any individual patient, however, is often unpredictable.

The Lukes-Butler system of classification for Hodgkin's disease has gained a large measure of acceptance, chiefly because it is clinically useful in terms of prognosis and management (Table 5–4). The presence of the Reed-Sternberg cell is a sine qua non for the diagnosis in any of the subgroups. Whether lymphocytes are preserved or depleted within the biopsied lymph node determines the favorable or unfavorable extremes of prognosis.

The evaluation of the extent of the disease by means of physical examination, radiographic procedures, and even exploratory laparotomy (or "staging") is essential in order to design a program of treatment properly. The stages into which Hodgkin's lymphoma is classified are shown in Figure 5–15. The presence of symptoms increases the probability that the disease is more disseminated. Splenic involvement increases the likelihood that the liver is also involved.

Extended field radiotherapy is the treatment of choice for patients with involvement confined to lymphatic tissue. When extralymphatic structures are involved, chemotherapy is preferred. Combined programs of radiotherapy plus chemotherapy are now under investigation. Although localized palliative radiotherapy occasionally is necessary, the major goal of radiotherapy is the cure of the patient. Chemotherapy has been traditionally considered to offer nothing more than temporary, although often very effective, palliation. Following in the footsteps of the experience gained with acute lymphatic leukemia, the chemotherapy of Hodgkin's disease has recently utilized combinations of agents, rather than single agents, given for a number of months to "induce" remission. The chemotherapeutic agents of greatest value are the alkylating agents (nitrogen mustard, cyclophosphamide, and chlorambucil); the vinca alkaloids (vincristine and vinblastine); the nitrosourea and anthracycline derivatives; procarbazine; bleomycin; and adrenal glucocorticoids. When these principles of chemotherapy are

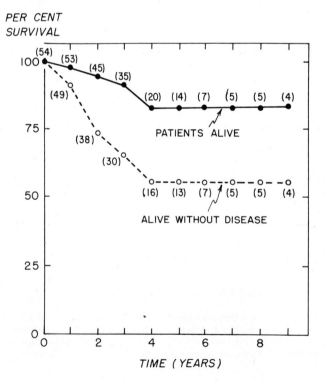

PER CENT SURVIVAL

Figure 5–14 Survival in patients with localized Hodgkin's disease treated with radical radiation therapy. Most of the deaths and recurrences occurred within 3 years. A similar group of patients not treated radically had a 5-year survival of 35 per cent, but no survivor was free of disease. (Redrawn from Prosnitz, L. R., et al.: Amer. J. Roentgenol., 105:618, 1969. Courtesy of Charles C Thomas, Publisher.)

TABLE 5–4 LUKES-BUTLER NOMENCLATURE: HODGKIN'S LYMPHOMA

Subgroup	Median Survival (Years)*	General Histologic Features
Lymphocyte predominant	9.2	Reed-Sternberg cells are seen in the midst of a sea of small mature lymphocytes arranged into a nodular or diffuse pattern.
Nodular sclerosis	4.2	A nodular pattern with the nodules separated by broad fibrous bands containing collagen bundles. The cellular pattern in the nodules may vary considerably, resembling that in any of the other three subgroups.
Mixed cellularity	2.5	A heterogeneous, usually diffuse cellular pattern containing lymphocytes, plasma cells, eosinophils, neutrophils, histiocytes, and fibroblasts, along with Reed-Sternberg cells, sometimes very numerous. Collagen bundles are absent.
Lymphocyte depletion	1.3	Undifferentiated histiocytes (or "reticulum cells") usually predominate in a diffuse pattern; at times Reed-Sternberg cells are very numerous. Fibrous obliteration of the entire lymph node is another variant of this subgroup.

*Lukes, R. J.: J.A.M.A., *222*:1294, 1972.

properly applied, as many as 40 per cent of patients with relatively advanced disease are alive and well for five years, a finding that encourages the hope that chemotherapeutic cure is being achieved in some cases.

Malignant Lymphoma Other Than Hodgkin's Type. Equally diverse in clinical manifestations and just as obscure etiologically, the non-Hodgkin's lymphomas are distinct from the Hodgkin's type and the principles of management and therapy differ (Patchevsky and associates, 1974). The most important difference is the greater tendency for the disease to be disseminated at the time of initial diagnosis by lymph node biopsy or histologic examination of an adequate piece of tissue from some extranodal site. Indeed, 90 per cent of patients with apparent Stage I or II disease show retroperitoneal node involvement by lymphography. This important point of difference no doubt explains why extended field radiotherapy does not clearly produce better results than more limited fields, as it does in patients with Stage I or II Hodgkin's disease. There is a slight male predominance. Most patients are older than 45 years of age. Systemic symptoms resemble those of Hodgkin's disease, but temperature elevations tend not to run as high. Their presence bears a similar poor prognostic significance.

A time-honored classification much used by cli-

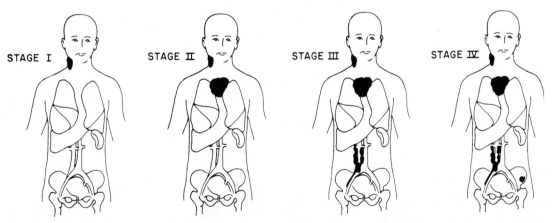

Figure 5–15 Stages of Hodgkin's disease. I to III represent progressively greater degrees of lymphatic involvement, while IV represents spread to extralymphatic structures.

nicians included three major categories: reticulum cell sarcoma, lymphosarcoma, and giant follicular lymphoma. This breakdown has been very useful from the clinical point of view because of the prognostic differences between these major groups. However, histologic classification has often proved difficult and even contradictory. This has been especially true for reticulum cell sarcoma because of the lack of uniform criteria and of a generally accepted nomenclature. The system of Rappaport has gained some measure of acceptance in recent years (Table 5–5). This system classifies the over-all node architecture as "diffuse" or "nodular" and the predominant cell type as a "well differentiated lymphocyte," a "poorly differentiated lymphocyte," or a "histiocyte." Controversy still surrounds the origin of the "histiocyte." Some consider it a close relative of the tissue macrophage and/or of cells capable of secreting reticulin fibers demonstrable by special silver stains. By the application of techniques for identifying surface markers, most "histiocytes" actually appear to be B lymphocytes, although many have no surface markers at all and a few are T cells. A nodular pattern and a well differentiated cell type are indicators of more favorable prognosis.

Traditional lymphoma histopathology has used the term "undifferentiated" to mean either a large transformed lymphoid blast cell, a lymphoid cell with an irregular or deeply cleaved nucleus, or both. The newer usage of the terms "undifferentiated" and "differentiated" refers to the level of functional development of the lymphoid cell, with allowance that a cell line derived from any level of functional development may enlarge and undergo transformation. Thus, for example, Burkitt's lymphoma arises from a B cell line that is moderately differentiated along functional lines, but the neoplastic cell population has transformed into blasts which traditional histopathology would consider morphologically "undifferentiated." Such differences of word usage are responsible for a certain amount of confusion in the current literature.

A life expectancy of eight to ten years is not an unreasonable hope for the majority of patients with nodular lymphoma. The course of this lymphoma may continue to follow a remarkably benign pattern even after the lymphatic system is rather generally involved. Lymph node enlargement may occur in very erratic fashion, first in one body region and then later in another near or distant region. The symptoms are often those of mechanical obstruction or of compression caused by the enlarged lymph nodes. After several years of disease the histologic pattern may change to a less differentiated cytologic type. Systemic symptoms intervene, relapses become more frequent, and resistance to treatment increases as the malignant cells spill beyond the confines of the lymphatic system. A fatal outcome is the ultimate rule, despite the initial symptom-free years.

The diffuse lymphocytic lymphomas are somewhat less benign, although individual cases may well follow a benign and protracted course (Pangalis and associates, 1977). About 50 per cent succumb within two years but 25 per cent are still alive after five years, and a significant number survive well beyond that. Focal or diffuse involvement of the marrow can be demonstrated in about one third of cases. When significant numbers of malignant cells infiltrate the circulating blood, the disorder is called lymphosarcoma cell leukemia, a condition which rather closely resembles chronic lymphatic leukemia. Lymphosarcoma cells have a more immature lacy nuclear chromatin pattern, a folded nucleus, and often irregular cytoplasmic outlines, but the distinction from chronic lymphatic leukemia may be difficult. A lymph node biopsy is not useful in the diagnosis of chronic lymphatic leukemia, but if one is obtained it will show a pattern indistinguishable from that of diffuse lymphocytic lymphoma.

Histiocytic lymphoma is the most malignant; 60 to 80 per cent of patients succumb within one year. However, even in this category individual patients not uncommonly defy over-all statistics and survive for five years or longer. Modern combination chemotherapy appears to have improved the over-all prognosis, and Fisher and co-workers report a five-year survival of 38 per cent of all patients treated. The tendency for the disease to first become apparent in extranodal sites — especially the gastrointestinal tract and bone — is most striking. Extensive involvement of the gastrointestinal tract or of the bone marrow predicts

---

TABLE 5–5   CLASSIFICATION OF
NON-HODGKIN'S LYMPHOMA

Nodular Lymphoma (Follicular Lymphoma)
   Poorly differentiated lymphocytic
   Mixed histiocytic-lymphocytic
   Histiocytic

Diffuse Lymphoma
   Well differentiated lymphocytic (lymphosarcoma)
   Poorly differentiated lymphocytic (lymphosarcoma)
   Mixed histiocytic-lymphocytic
   Histiocytic (reticulum cell sarcoma)
   Lymphoblastic
   Undifferentiated
      Burkitt's
      non-Burkitt's

(Modified from Rappaport, with more traditional terms in parenthesis. (From Byrne, G. E., Jr.: Cancer Treat. Rep., *61*:935, 1977.)

a poorer outcome for the patient. Marked weight loss with little overt manifestation of tumor growth, occult hepatosplenomegaly, or an infiltrating tumor of the muscle, brain, or almost any tissue may be the presenting sign. A leukemic phase of the illness occurs much more rarely than in diffuse lymphocytic lymphoma.

For the most part pathogenetic mechanisms in non-Hodgkin's lymphomas resemble those in Hodgkin's. Although chronologic patterns of progression may be capricious, spread usually occurs from the lymphatic system to the liver, spleen, and other tissues. Death may be caused by the tumor itself or it may come as a result of infectious complications which follow in the footsteps of the damage done to the immunologic system. Autoimmune phenomena, such as hemolytic anemia or thrombocytopenia, occur in a minority of patients before, concomitant with, or following the first overt sign of lymphoma. About 5 per cent of sera from non-Hodgkin's lymphoma have an IgM or IgG M-component, a finding which is rare in Hodgkin's. Other abnormalities of immunoglobulin production, such as Bence Jones proteinuria or hypogammaglobulinemia, are observed in some patients with non-Hodgkin's lymphoma but not as a rule in Hodgkin's. The several principles of staging outlined in the management of Hodgkin's lymphoma appear also to represent sound approaches to the patient with non-Hodgkin's types.

Other non-Hodgkin's lymphomas with distinctive clinical and morphologic features include lymphoblastic T cell lymphoma and Burkitt's lymphoma. Lymphoblastic T cell ("convoluted cell") lymphoma is a close relative of T cell ALL. It affects younger adults with rapidly growing tumors, usually affecting the mediastinum, with early transition to a leukemic phase and central nervous system involvement. The neoplastic cells are positive for terminal transferase. Most are also positive for T cell surface markers. Some also have complement receptors. The term "convoluted cell" refers to the surface contour of the cell nuclei as seen in fixed preparations. This appearance however cannot be relied upon as a marker of T cell origin (Greenberg and co-workers, 1976). Burkitt's lymphoma also has a rapid rate of cell proliferation. It commonly forms jaw tumors in the endemic African variety, although in the U.S.A. intra-abdominal presentation is more the rule. Despite the blastic appearance of the neoplastic cells they are heavily coated with surface IgM, identifying this lymphoma as a B cell type (Mann and associates, 1976).

M-Component Disorder. An "M-component" is the secretory product of a single monoclonal line of immunoglobulin-producing immunocytes. The abnormal protein is recognized as a narrow homogeneous band or "spike" in the electrophoretic pattern of serum or concentrated urine. It is the product of a cellular clone which has undergone an unusual degree of proliferation, often of a neoplastic character. The absolute production rate of the M-component can be used as a measure of the mass of the abnormal cell line, assuming that each cell produces a fixed quantity of immunoglobulin per unit time. The production rate can be estimated from measurement of its concentration and a knowledge of its turnover rate. An imbalance in the production rates of the subunits which combine to make up the immunoglobulin molecule causes overproduction of one of the subunits, usually L chains, which spill out readily into the urine because of their low molecular weight. The L chains, called "Bence Jones protein" in the premolecular era, are either κ or λ in type, but not both, a further demonstration of the monoclonal character of the cell of origin. Excesses of H chains in the serum and urine are a much more seldom observed event.

The presence of these abnormal proteins is sometimes uncovered by sheer diligence on the part of physicians, but increasingly they are discovered accidentally because of the frequency with which serum electrophoresis is used as a routine test. The heat test for Bence Jones protein in the urine is unreliable and should be replaced by electrophoresis of sufficiently concentrated urine. Paper dip techniques in common use for the routine detection of albuminuria are not sensitive to the presence in the urine of other proteins, such as L chains. L chains may be detected in the serum, but since they are so rapidly excreted by the kidney, their concentration is very low unless there is renal insufficiency. The concentration of the serum M-component varies from the range of 1 gram per 100 ml. to more than 10 grams per 100 ml. The daily urinary excretion of L chains may vary from less than 1 gram per day to 15 to 20 grams per day. Immunoelectrophoretic techniques are now in common use to classify the M-components of the serum and urine. Quantitation of immunoglobulins show depressed serum concentrations of the uninvolved types. The ability to produce specific antibody is often impaired. Recurrent bacterial pneumonia and other infectious complications then appear.

M-components in the serum sometimes confer strange properties upon it which may be of pathophysiologic significance. Reversible precipitation or gelation in the cold (i.e., the M-component is a "cryoglobulin") may cause circulatory embarrassment in exposed body parts. Red cells readily aggregate into "rouleaux," and the erythrocyte sedimentation rate is often rapid, but significant hemolysis usually does not occur. Bleeding may stem from antagonistic effects on plasma coagulation factors, fibrin polymerization, and platelet function. The M-component, especially if it is an

IgM type, may increase plasma viscosity by eight- to tenfold. Block and Maki have reviewed the "hyperviscosity syndrome" that may develop, with visual disturbances, retinal venous congestion and a sausage-like periodicity of the vein walls ("boxcar effect"), mental confusion, stupor, and even coma. Since the patients are usually aged, prompt recognition is not always achieved. Symptoms are quickly ameliorated by plasmapheresis. The excretion in the urine of large amounts of L chains is significantly related to the development of renal insufficiency, presumably through tissue deposition of L chains as amyloid, or by a direct toxic effect of this small protein on the renal tubule epithelial cells (Stone and Frenkel, 1975). Hypercalcemia and hyperuricemia also contribute to the multifactorial renal disease which complicates plasma cell myeloma.

Plasma cell myeloma is a malignant proliferation of plasma cells, usually in the bone marrow, sometimes forming solitary or multiple tumors, but almost always going on to widespread dissemination as diffuse "myelomatosis." Destructive bone disease is the major pathologic consequence, possibly because of the secretion locally of an osteoclast-stimulating factor (Mundy and associates, 1974). Localized osteolytic punched-out lesions affecting the skull, ribs, pelvis, or proximal portions of the long bones, as well as diffuse osteoporosis of the whole skeletal system, are common. Extramedullary myelomas may rarely form almost anywhere. Lymphatic involvement is not a feature of the disease, and hepatosplenomegaly is generally not detected. Localized bone pain and pathologic fractures are the most fearsome consequences. Symptomatic hypercalcemia, apparently related to bone dissolution, is common and may require emergency treatment.

Amyloidosis associated with plasma cell myeloma usually assumes the clinical features of the primary rather than the secondary form. Fragments of the L chains are invariably found in the tissue deposits. Musculoskeletal involvement is impressive and causes symptoms of arthritis, carpal tunnel syndrome, myocardial weakness, and macroglossia.

A mild normocytic and normochromic anemia is common, and about one third of patients have pancytopenia related to replacement of the marrow by the neoplastic plasma cells. Morphologic confirmation of the diagnosis is always necessary, either by biopsy of a plasma cell tumor or by random aspiration of bone marrow. If sheets of immature plasma cells replace the normal marrow cellular elements, the morphologic picture is diagnostic, but if the plasma cells are fewer, great care must be exercised in morphologic interpretation. Reactive plasmacytosis may increase the marrow plasma cells to 25 to 30 per cent of the total, although usually a reactive plasmacytosis is not in excess of 10 to 15 per cent. "Benign monoclonal gammopathy" and *primary amyloidosis* must also be distinguished from plasma cell myeloma. Increasing degrees of plasma cell immaturity along with frequent polyploid forms favor the latter diagnosis.

Depressed concentrations of the normal serum immunoglobulins are a constant feature of plasma cell myeloma. For quite some time this has been explained mechanistically as a "crowding out" of normal plasma cells by the neoplastic clone. Modern immunology has offered more plausible theories. These include the possibility of deficiencies of B cell surface receptors for antigen; excessive negative feedback from the high level of monoclonal protein and/or plasma cell mass; and depression of humoral immunity by a population of suppressor cells (Broder and associates, 1975).

Three fourths of plasma cell myeloma patients have either an IgG or an IgA M-component in the serum, IgG occurring twice as commonly as IgA. Almost all the remaining one fourth who lack such a serum component will have an M-component in the urine, with decreased serum immunoglobulin concentrations. In all, about one half to two thirds have demonstrable L chains in the urine. Rare cases of IgD and IgE myeloma have been reported. A few plasma cells are commonly seen in the peripheral blood in myeloma, but overt plasma cell leukemia is a rare and rapidly fatal variant.

Primary macroglobulinemia of Waldenström typically affects older people in their eighth decade. The clinical picture overlaps that of chronic lymphatic leukemia and lymphocytic lymphoma, in which about 5 per cent of patients have an M-component, usually IgM. The typical presentation of primary macroglobulinemia is one of a dense infiltration of the bone marrow with small mature lymphoid cells, many of which have plasmacytoid features. A number of typical plasma cells may also be seen. There is no leukemic infiltration of the blood; generalized lymphadenopathy and splenomegaly are present but are not marked. The diagnosis is confirmed by demonstrating the presence in the serum of an IgM M-component in excess of 2 grams per 100 ml. L chains may be found in the urine. Anemia is common and may be severe. Pancytopenia is not uncommon. Osteolytic bone lesions are exceptionally rare.

Finding an M-component in the serum or urine alone cannot be considered diagnostic of either of the above immunoproliferative conditions without the assistance of supporting information. The term *"benign monoclonal gammopathy"* has been applied to those patients with an M-component in the serum, usually less than 2 grams per 100 ml., without decreases in the other serum immuno-globulins, significant abnormalities in blood counts, bone disease, or more than a minority of mostly mature plasma cells in the marrow as reviewed by Abramson and Shattil. In some instances the M-component spontaneously disappears, suggesting that it may have been evoked as a physiologic but monoclonal response to some undetermined but highly specific antigen. About 15 per cent of these patients are discovered to have an associated carcinoma. A low concentration of monoclonal IgM occurs with cold agglutinin hemolytic anemia. Amyloidosis is thought to bear some relationship to an underlying process of plasma cell proliferation either of a secondary reactive nature, as in chronic infections, Hodgkin's lymphoma, or rheumatoid arthritis, or of a primary nature (Glenner and associates, 1973). Indeed one school of thought contends that primary amyloidosis is an expression of plasma cell myeloma, even in the absence of osteolytic bone disease and other diagnostic criteria of myeloma. M-components and marrow plasmacytosis are common findings in primary amyloidosis, the diagnosis of which is most readily confirmed by biopsy of the gum or rectal mucosa. In the absence of these associated conditions, patients with "benign monoclonal gammopathy" commonly remain stable and asymptomatic for many years and require no treatment, but in some instances the condition exists as the asymptomatic preclinical stage of plasma cell myeloma.

Heavy chain diseases are rare, having been first described by Franklin, who observed γ type H chains in the serum and urine of a patient with a lymphoma-like illness. A peculiar variant of H chain disease is the α type, which presents as a lymphoma of the small intestine in association with the signs and symptoms of sprue (Seligmann, 1975). The relationship is particularly intriguing because of the known abundance of IgA-secreting plasma cells in the normal gastrointestinal tract.

Therapy of the symptomatic M-component disorders is often successful and may arrest progression of the disease for years (Alexanian and co-workers, 1975). The chemotherapeutic agents of greatest utility have been alkylating agents (melphalan and cyclophosphamide) and adrenal glucocorticoids. Palliative radiation therapy is helpful for local bone pain and for such dread complications as spinal cord compression, for which surgical decompression may also be necessary.

Other Variants. *"Leukemic reticuloendotheliosis"* is now often considered a variant of lymphocytic lymphoma or chronic lymphatic leukemia, although as the name implies the abnormal cell was originally perceived as a reticuloendothelial cell, or macrophage (Naeim and Smith, 1974).

Because of the characteristic fringed cytoplasm of the neoplastic lymphoid cell seen by conventional microscopy, the disorder has earned the nickname *"hairy cell leukemia."* The neoplastic lymphoid cells infiltrate the bone marrow, spleen, and peripheral blood, but lymph node enlargement is not prominent. Splenectomy may be helpful. Resistance to chemotherapy has been the rule.

Mycosis fungoides and *Sézary syndrome* are two cutaneous variants of T cell lymphoma, the former characterized by a distinctive histologic feature of the skin (the "Pautrier abscess") and the latter by the presence in the peripheral blood of somewhat atypical convoluted lymphocytes containing a rim of PAS positive vacuoles surrounding the nucleus (Long and Mihm, 1974). Broder and co-workers have found that the Sézary syndrome is a neoplasia of functionally differentiated helper T cells which, as expected, are no longer positive for terminal transferase but do retain the characteristic surface markers. The cutaneous predilection may be the result of a "homing" instinct of this T cell subpopulation for the skin. Therapeutic responses to topical applications of nitrogen mustard have been explained by the hypersensitivity reaction evoked in the skin.

Pseudolymphoma. Some patients present clinical syndromes that lie in a twilight zone between lymphoma and chronic inflammatory states. These may be of a chronic autoimmune nature with an occasional subsequent lymphomatous transformation (e.g., *Sjögren's syndrome*). Others are idiopathic or drug-induced hypersensitivity states. Both clinicians and pathologists are faced with confusion and consternation in trying to arrive at a definite decision that only time will resolve. The term *"pseudolymphoma"* conveys the uncertainty. Lukes and Tindall have described the syndrome of *"immunoblastic lymphadenopathy,"* with lymph node enlargement, fever, sweats, an increase in polyclonal immunoglobulin, and a characteristic histopathologic picture. They postulate that it is a hypersensitivity state but allow that neoplastic transformation occasionally takes place. Chronic pulmonary lymphocytic infiltrates also fall in this general category (*lymphomatoid granulomatosis, lymphoid interstitial pneumonitis*) (Israel and associates, 1977). Similarly, lymphocytic infiltrations in the stomach, parotid, thyroid, or orbit may occasionally cause confusion in correctly distinguishing between a chronic inflammatory state and a lymphocytic lymphoma. Immunofluorescent staining of tissue sections to determine whether the lymphocyte population bears monoclonal or polyclonal surface immunoglobulin may help in sifting out the neoplastic conditions (Warnke and Levy, 1978).

REFERENCES

Abramson, N., and Shattil, J. J.: M-components. J.A.M.A., 223:156, 1973.

Alexanian, R., Balcerzak, S., Bonnet, J. D., Gehan, E. A., Haut, A., Hewlett, J. S., and Monto, R. W.: Prognostic factors in multiple myeloma. Cancer, 36:1192, 1975.

Belpomme, D., Mathé, G., and Davies, A. J. S.: Clinical significance and prognostic value of the T-B immunological classification of human primary acute lymphoid leukaemias. Lancet, i:555, 1977.

Block, K., and Maki, D.: Hyperviscosity syndromes associated with immunoglobulin abnormalities. Seminars Hematol., 10: 113, 1973.

Bortin, M. M., and Rimm, A. A.: Severe combined immunodeficiency disease. Characterization of the disease and results of transplantation. J.A.M.A., 238:591, 1977.

Broder, S., Edelson, R. L., Lutzner, M. A., Nelson, D. L., MacDermott, R. P., Durm, M. E., Goldman, C. K., Meade, B. D., and Waldman, T. A.: The Sézary syndrome. A malignant proliferation of helper T cells. J. Clin. Invest., 58:1297, 1976.

Broder, S., Humphrey, R., Durm, M., Blackman, M., Meade, B., Goldman, C., Strober, W., and Waldman, T.: Impaired synthesis of polyclonal (non-paraprotein) immunoglobulins by circulating lymphocytes from patients with multiple myeloma. Role of suppressor cells. N. Engl. J. Med., 293:887, 1975.

Byrne, G. E., Jr.: Rappaport classification of non-Hodgkin's lymphoma. Histologic features and clinical significance. Cancer Treat. Rep., 61:935, 1977.

David, J. R.: Lymphocyte mediators and cellular hypersensitivity. N. Engl. J. Med., 288:143, 1973.

Fauci, A. S., and Dale, D. C.: The effect of hydrocortisone on the kinetics of normal human lymphocytes. Blood, 46:235, 1975.

Fisher, R. I., DaVita, V. T., Johnson, B. L., Simon, R., and Young, R. C.: Prognostic factors for advanced diffuse histiocytic lymphoma following treatment with combination chemotherapy. Am. J. Med., 63:177, 1977.

Franklin, E. C.: Some impacts of clinical investigation on immunology. Surface IgD, IgE, and heavy-chain variants. N. Engl. J. Med., 294:531, 1976.

Fudenberg, H. H., Pink, J. R. L., Wang, A. C., and Douglas, S. D.: Basic Immunogenetics, 2nd ed. Oxford University Press, New York, 1978.

Geha, R. S., Schneeberger, E., Merler, E., and Rosen, F. S.: Heterogeneity of "acquired" or common variable agammaglobulinemia. N. Engl. J. Med., 291:1, 1974.

Glenner, G. G., Terry, W. D., and Isersky, C.: Amyloidosis: its nature and pathogenesis. Seminars Hematol., 10:65, 1973.

Gralnick, H. R., Galton, D. A. G., Catovsky, D., Sultan, C., and Bennett, J. M.: Classification of acute leukemia. Ann. Int. Med., 87:740, 1977.

Greenberg, B. R., Peter, C. R., Glassy, F., and MacKenzie, M. R.: A case of T-cell lymphoma with convoluted lymphocytes. Cancer, 38:1602, 1976.

Greenwood, M. F., Coleman, M. S., Hutton, J. J., Lampkin, B., Krill, C., Bollum, F. J., and Holland, P.: Terminal deoxynucleotidyl transferase activity in neoplastic and hematopoietic cells. J. Clin. Invest., 59:889, 1977.

Holland, J. F., and Glidewell, O.: Oncologists reply: survival expectancy in acute lymphocytic leukemia. N. Engl. J. Med., 287:769, 1972.

Israel, H. L., Patchevsky, A. S., and Saldana, M. J.: Wegener's granulomatosis, lymphomatoid granulomatosis, and benign lymphocytic angitis and granulomatosis of lung. Ann. Int. Med., 87:691, 1977.

Jaffe, E. S., Braylan, R. C., Nanba, K., Frank, M. M., and Berard, C. W.: Functional markers: a new perspective on malignant lymphoma. Cancer Treat. Rep., 61:953, 1977.

Klein, G.: The Epstein-Barr virus and neoplasia. N. Engl. J. Med., 293:1353, 1975.

Lai, P. K.: Infectious mononucleosis: recognition and management. Hosp. Pract., 12:8, 47, 1977.

Levine, A. S., Graw, R. G., Jr., and Young, R. C.: Management of infections in patients with leukemia and lymphoma. Cur-

rent concepts and experimental approaches. Seminars Hematol., 9:141, 1972.

Long, J. C., and Mihm, M. C.: Mycosis fungoides with extracutaneous dissemination; a distinct entity. Cancer, 34:1745, 1974.

Lukes, R. J., and Tindle, B. H.: Immunoblastic lymphadenopathy. A hyperimmune entity resembling Hodgkin's disease. N. Engl. J. Med., 292:1, 1975.

Mann, R. B., Jaffe, E. S., Braylan, R. C., Nanba, K., Frank, M. M., Ziegler, J. L., and Berard, C. W.: Non-endemic Burkitt's lymphoma. A B-cell tumor related to germinal centers. N. Engl. J. Med., 295:685, 1976.

Mauer, A. M., Saunders, E. F., and Lampkin, B. C.: Possible significance of nonproliferating leukemic cells. In Perry, S. (ed.): Human tumor cell kinetics. Natl. Cancer Inst. Monogr. 30:63, 1969.

Moran, E. M., and Ultman, J. E.: Clinical features and course of Hodgkin's disease. Clin. in Haematol., 3:91, 1974.

Mundy, G. R., Raisz, L. G., Cooper, R. A., Schechter, G. P., and Salmon, S. E.: Evidence for the secretion of an osteoclast stimulating factor in myeloma. N. Engl. J. Med., 291:1041, 1974.

Mundy, G. R., Raisz, L. G., Shapiro, J. L., Bandelin, J. G., and Turcotte, R. J.: Big and little forms of osteoclast activating factor. J. Clin. Invest., 60:122, 1977.

Naeim, F. and Smith, G. S.: Leukemic reticuloendotheliosis. Cancer, 34:1813, 1974.

Pangalis, G. A., Nathwani, B. N., and Rappaport, H.: Malignant lymphoma, well differentiated lymphocytic. Its relationship with chronic lymphocytic leukemia and macroglobulinemia of Waldenström. Cancer, 39:999, 1977.

Parkman, R., Gelfand, E. W., Rosen, F. S., Sanderson, A., and Hirschhorn, R.: Severe combined immunodeficiency and adenosine deaminase deficiency. N. Engl. J. Med., 292:714, 1975.

Patchevsky, A. S., Brodovsky, H. S., Menduke, H., Southard, M., Brooks, J., Nicklas, D., and Hoch, W. S.: Non-Hodgkin's lymphoma: a clinico-pathologic study of 293 cases. Cancer, 34:1173, 1974.

Paul, W. E., and Benacerraf, B.: Functional specificity of thymus dependent lymphocytes. Science, 195:1293, 1977.

Podleski, W. K.: Cytodestructive mechanisms provoked by lymphocytes. Am. J. Med., 61:1, 1976.

Polliack, A., Lampen, N., Clarkson, B. D., and De Harven, E.: Identification of human B and T lymphocytes by scanning electron microscopy. J. Exp. Med., 138:607, 1973.

Prosnitz, L. R., Hellman, S., vonEssen, C. F., and Kligerman, M. M.: The clinical course of Hodgkin's disease and other malignant lymphomas treated with radical radiation therapy. Am. J. Roentgenol., 105:618, 1969.

Seligmann, M.: Immunochemical, clinical, and pathological features of α-chain disease. Arch. Int. Med., 135:78, 1975.

Simone, J. V.: Childhood leukemia: the changing prognosis. Hosp. Practice, 9:7, 59, 1974.

Stone, M. J., and Frenkel, E. P.: The clinical spectrum of light chain myeloma. A study of 35 patients with special reference to the occurrence of amyloidosis. Am. J. Med., 58:601, 1975.

Tomasi, T. B.: Secretory immunoglobulins. N. Engl. J. Med., 287:500, 1972.

Tsukada, M., Hanamura, K., Eguchi, M., Komiyama, A., and Akabane, T.: Scanning electron microscopic study of peripheral blood lymphocytes, thymic cells, and acute lymphoblastic leukemic cells in children. Acta Haematol. Jap., 39:43, 1976.

Uhr, J. W.: The membranes of lymphocytes. Hosp. Pract., 10:3, 113, 1975.

Waldman, T. A.: Disorders of suppressor cells in the pathogenesis of immunodeficiency, autoimmune and allergic diseases: human disease associated with disorders of an immunological breaking system. Ann. Allergy, 39, 79, 1977.

Walker, W. A., and Isselbacher, K. J.: Intestinal antibodies. N. Engl. J. Med., 297:767, 1977.

Warnke, R., and Levy, R. Immunopathology of follicular lymphomas. A model of B-lymphocyte homing. N. Engl. J. Med., 298:481, 1978.

6

Thrombocytes

STRUCTURE

In 1906, Wright first proposed that the megakaryocyte, a well-known but mysterious bone marrow giant cell, produced blood platelets. Numerous subsequent morphologic and kinetic studies have supported this proposal and shown that this cell plays a key role in hemostasis. The average megakaryocyte measures about 5000 μ^3 in volume (Fig. 1–11) but cells almost twice that size and with diameters of more than 100 μ are often seen. Like other differentiated precursor cells, the megakaryocyte descends from a committed stem cell (CFU-M) programmed to undergo blast transformation to a megakaryoblast. This blast cell is morphologically similar to other blast cells, but the nucleus is engaged in rapid DNA synthesis without cell cleavage, so-called endomitosis. Within a few days, the blast cell has grown considerably in size, and the single dense nucleus may contain 2, 4, 8 or even 16 times the normal diploid content of DNA. At that time, further DNA synthesis and nuclear endomitosis cease and cellular maturation commences. The nucleus becomes lobulated and the cytoplasm increases in volume, both processes occurring in rough proportionality to the ploidy of the cell. Specific cytoplasmic organelles appear and the cytoplasm takes on a pale blue granular appearance. At this stage the cytoplasm becomes burrowed out by invaginated surface membrane which transforms the cytoplasm into a honeycomb of granulated fragments. These are then peeled off in long ribbons into the bone marrow sinusoids where they finally break up into individual platelets. After the lobulated megakaryocytic nucleus has become depleted of cytoplasm it is rapidly disposed of by macrophages.

As is true for the red blood cells, the newly formed platelets are larger than more mature forms, and careful sizing of blood platelets on a peripheral blood smear may provide information about the rate of platelet production. The mature platelets are disk-shaped, measure about 2 to 3 μ in diameter and are pale blue with a granular core. On electron microscopy (Fig. 6–1), the core is found to consist of glycogen granules, mitochondria, vacuoles, and various dense particles. The glycogen and mitochondria provide energy essential for viability and function. The vacuoles appear to be part of a spongelike canalicular system covered by interiorized phospholipid-containing surface membrane. This system facilitates the absorption of and interaction with various coagulation factors and also serves as a conduit for substances released from cytoplasm. Some of the dense particles, are enzyme-containing lysosomes, whereas others contain ADP and serotonin, which are released during aggregation. The platelets also contain a network of microfilaments which are organized into microtubules under the platelet membrane. These structures contain contractile proteins and may be responsible for the conversion from discoid to spherical shape which takes place during aggregation and subsequent clot retraction.

FUNCTION

Platelets constitute our first and foremost line of defense against accidental blood loss. They accumulate almost instantaneously at the site of a vascular injury and attempt first to provide a temporary seal by plugging the vascular leak and second to promote the formation of a permanent seal by making available an essential coagulation factor. The aggregation of non-sticky, circulating platelets into a firm platelet plug is a remarkable feat which is triggered by contact of the platelets to exposed subendothelial tissue, resulting in turn in phospholipase activation, prostaglandin and thromboxane synthesis, and the release of ADP. Observations in vitro, summarized by Zucker and by Deykin, have shown that the addition of small amounts of ADP to platelet-rich suspensions causes a change in the suspension stability, with smooth disk-shaped

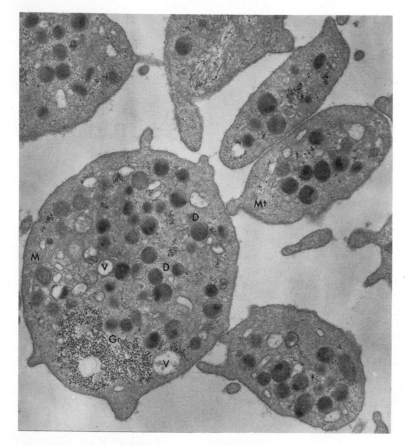

Figure 6–1 Electron microscopic picture of normal platelets showing dense particles (*D*), vacuoles (*V*), mitochondria (*M*), micro-tubules (*Mt*), and glycogen granules (*Gr*). (Courtesy of Dr. D. Zucker-Franklin.)

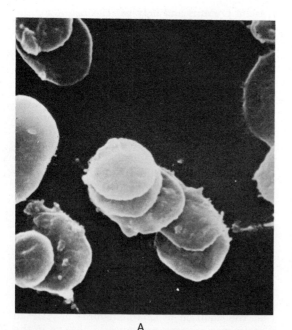

A

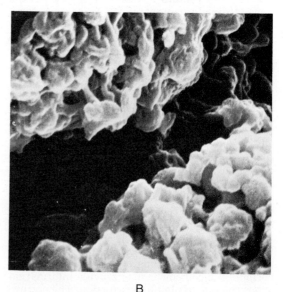

B

Figure 6–2 Pictures made by the scanning electron microscope of free disk-shaped platelets (*A*) and aggregates of spiny transformed platelets (*B*). (From Hovig, T.: Series Hematologica, *3*:47, 1970.)

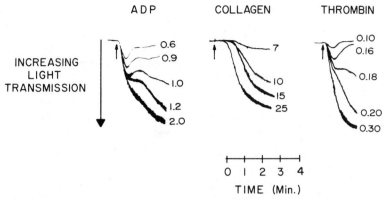

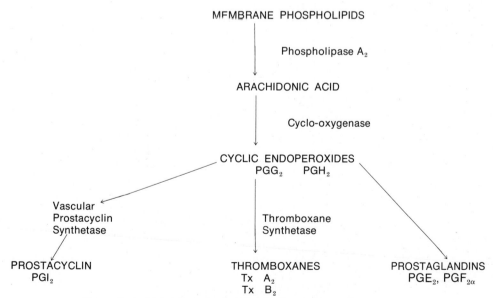

ADP COLLAGEN THROMBIN

INCREASING LIGHT TRANSMISSION

TIME (Min.)

Figure 6–3 Aggregation of human platelets in citrated platelet-rich plasma at 37° C. ADP, collagen suspension, or thrombin was added (arrow) to give the fluid concentrations shown (μ moles/liter, μ liter/ml., or units/ml., respectively). Photometric recordings indicate the increase in light transmission as the platelets aggregate over a period of about 3 minutes. (Courtesy of Dr. D. C. B. Mills.)

granulated platelets being transformed reversibly into aggregates of spiny, sticky degranulated spheres (Fig. 6–2). Large amounts of ADP will result in an irreversible aggregation of platelets, whereas intermediate amounts cause a characteristic biphasic response with aggregation, disaggregation, and renewed aggregation (Fig. 6–3). The second wave of aggregation is believed to be induced by endogenous ADP released from storage granules in the platelet. The addition of collagen to a platelet-rich suspension causes degranulation but only one wave of aggregation corresponding in time to the second ADP wave and believed to be due in part to collagen-induced release of endogenous ADP from platelets.

Prostaglandins E_2 and $F_{2\alpha}$ are formed during platelet aggregation, and the addition of aspirin or indomethacin will impair both prostaglandin formation and platelet aggregation (Smith and Willis, 1971). This basic observation has led to extensive studies, reviewed by Smith and Silver, of the role of prostaglandins in platelet function. It has been found that platelet aggregation activates a phospholipase which makes free arachidonic acid available to a platelet cyclo-oxygenase, transforming it to the short-lived but potent aggregating cyclic endoperoxides PGG_2 and PGH_2 (Fig. 6–4). This enzymatic transformation is inhibited by aspirin or indomethacin. The cyclic endoperoxides are either transformed to very small amounts of inactive prostaglandin PGE_2 or $PGF_{2\alpha}$ or by means of thromboxane synthetase to large amounts of another short-lived but potent aggregating agent, thromboxane TXA_2. These observations of in vitro activity provide the framework for our current concept of the mechan-

MEMBRANE PHOSPHOLIPIDS

Phospholipase A_2

ARACHIDONIC ACID

Cyclo-oxygenase

CYCLIC ENDOPEROXIDES
PGG$_2$ PGH$_2$

Vascular Prostacyclin Synthetase

Thromboxane Synthetase

PROSTACYCLIN
PGI$_2$

THROMBOXANES
Tx A$_2$
Tx B$_2$

PROSTAGLANDINS
PGE$_2$, PGF$_{2\alpha}$

Figure 6–4 Platelet prostaglandin and thromboxane formation.

ism responsible for the formation of a hemostatic platelet plug.

The initiating event in hemostasis is vascular injury with exposure of otherwise concealed collagen fibers to circulating blood (Fig. 6–5). Within a few seconds platelets passing by will adhere to the raw collagen fibers, become degranulated, and release ADP, prostaglandin intermediates, and serotonin, which in turn cause aggregation of new platelets, further ADP release, and further platelet aggregation. In this fashion a chain reaction is established, with the formation of a firm platelet plug covering the vascular break. In addition, a phospholipoprotein, so-called platelet factor 3, is unmasked on the surface of the transformed platelets. This membrane-bound factor augments thrombin formation and results in the coating of the platelet plug with resilient fibrin and the formation of a white thrombus. Thrombin also causes platelet aggregation, prostaglandin synthesis, and ADP release and contributes to both the platelet and the fibrin phases in the formation of a hemostatic seal.

Recent studies by Moncada and co-workers have disclosed that normal vascular walls contain prostacyclin synthetase which transforms platelet endoperoxides into prostacyclin PGI_2 which actively inhibits platelet aggregation. The presence of this prostacyclin may provide a balance for the proaggregating endoperoxides and thromboxane A_2, and vessel injury could conceivably decrease the production of prostacyclin and thereby tilt the balance toward aggregation and

clotting. A certain amount of intravascular coagulation and red thrombus formation takes place before the flow of blood has diluted and dissipated ADP, thrombin, and other procoagulants. Final clot retraction and consolidation are caused by thrombosthenin, a contractile platelet protein. Similar to other contractile proteins, it acts as an ATPase and requires ATP as an energy source. The release of prostaglandins, serotonin, and lysosomal enzymes during the early phase of platelet adhesion and aggregation is in part also responsible for the inflammatory reaction that may occur around a newly formed thrombus.

In addition to sealing vascular breaks, platelets appear to play an almost continuous role in maintaining normal vascular integrity. Patients with thrombocytopenia have a decreased capillary resistance, and petechiae appear following the slightest trauma or change in blood pressure. It seems probable that these petechiae are caused by superficial endothelial desquamations which under normal conditions are sealed immediately by platelets but in patients with thrombocytopenia remain open and permit the escape of a small amount of blood.

KINETICS

Until recently, kinetic studies of megakaryocytes and thrombocytes have appeared quite forbidding because of difficulties in quantitating the rate of production of platelets, the size of the circulating platelet mass, and the life span of

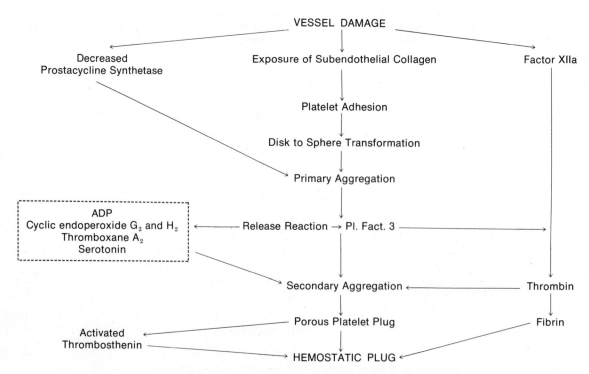

Figure 6–5 Formation of hemostatic platelet plug

individual platelets. However, careful planimetric measurements of megakaryocytes in bone marrow sections, the introduction of phase contrast microscopic measurements, automatic particle counting, and the use of random and cohort labeling with various isotopes have provided valuable and reproducible kinetic data. These data indicate that platelet production, like red cell production, is controlled by a feedback system which regulates the transformation of a committed but undifferentiated stem cell to a differentiated blast cell.

As previously emphasized, our current concept of the bone marrow stem cell pool is that it is made up of a multipotential compartment and several unipotential compartments, one of them committed to the megakaryocytic cell line (Fig. 1–7). The interrelationship between these compartments is not clear, but it appears that the multipotential stem cells are predominantly dormant (G_0) and are called into supportive action only if the committed stem cell compartments become depleted. Because increased erythropoiesis after blood loss or hemolysis is often associated with increased thrombopoiesis and under certain conditions with decreased granulocytopoiesis, questions have been raised, but not answered, about specific cooperation or competition among the committed stem cell compartments. In response to demands for platelets, the stem cells committed to megakaryocytes undergo blast transformation and differentiate to megakaryoblasts. During the next two to three days and before visible cytoplasmic maturation, the nucleus divides two to four times, resulting in the formation of a large blast cell. After the endomitotic division has ceased the nucleus becomes lobulated, the cytoplasm matures, granulated material segregates, and platelets are finally peeled off two to three days later. It has been estimated (Table 1–1) that the normal human bone marrow contains about 15×10^6 megakaryocytes per kg. body weight, with each megakaryocyte producing about 2000 to 7000 platelets. Since the average megakaryocytic volume is about $5000 \mu^3$, the total megakaryocytic mass is about $45 \times 10^9 \mu^3$ per kg. body weight, about one tenth the total mass of nucleated red cell precursors $(5 \times 10^9 \times 90 \mu^3)$. However, the daily production of platelets, about 2.5×10^9 per kg. body weight, is close to that of erythrocytes, about 3.1×10^9 per kg. body weight.

After the release from the bone marrow, the platelets will circulate for about eight to ten days before they are removed and destroyed by the macrophages, primarily in liver and spleen. During their circulating life span, the platelets are distributed between the spleen and the bloodstream. Aster has pointed out that, at any one time, about one third of the circulating platelets are present in the spleen, probably in a slow transit through the tortuous splenic cords rather than as trapped and starved cells. A transit time of merely 8 minutes would explain such a segregation of the total platelet mass between spleen and blood. It has been proposed that the youngest platelets are sequestered preferentially by the spleen but this may be due to a slower transit time of cells of larger size. Certainly, the sequestration of platelets in the spleen does not appear to last long enough to produce cellular injury, and splenic contraction induced by epinephrine will expel perfectly normal platelets into the circulation. The physiologic significance, if any, of the splenic pooling of platelets is not known, but its existence does explain that the platelet count almost invariably is higher in splenectomized than in normal individuals. In patients with splenomegaly, a significant proportion of the circulating platelets is slowly meandering through the large spleen, and although total platelet mass may be normal, the platelet count can be quite low. This splenomegalic thrombocytopenia is rarely as severe as thrombocytopenia caused by hypersplenic destruction of platelets. However, hemostasis depends on the number of circulating platelets, and if a large spleen cannot mobilize its content of platelets in time, the effect is the same as if the platelets had been permanently destroyed.

Since platelets are consumed during their function as hemostatic agents, it could have been anticipated that their destruction would be random rather than age-dependent. In other words, survival curves should be exponential rather than linear with time. Somewhat surprisingly, however, most studies of platelet life span utilizing random labels such as [51]chromium or cohort labels such as [32]phosphorus have indicated an age-dependent linear life span (Fig. 6–6). Furthermore, studies by Abrahamsen of individuals receiving anticoagulants have failed to show a change in the slope of the survival curve or a prolongation of the platelet life span. This would tend to rule out the existence of major continuous intravascular coagulation with random platelet utilization. However, the spread of the survival curve is wide enough to conceal the presence of some minor random utilization in addition to the major age-dependent destruction.

Under physiologic conditions, the platelet count and especially the platelet mass are kept constant, indicating the existence of a feedback system adjusting platelet production to platelet destruction. This feedback has a built-in delay that causes a considerable rebound thrombocytosis after induced thrombocytopenia and rebound thrombocytopenia after induced thrombocytosis (Fig. 6–7). The magnitude of this delay in humans can be estimated from careful measurements of the platelet count in patients who have undergone splenectomy. In such patients the platelet count tends to oscillate, with a period twice as long as the time it takes from the initia-

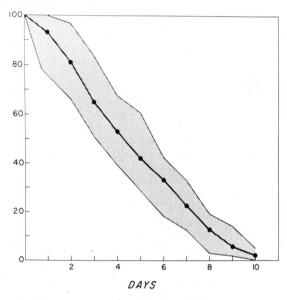

CIRCULATING PLATELET ⁵¹Cr
(% of Maximum Value)

DAYS

Figure 6–6 Survival of ⁵¹Cr-labeled human platelets. Shaded area from 30 normal subjects. (From Aster, R. H.: J. Clin. Invest., 45:645, 1966.)

tion of a signal for increased platelet production until the produced platelets have finished their life span. This oscillating pattern is occasionally very pronounced (Fig. 4–8), making it easy to discern a period which in most cases is quite uniform, about 28 days. Since the life span of platelets is about 10 days, the delay from the triggering effect of a stimulus until the platelet is released from the bone marrow must be around 4 days, which is about the time it takes for the megakaryoblast to mature into a megakaryocyte and release platelets. The stimulus could act either on the megakaryoblasts causing them to undergo additional endomitotic divisions, thereby increasing their volume, and producing more platelets, or it could act on committed stem cells causing the production of an increased number of megakaryoblasts. Since the megakaryocytes of

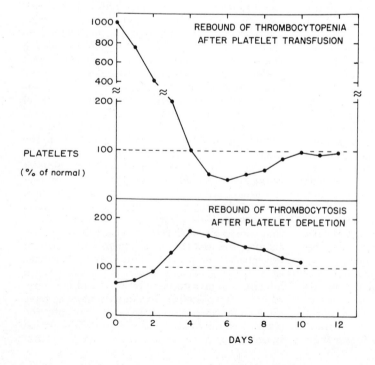

PLATELETS
(% of normal)

DAYS

Figure 6–7 Rebound thrombocytopenia after platelet transfusion and rebound thrombocytosis after platelet depletion in normal rats. (Adapted from Odell, T. T., Jr., et al.: Acta Haematol., 38:34, 1967, and Odell, T. T., Jr., et al.: Acta Haematol., 27:171, 1962.)

patients with thrombocytopenia due to increased platelet destruction are both larger and more numerous than normal, Harker concluded that the stimulus does both. It has also been suggested that the stimulus shortens maturation time, a suggestion more difficult to accept because the introduction of additional endomitotic divisions should lengthen the total maturation time, unless of course the generation time is cut way down.

Numerous investigators have suggested that the responsible stimulus is transmitted by a specific humoral factor, a so-called thrombopoietin (Adams, et al., 1978). Evatt and Levin, followed by McDonald, were the first, however, to provide convincing experimental data in support of this suggestion. Utilizing [75]selenium methionine to label megakaryocytic cytoplasm, Levin and co-workers showed that injection into normal animals of serum from donors with thrombocytopenia will cause a greater isotope incorporation into new platelets than injections of serum from normal donors. The difference becomes more pronounced if endogenous thrombopoiesis of the recipient is suppressed by platelet transfusions (Fig. 6–8). Although the technique is similar to the technique which has been used successfully in the study of erythropoietin, the logistic problems of maintaining a preparatory thrombocytosis are so large that very little additional information about thrombopoietin has been obtained.

If a thrombopoietin controls the production of platelets, what controls the production of thrombopoietin? Obviously platelets are needed for the maintenance of vascular integrity and it would seem likely that impaired hemostasis causes the release of a thrombopoietin in the same way as impaired oxygenation of the kidney causes the release of erythropoietin. However, as shown by the age-dependent life span of platelets, most platelets do not get involved in hemostatic activities. Furthermore, hemostatic function remains normal until the platelet count is reduced far below the level at which a compensatory increase in platelet production is initiated. Finally, the patients with congestive splenomegaly in whom up to 80 per cent of the total platelet mass is in the spleen fail to show a compensatory increase in platelet production despite low circulating platelet count and impaired hemostatic function. These observations suggest that it is the platelet mass rather than the platelet count which triggers the release of thrombopoietin. On the other hand, it is very difficult to envision a sensor which can perceive the size of the platelet mass, distributed as it is between the spleen and the circulating blood. Furthermore, it seems possible that rather than being the number or mass, it is the surface area which is involved in sensing and adjusting the concentration of thrombopoietin. The platelet surface is well known to act as a sponge and absorb a variety of plasma factors. Actually, deGabriele and Penington have shown that thrombopoietic activity of plasma could be removed by preincubation with normal platelets. Consequently, platelet function, mass, and surface have to be incorporated into the hypothetical model of the feedback circuit controlling platelet production and depicted in Figure 6–9.

PATHOPHYSIOLOGY

Classification and General Considerations

The thrombocytic disorders are usually classified according to number and function of platelets into "quantitative abnormalities" and "qualitative abnormalities" (Table 6–1).

In general, patients with platelets in inadequate numbers or with inadequate functional competence will have petechiae, hemorrhages, prolonged bleeding time, and impaired clot re-

Figure 6–8 Effect of plasma from thrombocytopenic donor rabbits upon incorporation of selenomethionine-75 ([75]SeM) into the platelets of rabbits previously transfused with platelet concentrates. The plasma, in volume from 20 ml. to 150 ml., was administered in three divided doses and [75]SeM was given 6 hours after the last infusion (solid lines). The broken line is the mean [75]SeM utilization in six platelet transfused control rabbits. (From Shreiner, D. P., and Levin, J.: J. Clin. Invest., *49*:1709, 1970.)

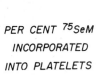

PER CENT [75]SeM
INCORPORATED
INTO PLATELETS

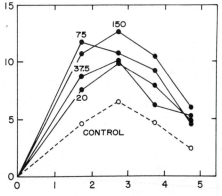

DAYS AFTER ADMINISTRATION OF [75]SeM

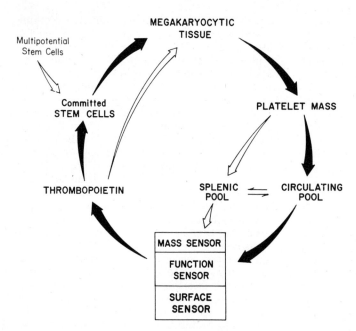

Figure 6–9 Model of a feedback control system for platelets. (Adapted from Erslev, A. J.: Am. J. Pathol., *65*:629, 1971.)

traction. Since platelets are primarily responsible for hemostasis in small superficial vessels, petechiae are the hallmark of platelet deficiency disorders. Local pressure from tissue tension will tend to diminish blood loss from deep vessels, and the presence of many petechiae and hemorrhages on the skin or visible mucous membrane does not necessarily mean that similar bleedings are present throughout the body. Actually, deep bleedings into tissues or joint spaces are much more characteristic of a deficiency in coagulation proteins than of a deficiency in platelets. The minimal number of platelets needed for normal hemostasis is usually considered to be about 50,000 per

cu. mm. However, spontaneous hemorrhages are rare until the platelet count is reduced to less than 20,000 per cu. mm. Observations by Karpatkin and others indicate that the hemostatic competence of young, large platelets is greater than that of old platelets, explaining that hemorrhagic problems tend to be less at a given platelet level for individuals with thrombocytopenia due to peripheral destruction than for those with thrombocytopenia due to decreased production.

Elevated platelet counts are usually tolerated well but may cause either thrombosis or bleeding. The thrombotic tendency is probably related to an excessive hemostatic response to minor vascular injury, but the reason for the bleeding tendency in face of an increased number of functional platelets is still unknown.

Quantitative Abnormalities

Thrombocytopenia. *Decreased platelet production* occurs in a bewildering collection of congenital and acquired disorders. In some the pathogenesis has been unraveled but in most the responsible dysfunction of the megakaryocytes awaits identification.

Of special interest among the many descriptions of individual cases is a report by Shulman and co-workers about a child with severe congenital thrombocytopenia who was found to respond to infusions of normal plasma with brief increases in platelet count and who for many years has been kept alive and functioning on regularly spaced plasma infusions. The responsible plasma factor was named thrombopoietin and was believed to cause maturation of existing mega-

TABLE 6–1 CLASSIFICATION OF THROMBOCYTIC DISORDERS

I. *Quantitative Abnormalities*
    Thrombocytopenia
        Decreased production
            Congenital
            Acquired
                Megakaryocytic disorders
                Bone marrow replacement
        Increased destruction
            Immune
            Consumptive
        Uneven distribution
            Hypersplenism
        Thrombocytosis
            Reactive
            Myeloproliferative disorders
II. *Qualitative Abnormalities*
    Congenital
    Acquired

karyocytes. Reevaluation of this case recently has suggested a link to thrombotic thrombocytopenic purpura and to the responsiveness of this disease to plasma.

Acquired abnormalities of megakaryocytes causing moderately severe thrombocytopenia are usually found in patients with megaloblastic anemia due to folic acid or B_{12} deficiency, and specific treatment causes a prompt return of platelet count to normal. Patients with chronic alcoholism also may have maturation problems of both nucleated red cells and megakaryocytes, but the cause is difficult to pinpoint, since such patients usually suffer from a multitude of nutritional deficiencies and hepatic abnormalities. Nevertheless, metabolic studies by Post and Des Forges have demonstrated that one cause may be alcohol itself, which apparently impairs megakaryocytic function directly. Although iron deficiency has been associated with thrombocytopenia, thrombocytosis is observed far more commonly. If decreased platelet production is found in iron-deficient patients, it is usually assumed that complicating deficiencies of folic acid or B_{12} are responsible.

Viral infections and exposures to certain drugs are often associated with megakaryocytic dysfunction and thrombocytopenia. During pregnancy, such infections and exposures may lead to neonatal thrombocytopenia, usually of short duration. However, if the bone marrow insult occurs during the first trimester, a specific syndrome characterized by *amegakaryocytic thrombocytopenia,* malfunction of the heart, and absence of the radius may occur. Since the megakaryocytes, heart, and radius all appear at about the sixth to eighth week of gestation, an infectious or toxic insult at that time may explain the development of this seemingly unrelated triad. In both children and adults, viral infections frequently cause thrombocytopenia. For example, inoculation with live measles vaccine will, as Oski and Naiman have shown, regularly cause a temporary decrease in platelet production. As a general principle, a self-limited viral infection should always be suspected as the etiology in every patient with unexplained thrombocytopenia. Despite this frequent association, drugs are actually the most common cause of defective platelet production. The many myelosuppressive agents used in the treatment of neoplastic and autoimmune disorders make up the majority of drugs causing thrombocytopenia. The anticipated response to such drugs is a general bone marrow suppression, but certain drugs such as cytosine arabinoside and busulfan have a reputation for causing particularly marked suppression of platelet production. More capricious and still unexplained is the mild megakaryocytic suppression which may follow the use of thiazide diuretics. It has recently been suggested that they may bring about a process of immunologic "rejection" of megakaryocytes akin to the "rejection" of nucleated red cells observed in patients with pure red cell aplasia. However, drug-induced immunologic injury of megakaryocytes is a far less common cause for thrombocytopenias than drug-induced, immunologic destruction of circulating platelets.

Among disorders of *increased destruction,* antibodies play a prominent role. Immunologic destruction of platelets can cause thrombocytopenia at any age. In the newborn the pathogenetic mechanism is similar to that causing erythroblastosis fetalis inasmuch as an antibody produced in the mother crosses the placenta and causes destruction of the infant's platelets. During pregnancy and at time of delivery, platelets from the fetus pass into the circulatory system of the mother, and if they contain antigens different from hers, they will evoke an antibody response. The subsequent transfer of the antibody across the placenta results in platelet destruction and thrombocytopenia. Such isoimmune thrombocytopenia does not depend on ABO or Rh incompatibility but on incompatibility in the platelet specific antigens (Pl^{A1}) or the more general HL-A tissue antigen system. Since tests for antigens and antibodies in this system are time-consuming and difficult, the diagnosis is usually made by exclusion. First, thrombocytopenia due to infections has to be ruled out immediately. Maternal viremia can cause changes in the fetal production and destruction of platelets, and bacteremia in the newborn may be associated with disseminated intravascular coagulation and thrombocytopenia. Other infectious etiologies to be excluded are congenital syphilis, toxoplasmosis, cytomegalic inclusion disease, and rubella. Second, the possibility that the mother has idiopathic thrombocytopenic purpura with an anti-platelet autoantibody crossing the placenta and non-specifically attacking the infant's platelets must be excluded by obtaining a thorough history and a platelet count on the mother. Finally, maternal drug ingestion must be looked into as a possible cause.

In children and adults, the cause for immunologic destruction of platelets is usually idiopathic, but the possibility that it is drug related should always be considered. Quinidine is the most widely recognized offender, and its mechanism of action is slowly being unraveled. When attached to a protein the drug acts as a hapten, causing the production of antibodies in sensitized individuals. It was first assumed that the hapten attached itself to a platelet protein and that this hapten-platelet complex elicited and responded to antibody. However, recent data suggest that the hapten is bound to a plasma protein carrier and that it is this complex which elicits and combines with antibody. The subsequent binding of the antigen-antibody complex to platelet membrane is due to a chance affinity between the immune complex and the membrane, and the platelet is actually an "innocent bystander" in the immunologic reaction (Fig. 6–10). Unfortunately for the platelets the coating with antigen-antibody complexes causes agglutination, complement-fixation, and destruction. A great number of drugs have been implicated in immunologic platelet destruction but only in a few instances have in-vivo and in-vitro testing convincingly shown a drug to be causative. (Miescher, 1973). In addition to quinidine, quinine, stibophen, digitoxin, methyldopa, sulfonamides, sedormid and gold have been so identified. The association of aspirin or birth control pills with thrombocytopenia has been of interest, but the possibility of a mere coincidence rather than a cause-effect relationship has not been ruled out. In order to establish a diagnosis of drug-induced thrombocytopenia several in-vitro tests have been developed. These are based on finding impaired platelet function after the addition of the drug to the patient's plasma. Inhibition of normal clot retraction is the easiest test (Fig. 6–11) but it is less sensitive than tests depending on agglutination, lysis, complement fixation, or release of platelet factor 3.

Idiopathic thrombocytopenic purpura (ITP) is a disorder characterized by increased platelet destruction in an otherwise healthy individual. In childhood, ITP is usually acute and time-limited, and many studies have related it immunologically to a preceding viral infection. In adults, ITP is usually chronic and, although also believed to be immunologically determined, its etiology is still truly idiopathic.

Acute thrombocytopenia may follow well-established viral infections such as rubella, rubeola, or chicken pox, but in most cases the preceding illness consists merely of a mild respiratory or gastrointestinal upset, so frequently experienced in childhood that it is often overlooked. The thrombocytopenia is usually first noticed after the "viral symptoms" have subsided, suggesting that the platelet injury is caused by antibodies rather than by the virus itself. It has been proposed that platelet antibodies are elicited by platelet membranes antigenetically altered by the attachment of viral particles. However, similar to the mechanism believed to operate in drug-induced thrombocytopenia, the platelets may merely be "innocent bystanders" with a fatal affinity for viral antigen-antibody complexes. In either case, the antibody production and action would depend on the presence of a circulating viral antigen, and the disease would be of limited duration. Complete recovery can be expected if the patient is carried through the dangerous thrombocytopenic period by the judicious use of careful observation, protection against trauma, platelet transfusions, and corticosteroids. Splenectomy, although undoubtedly effective, need

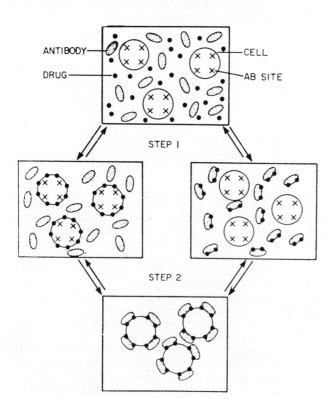

Figure 6–10 Possible mechanism for drug-induced and other immunologic thrombocytopenias. *Left,* the platelets are directly involved by initially being coated by antigen. *Right,* the platelets act as "innocent bystanders." (From Shulman, N. R.: Ann. Intern. Med., *60*:506, 1964.)

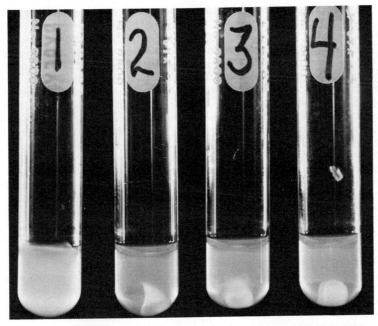

Figure 6–11 A positive clot retraction inhibition test in a patient with quinidine-induced purpura. The four test tubes were prepared as follows:

	Serum	Quinidine	Normal Platelet-Rich Plasma
(1)	Patient	+	+
(2)	Patient	−	+
(3)	Control	+	+
(4)	Control	−	+

After one hour of incubation, $CaCl_2$ was added, and the degree of clot retraction inhibition was observed one hour later. Inhibition of clot retraction is seen in tube 1.

rarely be contemplated in the acute time-limited ITP of childhood.

The chronic variety of ITP is a disease of adults, although children who fail to recover from acute ITP must be included. Like acute ITP, it is believed to be immunologically induced, but if a foreign antigen is involved, this antigen must be an almost permanent component of the body, since the disease despite remissions is rarely cured. The thrombocytopenia often found in association with disseminated lupus erythematosus is considered an ITP, since its pathogenesis is still clearly idiopathic.

The immunologic nature of this disorder was first suspected when Harrington and co-workers found that plasma or its gamma globulin fraction from patients with chronic ITP caused thrombocytopenia when infused into normal subjects. Supportive evidence for the existence of an autoimmune mechanism was provided by the fact that infants of mothers with chronic ITP often have transient thrombocytopenia at birth and that in-vitro immunologic tests indicate the presence of an antiplatelet antibody in plasma from a large number of patients with chronic ITP. So far the antibody has reacted with all platelets, re-gardless of antigenic composition, and it appears that it is directed against a common platelet component rather than a type-specific antigen. The agent responsible for the production of autoantibodies is unknown, but the life-long presence of certain viral antigens in tissue cells makes a viral etiology an attractive hypothesis.

The severity of chronic ITP and its response to splenectomy seems to be dependent on the amount of antibody coating the platelets. Heavy coating will cause agglutination with easy recognition, sequestration, and destruction by all macrophages, and splenectomy by removing merely a fraction of these will be of only moderate therapeutic benefit. Light coating, however, will not cause significant agglutination of circulating platelets, and only the spleen with its slow percolation of blood through vessels densely lined with macrophages will recognize, sequester and destroy coated platelets. In this condition, splenectomy will be of definite benefit, and the life span and function of lightly coated platelets will be almost normal after surgery. In a few cases the titer of antiplatelet antibodies has decreased after splenectomy, suggesting that the spleen preferentially produces these antibodies and that splenectomy not only removes a filter but also eliminates a major site of antiplatelet antibody production (McMillan, et al., 1974).

One of the most controversial findings in chronic ITP has been the presence of megakaryocytes of unusual morphologic appearance. Not only are they increased in number, as would be expected as a compensation for increased destruction of mature platelets, but many are immature, devoid of intracytoplasmic demarcations, and show no evidence of active platelet production (Fig. 6–12). It has been suggested that the antibody to circulating platelets also reacts with megakaryocytes and prevents platelet formation. However, platelet turnover studies show an increased rate of platelet production, and it seems more likely that accelerated thrombopoietic activity causes an early release of platelets from still immature cells and a shift to the left in the megakaryocytic series. The presence of unusually large platelets in the blood of patients with chronic ITP also suggests a hurried production with the release of unfinished pieces of megakaryocytic cytoplasm.

The clinical manifestations of chronic ITP are determined entirely by the number of available platelets, and the treatment is directed toward maintaining the number at an asymptomatic level. As expected, platelet transfusions are of very brief effect, since transfused platelets are destroyed as fast as endogenous platelets. Adrenocortical steroids are usually quite effective in increasing the platelet count in patients with chronic ITP. They may act by suppressing phagocytic activity, but the exact reason for their beneficial effect still has not been established (Claman, 1972). In patients who do not respond to steroids with an increase in platelet count, the bleeding manifestations are nevertheless reduced, as if the steroids in some way enhance capillary stability. In the treatment of chronic ITP, steroids usually are administered for a few months in the hope that the disease will remit spontaneously. If the thrombocytopenia recurs immediately after discontinuation of the drug or if the patient is only partly responsive, splenectomy is the treatment of choice. Splenectomy will result in a sustained improvement in 70 to 90 per cent of patients. In almost all, the operation will be followed by a brief thrombocytosis which reaches its peak at about the tenth day and then slowly decreases over the next few months (Fig. 6–13). This sequence corresponds well to the fact that in the absence of the spleen the platelets produced by the increased number of megakaryocytes live a normal 10-day life span, and it suggests that it must take some time to adjust the number of megakaryocytes in the bone marrow to the actual need for platelets in the circulation. Postsplenectomy thrombocytosis is of concern in patients in whom postoperative complications force them to rest immobile in bed, and in such patients the use of preventive anticoagulants or

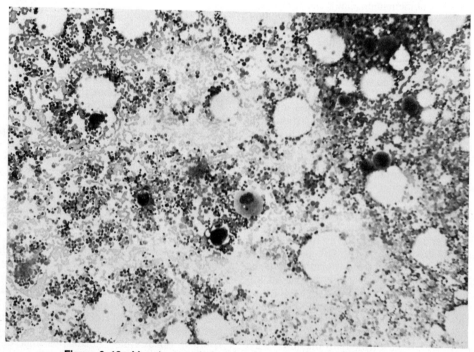

Figure 6–12   Megakaryocytic hyperplasia in patient with chronic ITP.

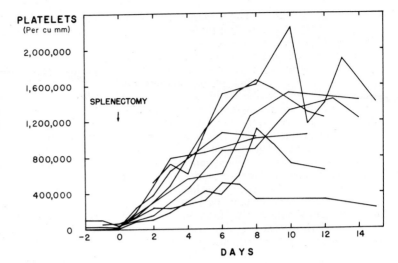

PLATELETS
(Per cu mm)

Figure 6–13 Thrombocytosis following splenectomy in patients with ITP.

platelet antiaggregating agents may be indicated. It is assumed that platelets of patients who do not derive lasting benefit from splenectomy are so heavily coated with antibody that they are removed by the total mononuclear phagocyte system, not merely by the spleen. In such patients, immunosuppression has been attempted using drugs developed for the treatment of neoplastic disorders. In some patients gratifying remissions have been obtained especially after the use of vincristine, but the decision to use these potentially leukemogenic agents certainly has to be made with great reluctance and only if other methods of treatment fail.

Post-transfusion purpura is an unusual syndrome consisting of a temporary period of thrombocytopenia with onset about a week after blood transfusion. The disorder occurs only in individuals lacking the platelet-specific antigen (Pl^{A1}), a circumstance found in only 1 to 2 per cent of the population. The presence of this antigen in platelet material present in the transfused blood evokes the production of an antibody in the recipient. Immune complexes adhere to the patient's own platelets ("innocent bystanders") bringing about their destruction as in quinidine purpura. Spontaneous remission occurs when the immune complexes are cleared from the circulation.

Non-immunologic destruction of circulating platelets in bacterial or viral infections is often difficult to separate from immunologic destruction since these infections may be associated with both. However, non-immunologic destruction usually occurs at the height of the infectious illness and is accompanied by decreased levels of several coagulation proteins such as fibrinogen and Factors V and VIII. The pathogenesis is believed to be increased platelet consumption due to *disseminated intravascular coagulation* (DIC) (Deykin, 1970). Despite the presence of purpura

and increased bleeding tendency, heparin may be the treatment of choice whenever laboratory studies indicate an increased rate of consumption of platelets and coagulation proteins. The thrombocytopenia characterizing *"thrombotic thrombocytopenic purpura"* or the *"hemolytic uremic syndrome"* is probably caused by excessive intravascular deposition of platelets in cerebral and renal vessels. However, there is little evidence of excessive consumption of coagulation proteins and it appears that these diseases are caused by a platelet or vascular wall dysfunction due to the absence of a plasma factor. The recent therapeutic use of exchange transfusions and of plasma infusions appears most promising in these otherwise highly fatal diseases (Byrnes and Khurana, 1977).

Thrombocytopenia is observed regularly in patients with splenomegaly, and in the past many explanations were given for the development of this *hypersplenic thrombocytopenia*. The most obvious explanation for the thrombocytopenia would appear to be increased platelet destruction by the large spleen, but this explanation was made untenable some years ago when Cohen, Gardner, and Barnett found that the platelet life span in patients with hypersplenic thrombocytopenia was normal. The alternate explanation, that platelet production was decreased owing to the effect of megakaryocytic inhibitors released by the large spleen, was also found to be untenable because platelet turnover studies did not suggest a decreased rate of platelet production. Recent studies by Aster of platelet kinetics have provided a third and much more likely explanation.

As described earlier, the spleen, because of its tortuous vascular channels, always contains a considerable number of platelets in slow transit. In patients with splenomegaly, the transit time becomes longer, and instead of containing about 30 per cent of all circulating platelets, a large spleen may contain up to 80 per cent of the platelets. Since platelet production appears to be aimed at maintaining a constant total platelet mass, the uneven distribution of platelets between spleen and circulating blood is not being compensated for by an increased rate of platelet production, and the splenomegalic patient will stay thrombocytopenic. This explanation is supported by the observation that the infusion of platelets to patients with hypersplenic thrombocytopenia results in lower peripheral recovery than normal (Fig. 6–14) and that large numbers of viable platelets can be mobilized from an intact spleen by giving epinephrine and from an excised spleen by flushing its vascular system with saline. Supporting evidence is also provided by the fact that hypersplenic thrombocytopenia is not always proportional to the size of the spleen but is more closely related to its vascularity. For example, congestive splenomegaly secondary to liver cirrhosis is usually associated with lower platelet counts than "meaty" splenomegaly secondary to lymphomas or lipidosis. The potential availability of splenic platelets and the distributional limits to the number of platelets which can be present in the spleen make this thrombocytopenia rather mild and rarely in need of treatment per se.

Thrombocytosis. Thrombocytosis occurs as an obscure reactive response to a number of ill-

nesses and as a manifestation of the myeloproliferative syndrome. A high platelet count is a useful diagnostic clue in patients with anemia, since iron deficiency regularly causes an increase in platelet production, and counts in excess of one million per cu. mm. may be found in children with nutritional iron deficiency anemia. Other conditions in which a high platelet count may be of diagnostic help are Hodgkin's disease, disseminated malignant diseases, and chronic inflammatory disorders (Schloesser, et al., 1965; Tranum and Haut, 1974; and Marchasin, et al., 1964). Pronounced thrombocytosis with levels of several millions per cu. mm. is usually seen only after splenectomy or in myeloproliferative disorders, such as polycythemia vera, myelofibrosis, chronic myelogenous leukemia, or essential thrombocytosis. The clinical manifestations of very high platelet counts consist of a capricious combination of thrombotic episodes and increased bleeding tendency. The thromboses are probably caused by aggregation and platelet factor 3 release by the expanded platelet mass, but the bleeding tendency is more difficult to explain. Cardamone and co-workers have found a platelet dysfunction in some cases, but in most cases the only abnormality found has been an increase in the number of circulating platelets.

Qualitative Abnormalities

Qualitative abnormalities of platelet function have been found in a confusing collection of rare hereditary disorders and more commonly in uremia or after ingestion of certain drugs such as aspirin, antihistamines, and antiinflammatory agents. The inherited disorder most often found is *von Willebrand's disease* described in the next chapter. *Glanzmann's thrombasthenia* is seen more rarely and is characterized by a prolonged bleeding time, impaired clot retraction, and absent ADP-induced aggregation. The number and morphology of platelets and megakaryocytes are normal, but the patients suffer from a mild, lifelong increased bleeding tendency. Impaired platelet glycolysis with decreased ATP production and decreased reductive capacity has been found in some cases (Karpatkin and Weiss, 1972), whereas in others the adsorption of fibrinogen to platelets appears to be defective. *Storage pool disease* is a recently recognized congenital disorder of platelet formation (Holmsen and Weiss, 1972). The platelets respond to exogenous ADP with a normal first-phase aggregation, but fail to release endogenous ADP in response to collagen (second-phase aggregation). The number of ADP-containing dense particles is diminished, suggesting that the basic abnormality is a defect in the production, packaging, or storing of ADP. The clinical consequences are mild, and consist pri-

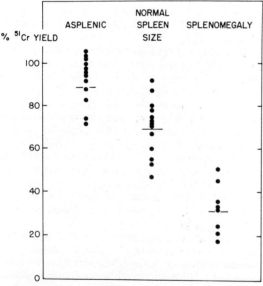

Figure 6–14   Recovery of transfused platelets in the circulating blood of asplenic patients, normal patients, and patients with congestive splenomegaly. (Gardner, F.: Clin. Haematol., *1*:307, 1972.)

marily of increased bruising and excessive bleeding after trauma or surgery. The so-called *thrombopathies* are congenital platelet disorders with even less of a common metabolic denominator than the thrombasthenias. The platelets may be larger than normal in size, so-called *Bernard-Soulier syndrome,* or they may be defective in platelet factor 3 activity, in ADP release, in adhesive capacity, and so on, but so far the cases are collectors' items and have failed to provide unifying clues.

Of the acquired disorders of platelet function, the clinically most important is the disorder found associated with chronic renal failure. Purpura and increased bleeding tendency are important manifestations of uremia and occur regularly despite normal platelet counts. Platelets from affected individuals have been found to be lacking in platelet factor 3 activation. However, of probably greater significance is the finding that these platelets fail to aggregate normally in response to ADP. Intensive dialysis rectifies this

response and also normalizes the bleeding time, and it seems most likely that a retention product of small molecular size is responsible for the platelet defect. Horowitz has proposed that this chemical is guanidinosuccinic acid, a metabolite of urea, but definite proof is still lacking. The effect of aspirin on in-vitro platelet function is quite remarkable. The ingestion of only one to two aspirin tablets will cause a week-long impairment in the release of platelet ADP in response to collagen or other aggregating agents such as epinephrine. Studies by Roth and Majerus suggest that this impaired ADP release may be caused by irreversible aspirin-induced acetylation of platelet cyclo-oxygenase necessary for the transformation of arachidonic acid to prostaglandin endoperoxides. Although aspirin clinically has been associated with an increased bleeding tendency, it must be conceded that bleeding problems, despite the striking in-vitro changes, are rare among the millions who daily consume aspirin preparations.

REFERENCES

Abrahamsen, A. F.: Platelet survival studies in man — with special reference to thrombosis and atherosclerosis. Scand. J. Haematol., Suppl. 3, 1968, p. 7.

Adams, W. H., Liu, Y. K., and Sullivan, L. W.: Humoral regulation of thrombopoiesis in man. J. Lab. Clin. Med., 91:141, 1978.

Aster, R. H.: Pooling of platelets in the spleen: Role in the pathogenesis of "hypersplenic" thrombocytopenia. J. Clin. Invest., 45:645, 1966.

Byrnes, J. J., and Khurana, M.: Treatment of thrombotic thrombocytic purpura with plasma. N. Engl. J. Med., 297:1386, 1977.

Cardamone, J. M., Edson, J. R., McArthur, J. R., and Jacob, H. S.: Abnormalities of platelet function in the myeloproliferative disorders. J.A.M.A., 221:270, 1972.

Claman, H N,: Corticosteroids and lymphoid cells. N. Engl. J. Med., 287:388, 1972.

Cohen, P., Gardner, F. H., and Barnett, G. O.: Reclassification of the thrombocytopenias by the ⁵¹-Cr-labeling method for measuring platelet lifespan. N. Engl. J. Med., 264:1294, 1961.

deGabriele, G., and Penington, D. G.: Regulation of platelet production: "thrombopoietin." Br. J. Haematol., 13:210, 1967.

Deykin, D.: The clinical challenge of disseminated intravascular coagulation. N. Engl. J. Med., 283:636, 1970.

Deykin, D.: Emerging concepts of platelet function. N. Engl. J. Med., 290:144, 1974.

Erslev, A. J.: Feedback circuits in the control of stem cell differentiation. Am. J. Path., 65:629, 1971.

Evatt, B. L., and Levin, J.: Measurements of thrombopoiesis in rabbits using ⁷⁵selenomethionine. J. Clin. Invest., 48:1615, 1969.

Gardner, F. H.: Platelet kinetics and lifespan. Clin. Haematol., 1:307, 1972.

Harker, L. A., and Finch, C. A.: Thrombokinetics in man. J. Clin. Invest., 48:963, 1969.

Harrington, W. J., Minnich, V., Hollingsworth, J. W., and Moore, C. V.: Demonstration of a thrombocytopenic factor in the blood of patients with thrombocytopenic purpura. J. Lab. Clin. Med., 38:1, 1951.

Holmsen, H., and Weiss, H. J.: Further evidence for a deficient

storage pool of adenine nucleotides in platelets from some patients with thrombocytopathia — "storage pool disease." Blood, 39:197, 1972.

Horowitz, H. J.: Uremic toxins and platelet function. Arch. Intern. Med., 126:823, 1970.

Hovig, T.: Influence of various compounds on blood platelets and platelet aggregation. A scanning electron microscopic study. Series Haematol., 3:47, 1970.

Karpatkin, S.: Heterogeneity of human platelets. II. J. Clin. Invest., 48:1083, 1969.

Karpatkin, S., and Weiss, H. J.: Deficiency of glutathione peroxidase associated with high levels of reduced glutathione in Glanzmann's thrombasthenia. N. Engl. J. Med., 287:1062, 1972.

McMillan, R., Longmire, R. L., Yelenosky, R., Donnell, R. L., and Armstrong, S.: Quantitation of platelet-binding IgG produced in vitro by spleens from patients with idiopathic thrombocytopenic purpura. N. Engl. J. Med., 291:812, 1974.

Marchasin, S., Wallerstein, R. D., and Aggeler, P. M.: Variation of the platelet count in disease. Calif. Med., 101:95, 1964.

Miescher, P. A.: Drug-induced thrombocytopenia. Seminars Hematol., 10:311, 1973.

Moncada, S., Gryglewski, S., Bunting, S., and Vane, J. R.: An enzyme isolated from arteries transforms prostaglandin endoperoxides to an unstable substance that inhibits platelet aggregation. Nature, 263:663, 1976.

Odell, T. T., Jr., Jackson, C. W., and Reiter, R. S.: Depression of the megakaryocyte platelet system in rats by transfusion of platelets. Acta Haematol., 38:34, 1967.

Odell, T. T., Jr., McDonald, T. P., and Asano, M.: Response of rat megakaryocytes to bleeding. Acta Haematol., 27:171, 1962.

Oski, F. A., and Naiman, J. L.: Effect of live measles vaccine on the platelet count. N. Engl. J. Med., 275:352, 1966.

Post, R. M., and Des Forges, J. F.: Thrombocytopenia and alcoholism. Ann. Intern. Med., 68:1230, 1968.

Roth, G., and Majerus, P.: The mechanism of the effect of aspirin on human platelets. I. Acetylation of a particulate fraction protein. J. Clin. Invest., 56:624, 1975.

Schloesser, L. L., Kipp, M. A., and Wenzel, F. J.: Thrombocytosis in iron-deficiency anemia. J. Lab. Clin. Med., 66:107, 1965.

Shreiner, D. P., and Levin, J.: Detection of thrombopoietic activity in plasma by stimulation of suppressed thrombopoiesis. J. Clin. Invest., *49*:1709, 1970.

Shulman, I., Pierce, M., Lukens, A., and Currimbhoy, Z.: Studies on thrombopoiesis. I. A factor in normal human plasma required for platelet production; chronic thrombocytopenia due to its deficiency. Blood, *16*:943, 1960.

Shulman, N. R.: A mechanism of cell destruction in individuals sensitized to foreign antigens and its implications in autoimmunity. Ann. Intern. Med., *60*:506, 1964.

Smith, J. B., and Silver, M. J.: Prostaglandin synthesis by platelets and its biologic significance. *In* Gordon, J. L. (ed.): Platelets in Biology and Pathology. North Holland Pub. Co., Amsterdam, 1976, p. 331.

Smith, J. B., and Willis, A. L.: Aspirin selectivity inhibits prostaglandin production in human platelets. Nature, *231*:235, 1971.

Tranum, B. L., and Haut, A.: Thrombocytosis: Platelet kinetics in neoplasia. J. Lab. Clin. Med., *84*:615, 1974.

Wright, J. H.: The histogenesis of the blood platelets. J. Morphol., *21*:263, 1910.

Zucker, M. B.: Platelet function. *In* Williams, W. J., et al. (eds.): Hematology, 2nd ed. McGraw-Hill Book Co., New York, 1977, p.1200.

7

Plasma Coagulation Factors

NORMAL STRUCTURE AND FUNCTION

WHITE AND RED THROMBI

The circulatory system is self sealing, thanks to the clotting ability of the blood and the contractility of the vascular wall. Leakages ranging from pinpoint hemorrhages to life-threatening exsanguination may occur when the coagulation mechanism breaks down. On the other hand, the pathologic formation of clots within the intact circulatory system is equally serious. The cause and nature of clot formation within the circulatory system vary with the site. The "white thrombus," consisting of platelets trapped in a fibrin meshwork, forms in rapid-flow arterial systems at points where the continuity of the endothelial lining is interrupted. The "red thrombus" has a white head with growth downstream of a red tail and is found in the venous system as a result of stasis of blood flow. Clots in large vessels are likely to undergo fibrous organization and recanalization, whereas those formed in the microvasculature are dissolved by virtue of the presence in the vascular wall of potent activators of the fibrinolytic system.

Although platelets are the "prime movers" in the formation of the white thrombus, the substance and strength of the clot, whether white or red, lie in the physical nature of the fibrin polymer which is formed as the end-product of a complex and controlled series of sequential reactions of the plasma coagulation factors. The nomenclature of the plasma coagulation factors has undergone revision over the years. Current and past usage is summarized in Table 7–1. Factors V and VII through XIII are in fact most commonly designated by their numbers today, while Factors I and II are generally called fibrinogen and prothrombin, respectively. There is no Factor VI. Factor III is tissue thromboplastin and should not be confused with platelet factor 3.

The cascade hypothesis has provided a conceptual framework that pictures the coagulation factors existing in an inactive (or procoagulant) and active state. The active form of one factor specifically activates the next one in line in a sequential series of controlled reactions, giving rise to a cascade, or "waterfall" effect. The process of activation is accomplished for most of the factors by the enzymatic splitting off of a small piece of the inactive procoagulant. There is progressive acceleration and amplification of the chain of reactions culminating in the formation of the fibrin clot. Most of the activated clotting factors (designated "a") are serine proteases, which are a family of protein-cleaving enzymes with serine at their active centers. Factors V, VIII, XIII, and fibrinogen are notable exceptions. Coagulation factor serine proteases have a high degree of substrate specificity. Plasmin is also a serine protease with the major function of cleaving fibrin and fibrinogen.

Fibrinogen

Fibrinogen, the raw material for the production of the clot, is a major constituent of the plasma, with a normal concentration of 200 to 400 mg. per

TABLE 7–1 PLASMA COAGULATION FACTORS AND THEIR SYNONYMS

Factor I	Fibrinogen
Factor II	Prothrombin
Factor III	Tissue thromboplastin
Factor IV	Calcium
Factor V	Proaccelerin
Factor VII	Proconvertin; SPCA
Factor VIII	Antihemophilic Factor (AHF)
Factor IX	Plasma thromboplastin component (PTC), Christmas factor
Factor X	Stuart-Prower factor
Factor XI	Plasma thromboplastin antecedent (PTA)
Factor XII	Hageman factor
Factor XIII	Fibrin stabilizing factor

100 ml. The other plasma factors, present in much lower concentration, stand poised as the parts of a loaded gun with trigger cocked, aimed at fibrinogen. Most of the body pool of fibrinogen circulates in the plasma with a catabolic rate having a half-life of four days. The plasma concentration readily increases secondary to a large number of stimuli, including pregnancy, acute or chronic inflammatory states, and injury or surgical operation. The increase is entirely accounted for by increased synthesis, which takes place in the liver.

Fibrinogen spends an uneasy existence in the plasma, circulating between the forces of clot promotion, represented by thrombin, and those of clot dissolution, represented by plasmin. Its molecular weight of 340,000 is equally divided between two identical subunits centrally bound together to give the molecule a symmetrical mirror-image structure (Fig. 7–1). Each of the subunits consists of an Aα, a Bβ, and a γ polypeptide chain, the N-terminal ends of which are bound together into a "disulfide knot." Thrombin acts enzymatically on fibrinogen at arginyl-glycyl bonds by splitting off small pieces from the N-terminal ends of the Aα and Bβ chains amounting to about 3 per cent of the total molecular weight. The pieces split off are called fibrinopeptides A and B, respectively, with fibrinopeptide A released at a more rapid rate than B. Their cleavage from the parent molecule leaves behind "fibrin monomer," which then rapidly undergoes intermolecular association to form hydrogen-bonded polymers. The clot is finally strengthened by the action of Factor XIIIa. This causes strong linkage between adjacent fibrin strands through crosslinking peptide bonds which join γ and α chains in an intermolecular association. Such "stabilization" renders the clot insoluble in 5 M urea and rather more resistant to plasmin digestion.

Certain snake venoms resemble thrombin in their action on fibrinogen. Pit viper venom hydrolyzes only the Aα polypeptide chains, releasing fibrinopeptide A. The parent molecule, like fibrin monomer, polymerizes into a clot. However, the clot is weak and is readily dissolved through the action of plasmin.

In contrast to the limited fibrinogen degradation which sets off its polymerization into a firm clot, the degradative process of clot dissolution by plasmin involves a much more aggressive attack upon the molecule at multiple points in its structure. Plasmin (or "fibrinolysin") is an enzyme which resembles trypsin in its breadth of action as an endopeptidase which splits lysine and arginine bonds. Like trypsin, it attacks a variety of proteins, including plasma proteins. It is active at neutral pH; trypsin has a more alkaline pH optimum. The circulating plasma proteins are not physiologically exposed to its broadly destructive propensity, since it circulates as an inactive precursor, plasminogen, which is activated locally at the site of clot deposition. Plasmin attacks fibrinogen with the same fervor that characterizes its assault upon fibrin. The degradation products of the two cannot be distinguished and therefore are referred to as fibrinogen-fibrin degradation products, or "split products."

During the initial degradation of fibrinogen by plasmin, its molecular weight is reduced from 340,000 to 270,000 with the release of low molecular weight fragments from the carboxy-terminal ends of the Aα chains and the amino terminal ends of the Bβ chains (Fig. 7–2). The latter fragments contain the B fibrinopeptides. The macromolecular structure which remains, called fragment X, retains the property of engaging in clot formation after exposure to thrombin. However, in comparison to fibrin monomer, it clots slowly and its presence weakens the clot structure. Fragment X undergoes additional cleavage by

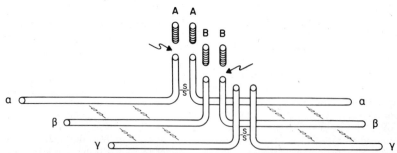

Figure 7–1 Schematic illustration of the molecular structure of fibrinogen. Three pairs of polypeptide chains (Aα, Bβ, and γ) are symmetrically arranged with their N-terminal regions joined in the "N-terminal disulfide knot." The C-terminal regions are represented here at opposite ends of the molecule, although they may actually be juxtaposed in the three dimensional orientation of the globular molecule. Thrombin cleavages release fibrinopeptides A and B, as shown by the arrows. Thus, the structure of fibrinogen is (AαB$\beta\gamma$)$_2$ and that of fibrin monomer is ($\alpha\beta\gamma$)$_2$. Disulfide bonding is symbolically represented; the N-terminal disulfide knot alone has 12 bonds. (Adapted from Marder, V. J., and Budzynski, A. Z.: Schweiz. Med. Wochenschr. *104*:1338, 1974.)

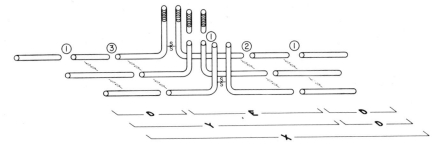

Figure 7–2 The degradation of fibrinogen by plasmin. The first stage (1) releases small fragments, including fibrinopeptide B, leaving behind fragment X. In the second stage (2) fragment X is asymmetrically reduced to fragments D and Y. The third stage (3) results in further breakdown of fragment Y to fragments D and E. The latter contains the N-terminal disulfide knot.

plasmin, with further reduction of molecular weight to derivatives designated fragment Y (MW 155,000) and fragment D (MW 90,000). Both of these fragments are nonclottable, but they interfere with fibrin strand formation and are potent anticoagulants. As degradation goes on to completion, fragment Y is further reduced to fragments D and E. The latter contains the N-terminal disulfide knot, has a MW of 55,000, and is relatively less active with regard to its anticoagulant effect.

Excessive action of plasmin in vivo is best detected by demonstrating elevated levels of fibrinogen-fibrin degradation products in serum from which all clottable material has been completely removed in the presence of a fibrinolytic inhibitor. Although excess plasmin activity most commonly occurs secondary to abnormal clotting, a high level of "split products" does not distinguish primary from secondary fibrinolysis. The presence of soluble complexes of fibrin monomer polymerized with fibrinogen-fibrin degradation products into higher molecular weight derivatives clearly signals that the increased plasmin activity was preceded by excessive action of thrombin on fibrinogen. These soluble complexes are demonstrated in plasma by tests for "paracoagulation." These include precipitation after addition of protamine sulfate, reversible insolubility in the cold (hence the term "cryofibrinogen"), and gelation after addition of ethanol. Nossel has proposed that excessive action of thrombin on fibrinogen in vivo might also be detected by an assay of the plasma for its content of fibrinopeptide A.

Plasminogen

Plasminogen is present in the plasma at a concentration of 10 to 20 mg. per 100 ml. Potent and specific plasminogen activators are present in many tissues and body fluids. As an example, the plasminogen activator of the urinary tract keeps this system free of clots and the potential disaster they could cause by obstructing the flow of urine. Especially large quantities of plasminogen activators are found in white cell lysosomes, from which they are released with difficulty, and also in the endothelial cells which line the vascular walls, from which release easily occurs. The development of a fibrin clot causes a rapid release of plasminogen activator into the clot, where it converts plasminogen to plasmin (Fig. 7–3). Plasmin thus appears mostly at the site of the clot, with relatively little spilling over into the general circulation. Plasmin is unstable and its activity soon disappears. Circulating plasmin inhibitors also contribute to the systemic protection of fibrinogen and other plasma proteins. Since the ratio of surface endothelium to cross-sectional area is greatest in the microcirculation, this is the site within the circulatory system with the greatest potential for plasminogen activation and complete clot dissolution.

A variety of influences other than fibrin deposition also bring about the release of plasminogen activators from the endothelium. These include exercise, acute stress of almost any kind, and pharmacologic and other kinds of vasoreactive stimuli. The increase in plasma fibrinolytic activity, however, is transient and mild, since the plasminogen activators are rapidly cleared from the plasma by the liver with a half-life of only 13 minutes. The impairment of this clearing mechanism will lead to somewhat less transient and less mild degrees of systemic fibrinolysis, a situation which arises in shock or in the presence of liver disease, as described by Hillenbrand and associates.

Surface Activation

Rupture of the endothelial lining of blood vessels exposes collagen and initiates thrombus formation. The fibrin clot is laid down as the end result of the recognition of the altered surface by Factor XII, which then becomes activated. Beyond its role in initiating clot formation, Fac-

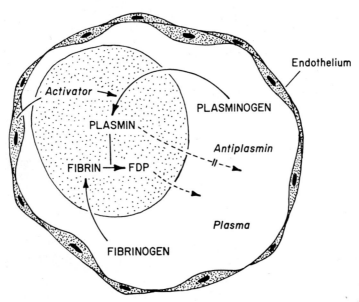

Figure 7–3   The local activation of plasminogen at the site of fibrin clot within a small blood vessel. (*FDP* = fibrin degradation products.)

tor XIIa also initiates reactions leading to the formation of vasoactive peptides (kinins) and plasmin and to the activation of the complement system. Despite the fact that Factor XII stands at the central point of this variety of events important to the defensive inflammatory response, inherited deficiency of this factor produces no clinical consequences, even though laboratory parameters such as the partial thromboplastin time are abnormal. A possible explanation may lie in the existence of "back-up" systems and "built-in safeguards," requirements of any skillfully engineered system which must be free from

failure. But the nature of these safeguards is still not understood.

Normal clotting in vitro is dependent on the kallikrein-kinin system, since deficiency of prekallikrein (Fletcher factor) or of high molecular weight kininogen (Fitzgerald factor) causes an abnormal prolongation of the partial thromboplastin time (Figure 7–4) (Donaldson and coworkers, 1976). Like Factor XII deficiency, lack of either of these factors causes no abnormal clinical effects, including bleeding. Although evidence indicates that kallikrein amplfies Factor XII activation in a feedback reaction, most of the details

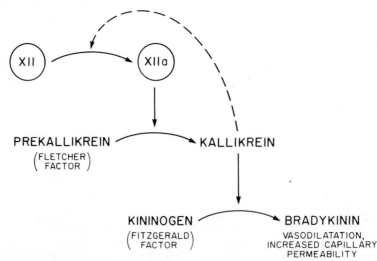

Figure 7–4   The interrelationship of Factor XII (Hageman factor), prekallikrein (Fletcher factor), and kininogen (Fitzgerald factor).

relating the kallikrein-kinin system to the initiation of the plasma coagulation factor cascade remain to be filled in.

Vitamin K Dependent Factors

The biologic activities of Factor II, VII, IX, and X depend upon an adequate supply of vitamin K, which comes mostly from the diet with a smaller proportion from bacterial synthesis in the gastrointestinal tract. These four factors share similar amino acids in certain areas of their structure and this homology has suggested a common genetic locus of origin early on in evolution, even though Factor IX is X-linked while the other three factors are autosomal. Vitamin K is not involved in the assembly of the amino acid backbones of these factors, but rather plays a key role in their post-synthetic transformation in the hepatocytes, as summarized by Davie and Fujikawa. This modification converts the factors from inert proteins to the biologically active forms present in normal plasma. Most of the investigations have dealt with prothrombin, but it is likely that the same mechanism applies to the others. Vitamin K mediates the carboxylation of ten glutamic acid residues clustered near the amino terminal end of the molecule. The carboxylation occurs at the γ position yielding γ-carboxyl glutamic acid derivatives. Calcium binding is dependent upon this cluster of carboxyl groups; without calcium binding the factor has no activity. In the vitamin K-depleted individual, prothrombin and presumably Factors VII, IX, and X in the plasma cannot be detected by their usual functional properties. However, they are present in adequate quantities if measured by their immunochemical properties.

Certain adsorbents, such as barium sulfate, selectively remove the vitamin K-dependent factors from plasma. This process, like calcium binding, is also dependent on carboxylation. Adsorption is useful in preparing test plasma deficient in the vitamin K-dependent factors for use in laboratory diagnosis. Elution from the adsorbent yields factor concentrates therapeutically useful in the management of patients with hemophilia B as well as in certain other hemorrhagic circumstances.

The coumarin anticoagulants compete with vitamin K in the body to bring on a deficiency of the vitamin K-dependent factors. They are of therapeutic value in the prevention of thrombosis. It takes about six hours before the effect is counteracted by the administration of vitamin K. Obviously, the coumarins are not active when added to plasma in vitro.

Factor VIII

The structure of Factor VIII has remained elusive for a long time, but recently the mystery has begun to unravel, giving rise to a picture of a most unorthodox molecule — or complex of molecules. It has a molecular weight of at least 1,200,000 and consists of identical subunits each with molecular weight of about 230,000 (Fig. 7–5). Three separate and distinct structural loci

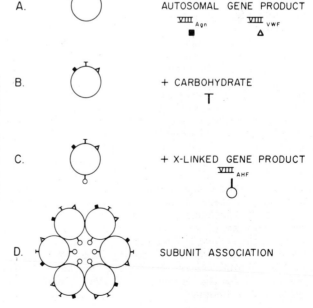

Figure 7–5 Conceptual diagram of the structure of Factor VIII. The autosomal gene product contains one region with the antigenic site (VIII$_{Agn}$) and another with the von Willebrand Factor (VIII$_{VWF}$). The addition of carbohydrate (CHO) appears to be necessary for proper function of the molecule. The procoagulant region, or "antihemophilic factor," (VIII$_{AHF}$) is added either directly or indirectly as a product of an X-linked gene. Subunits associate into a macromolecule. (Adapted from Grainick, H. R., et al.: Ann. Int. Med., 86: 598, 1977.)

of the molecule have been identified: (1) a low molecular weight procoagulant piece (VIII_{AHF}) which contains the antihemophilic factor deficient in patients with hemophilia A; (2) a high molecular weight portion which contains the antigenic site (VIII_{Agn}) to which precipitating antibodies are formed; and (3) another locus on the high molecular weight piece with an activity necessary for normal platelet adhesion to vascular walls, designated VIII_{VWF}, or von Willebrand factor because it is deficient in patients with von Willebrand's disease. Quantitation of VIII_{AHF} is done biologically by specifically measuring its activity in VIII_{AHF} deficient plasma, and VIII_{Agn} is measured immunochemically by a precipitating antibody. A method has recently been described for measuring VIII_{VWF}, depending on the empiric observation that the antibiotic ristocetin causes aggregation of washed normal platelets in a reaction that depends on the plasma concentration of VIII_{VWF}. This reaction occurs with a specific VIII_{VWF} receptor present on the platelet membrane.

Whether these three Factor VIII principles should be considered as a complex molecule or as a multimolecular complex is still uncertain. Under certain in-vivo experimental conditions, to be discussed subsequently, they exhibit different metabolic behavior patterns, suggesting processes of association within the body. There is no doubt that Factor VIII is the product of at least two different genes, since VIII_{AHF} is an X-linked trait and VIII_{VWF} is autosomal.

Intrinsic and Extrinsic Clotting Systems

The terms "intrinsic" and "extrinsic" refer to clotting inside and outside the vascular system, respectively. The intrinsic system is relatively slow and the extrinsic somewhat faster, thanks to the action of tissue thromboplastin. In either case the final common pathway is the conversion of prothrombin to thrombin, the active enzyme which acts upon fibrinogen as its substrate.

The sequential reaction of clotting factors which brings about this conversion involves aspects of the cascade hypothesis as well as the concept of complex formation on phospholipid micelles (Fig. 7–6). The first phase of the intrinsic system is the surface activation of Factors XII and XI. Factor XIa then triggers coagulation by activating IX to IXa, a potent procoagulant. A complex is then formed of Factors IXa and VIII with platelet phospholipid. The formation of this "Factor VIII complex" is accelerated by the presence of small quantities of thrombin. This complex then converts Factor X to Xa, which by itself has "prothrombinase" activity. Its reaction rate with prothrombin, however, is markedly accelerated by the presence of Factor V and platelet phospholipid.

The extrinsic system short-circuits the first two phases of the intrinsic system by directly activating Factor X through the formation of a complex between Factor VII and tissue thromboplastin, which is composed of phospholipid and protein. Tissue thromboplastin is found in many tissues, but brain, lung, and placenta are particularly rich sources.

Calcium is required for most of the coagulation reactions, a point of considerable laboratory importance. Citrate, which complexes calcium, is the most commonly used anticoagulant for sample collection in coagulation testing. However, it is virtually impossible for hypocalcemia to be of sufficient magnitude in vivo to cause abnormal bleeding.

The thrombin formed as the end-product of this accelerating series of reactions not only causes formation of fibrin monomer and activates Factor XIII, but it also engages in positive feedback by promoting platelet aggregation and by increasing the activities of Factors V and VIII. It also increases its own rate of formation by activating prothrombin. The activated forms of the coagulation factors are cleared from the circulation rapidly, thereby keeping the process of clot formation under physiologic control.

Control of Coagulation Reactions: Heparin Cofactor

The key to keeping the forward forces of clot formation under control lies in prompt removal of the activated coagulation factors from the circulation. One important means of achieving this goal is the maintenance of rapid blood flow to wash away local concentrations from the site of thrombus formation. Given an adequate perfusion, the liver rapidly clears the activated factors with a half-life of only a few minutes. There they are rapidly degraded.

There are at least two plasma inhibitors of the activated factors. One is an α-2 macroglobulin. The other, of greater importance, is antithrombin III, identified by Rosenberg as the "heparin cofactor." Antithrombin III is an anti-serine protease (Fig. 7–7). The serine proteases seek out arginine residues where they cleave their protein substrates. In like fashion, the active serine site has an affinity for an arginine site on the antithrombin III molecule, but in this instance the product of the reaction is a stable complex rather than a cleavage. Originally antithrombin III was thought to inhibit only thrombin, but now it is known that it inhibits other serine proteases as well, including Factors XIIa, XIa, Xa, and plasmin.

The combination of heparin with antithrombin III enhances its affinity for serine proteases about 100 fold. The effect is immediate. In the absence of antithrombin III heparin has no effect on clot

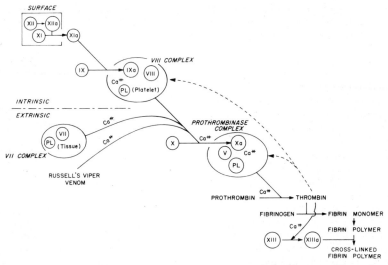

Figure 7–6   The sequence of reactions of the plasma coagulation factors. (PL = phospholipid)

formation, hence its identification as the "heparin cofactor." Heparin binds to a specific ϵ-amino lysyl group at a point on the molecule distant from the active arginine which forms the complex with serine proteases.

Heparin in plasma prolongs the prothrombin time by only a few seconds; its action on the activated partial thromboplastin time is much more pronounced. Its action is immediate and, in contrast to the coumarin anticoagulants, is present in vitro as well as in vivo. It is rapidly cleared from the circulation with a half-life of 90 minutes

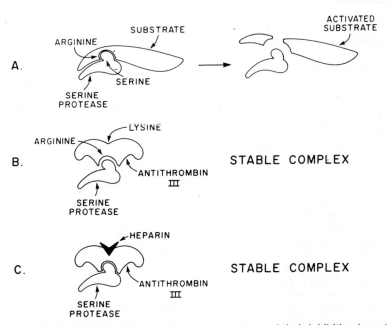

Figure 7–7   Conceptual diagram of the action of serine proteases and their inhibition by antithrombin III.
   A. Serine protease forms a complex with its specific substrate and cleaves it, producing activation (or degradation in the case of plasmin acting upon fibrin-fibrinogen).
   B. Serine protease forms a stable complex with antithrombin III.
   C. The binding of heparin with antithrombin III markedly enhances its affinity for serine protease, illustrated as a "better fit."

and its effect is dissipated within six hours. Although there is significant renal excretion, its metabolic fate is not thoroughly understood.

Synthesis and Turnover

Most of the coagulation factors are made in the liver, with the notable exception of Factor VIII. Jaffe has summarized evidence pointing to the endothelial cells as the source of Factors VIII_{Agn} and VIII_{VWF}, although not of VIII_{AHF}, the origin of which remains unknown. Fibrinogen and Factor VIII are "acute phase reactants," and their levels rise in response to inflammatory states, surgery, and pregnancy.

A significant proportion of the intravascular coagulation factor pool is associated with platelets, partly with the outer membrane and partly in the interior granules. The origin of the platelet coagulation factors is still open to question, but it has been suggested that the interior pool of Factor VIII_{Agn} and VIII_{VWF} is produced in megakaryocytes. If so, this would provide an intriguing functional link between the platelets and the vascular endothelium, which hitherto has often been looked upon as only an inert lining of the vasculature. An epinephrine response is rapidly followed by a transient rise in both the platelet count and the plasma Factor VIII level. The platelets are presumably released from the sequestered pool in the spleen. The mechanism of the Factor VIII increase is not clear.

The biologic half-lives of most of the clotting factors are relatively short (Table 7–2). Factor VII has the shortest and fibrinogen and Factor XIII have the longest. The disappearance of a plasma protein from the intravascular space is a complex function determined not only by its catabolism but also by its passage into extravascular spaces. Thus the meaning of "half-life" is open to considerable discussion. Nonetheless the value is useful in scheduling the frequency of replacement infusions in patients being treated for bleeding due to known factor deficiencies.

Coagulation Tests

Most of the tests of the clotting mechanism depend on the appearance of a fibrin clot in the test tube. The simplest of these is the whole blood clotting time, which is a crude measure of the intrinsic system. A much more convenient, accurate, and reproducible method of measuring the clotting time in the laboratory rather than at the bedside is to collect citrated plasma and subsequently measure the plasma clotting time in the laboratory by adding excess calcium. The normal "recalcification time" is about 100 to 240 seconds, compared to 5 to 15 minutes for the whole blood clotting time. The addition of various reagents to recalcified plasma gives considerable information

TABLE 7–2   BIOLOGIC HALF-LIVES OF PLASMA COAGULATION FACTORS

Factor VII	1.5 to 5 hours
Factor VIII	9 to 18 hours
Factor V	15 to 20 hours
Factor IX	20 to 24 hours
Factor X	1 to 2 days
Factor XI	1.7 to 3.5 days
Factor XII	2 days
Factor II	2.8 to 4.4 days
Factor I	3.2 to 4.5 days
Factor XIII	4.5 to 7 days

about the coagulation mechanism. The addition of a substitute for platelet phospholipid (a "partial thromboplastin") shortens the time to about 60 to 90 seconds; this is the "partial thromboplastin time," which reflects the status of the intrinsic system. The activation of Factors XII and XI by surface-active materials, such as kaolin, celite, or ellagic acid, shortens the time to about 25 to 40 seconds and gives a more reproducible test ("activated partial thromboplastin time"). If tissue (i.e., complete) thromboplastin is added, the plasma clotting time is about 13 seconds, and the corresponding test, somewhat erroneously called the "prothrombin time," is a measure of the extrinsic system. The addition of Russell's viper venom ("Stypven time") activates Factor X directly and thus eliminates Factor VII as a variable in the assessment of the extrinsic system. The addition of thrombin ("thrombin time") is a direct measure of the ability to form a fibrin clot in the test plasma and normally produces a clot so rapidly (about 6 seconds) that dilution of the thrombin is necessary in order to lengthen the time and thus to obtain more accurate and meaningful results. It is obvious that all tests which depend on the appearance of a fibrin clot require an adequate concentration of fibrinogen in the test plasma.

In summary, the initial evaluation of a hemostatic disorder requires an activated partial thromboplastin time (APTT) and a prothrombin time (PT) to evaluate the intrinsic and extrinsic systems. Deficiencies of Factors X, V, II, or fibrinogen, or the presence of heparin or "split products" prolong both the APTT and the PT. Factor VII lack prolongs the PT but not the APTT, while the reverse is true for deficiencies of Factors XII, XI, IX, or VIII. The thrombin time detects fibrinogen abnormalities, heparin, or "split products." Although the concentration of fibrinogen is readily measured, a rough index of fibrinogen level is easily obtained by inspecting the bulk of a retracted clot in a test tube. Rapid lysis of the incubated clot indicates pathologic fibrinolysis. The routine hemostasis evaluation is completed by a platelet count and sometimes by tests of platelet function, of which clot retraction and bleeding time are the most useful.

Tentative conclusions about the identity of a plasma factor deficiency are drawn from substitution tests in an "expanded" partial thromboplastin time. The reagents used for substitution are aged plasma (which lacks the labile Factors V and VIII), fresh adsorbed plasma (which lacks the vitamin K dependent Factors II, VII, IX, and X), and fresh serum (which lacks the consumable Factors II, V, VIII, and fibrinogen). For example, the prolonged APTT in a patient with VIII$_{AHF}$ deficiency (hemophilia A) is corrected by substitution of normal fresh adsorbed plasma, but not aged plasma or serum. In Factor IX deficiency (hemophilia B) the abnormality is corrected by normal serum or aged plasma, but not adsorbed plasma. Final confirmation and quantitation is accomplished by specific factor assays using a test plasma of known deficiency mixed with patient plasma.

ABNORMAL STRUCTURE AND FUNCTION

The hereditary abnormalities of the coagulation factors are readily classified because they are definable in terms of a single inherited abnormality in either the amount or the structure of a single protein. Acquired defects are more difficult to categorize in that they frequently affect many different aspects of the coagulation sequence as well as multiple coagulation factors (Table 7–3).

The general effects are those of bleeding and/or clotting. The clinical nature of the bleeding gives clues about its underlying cause. Intra-articular hemorrhage is highly characteristic of hemophilia and is only rarely seen in other disorders, while petechiae are strongly suggestive of thrombocytopenia. Ecchymoses and purpura are very nonspecific; deep hemorrhage into muscles or the retroperitoneum is more a feature of hemophilia or of adverse effects of anticoagulants. Intracranial hemorrhage, regardless of the underlying hemostatic defect, is the most dread complication. Bleeding from the umbilical stump or after circumcision may be the first sign of a hereditary disorder. Later in life, the onset of the menses, dental extraction, and surgical procedures are natural tests of hemostasis. Delayed hemorrhage several days after the completion of a procedure raises the index of suspicion that there is a disorder of plasma coagulation factors.

DISORDERS OF FIBRINOGEN AND RELATED FACTORS

A low level of circulating fibrinogen may be secondary to decreased production or more frequently to an increase in the rate of its degrada-

TABLE 7–3 CLASSIFICATION OF DISORDERS OF PLASMA COAGULATION AND VASCULAR FACTORS

I. *Disorders of Fibrinogen and Related Factors*
    Hereditary
        Afibrinogenemia
        Dysfibrinogenemia
        Factor XIII deficiency
    Acquired
        Disseminated intravascular coagulation
        Primary fibrinolysis
        Liver disease

II. *Disorders of the Intrinsic and Extrinsic Systems*
    Hereditary
        Hemophilia A
        Hemophilia B
        Deficiencies of surface active Factors XII or XI
        Other deficiencies: Factors VII, X, V, or II
        von Willebrand's disease
    Acquired
        Vitamin K deficiency
        Liver disease
        Hemorrhagic diseases of the newborn
        Exogenous anticoagulants
        Endogenous anticoagulants (antibodies to Factor VIII and other Factors)

III. *Vascular Disorders*
    Hereditary
        Hereditary hemorrhagic telangiectasia
        Ehlers-Danlos syndrome and other connective tissue disorders
    Acquired
        Superficial purpura
        Scurvy
        Cushing's syndrome
        Amyloidosis
        Allergic purpura

tion. The excess in fibrinogen consumption above its production rate is most often due to a process of intravascular coagulation. Rarely it is caused by the presence of a high level of circulating plasmin.

Several different terms have been used to describe the process of *extensive intravascular clotting,* none of them entirely satisfactory. "Consumption coagulopathy" emphasizes the depletion of the plasma coagulation factors, but not all the factors are consumed, and the "panel" of depressed factor levels is neither uniform nor predictable. "Disseminated intravascular coagulation" places major emphasis on the pathogenetic importance of the deposition of large quantities of fibrin throughout the microcirculation but does not fit those situations in which the fibrin deposition is extensive and yet mostly or entirely localized to the vascular beds of certain tissues.

If not fatal, the process may be acute and self-limited, subacute, or chronic, depending on the underlying cause as discussed by Colman and his associates. It may be set off by a pathologic activation of the extrinsic or the intrinsic clotting systems; in many circumstances the triggering mechanism is not known. The activation of the extrinsic system is caused by the entry into the circulation of large amounts of tissue thromboplastin. Examples are the hypofibrinogenemic states associated with pregnancy: abruptio placentae, amniotic fluid embolism, toxemia, and retained dead fetus. Since fibrinogen concentration normally increases in pregnancy, the finding of a plasma concentration within the normal range may be indicative of significant consumption if found late in pregnancy in association with one of the aforementioned complications. Widespread carcinoma may incite intravascular clotting, also presumably on account of the tumor content of tissue thromboplastin which finds its way into the circulation. The intrinsic system may be activated by bacterial septicemia and certain rickettsial and viral infections (Rocky Mountain spotted fever, epidemic hemorrhagic fever) which lay bare the vascular endothelium and expose collagen. Antigen-antibody complexes trigger intrinsic clotting by an unknown mechanism in massive transfusion reactions (although the thromboplastic properties of red cell membrane may play some role) and in anaphylactic reactions. It has been suggested that an immunologic mechanism underlies purpura fulminans, a serious and often fatal disorder primarily of children which characteristically follows shortly after recovery from a minor viral infection (Spicer and Rau, 1976). Properly timed injections of endotoxin given to animals have been experimentally used to produce the so-called generalized Shwartzman reaction, a disseminated intravascular coagulation syndrome, but in this model the precise initiating event also remains obscure. The classification of intravascular coagulation syndromes is given in Table 7–4.

Local factors may prepare the vascular bed of a certain organ or tissue for selective fibrin deposition. In pregnancy the kidney is particularly vulnerable, and the syndrome which may ensue is bilateral renal cortical necrosis with oliguric renal failure. In cavernous hemangiomas, a large vascular bed with a high ratio of endothelial surface area to vascular cross-sectional area accommodates a large volume of blood with static flow. This may be sufficient to set up a chronic process of extensive but localized fibrin deposition, the endothelium contributing high plasminogen activating activity and thus releasing fibrin degradation products into the circulation.

An adequate hepatic perfusion is necessary for rapidly clearing activated coagulation factors as well as fibrinogen-fibrin degradation products and their complexes from the circulation. Any impairment of this process will prolong and aggravate the severity of the coagulopathy. Clinical states of shock, whatever the underlying primary cause, lead to poor perfusion and may seriously

TABLE 7–4 CLASSIFICATION OF DISSEMINATED INTRAVASCULAR COAGULATION SYNDROMES

I. Pregnancy
  Abruptio placentae
  Amniotic fluid embolism
  Toxemia
  Retained dead fetus
  Saline abortion
  Septic abortion with septicemia
  Hydatidiform mole
II. Malignant Disease
  Metastatic carcinoma
  Acute leukemia (promyelocytic)
III. Infectious Disease
  Bacterial septicemia (meningococcal, other gram negative and gram positive)
  Rickettsial (Rocky Mountain spotted fever)
  Viral (epidemic hemorrhagic fever)
  Parasitic (malaria)
IV. Pediatric Syndromes
  Neonatal (respiratory distress syndrome, retained dead twin fetus, septicemia, rubella, abruptio placentae)
  Purpura fulminans
  Hemolytic uremic syndrome
V. Antigen-Antibody Complexes
  Anaphylactic reaction
  Massive transfusion reaction
VI. Miscellaneous
  Liver disease
  Aneurysm
  Vasculitis
  Postoperative (open heart and other thoracic surgery, prostatic surgery)
  Massive trauma (including burns)
  Heat stroke
  Drowning
  Snake bite
  Giant hemangioma

increase the magnitude of the syndrome. Macrophage blockade with substances such as Thorotrast contributes to the severity of intravascular coagulation syndromes experimentally in animals. A similar blockade may be of pathogenetic significance in septicemia or in massive hemolysis.

The ischemic consequences to local tissues of the blockage of the microcirculation are fortunately usually self-limited, owing to the local fibrinolytic efficiency, which rapidly removes the fibrin deposits. However, renal failure is one of the most dire of the ischemic effects. Cutaneous patches of gangrene and acrocyanosis are more externally visible effects seen in purpura fulminans and sometimes in septicemia. Erythrocyte fragmentation, occurring as red cells are forced through the obstructing fibrin meshwork, causes the morphologic appearance of microangiopathic hemolytic anemia on the peripheral blood film. The picture may be accompanied by clinical signs of hemolysis. Intravascular coagulation causing oliguric renal failure and erythrocyte fragmentation is therefore one of the "hemolytic uremic" syndromes.

Laboratory tests reflect the paradoxic circumstance that excessive intravascular clotting brings forth a hemorrhagic diathesis. The consumption of coagulation factors in vivo resembles the process of conversion of plasma to serum in vitro. The most consistent changes are decreases in the platelet count and in the levels of fibrinogen and Factors II, V, and VIII. Plasminogen activation releases fibrinogen-fibrin degradation products into the circulation. These form complexes with fibrin monomer and interfere with the normal polymerization of fibrin monomer during clot formation. The widespread derangements in the coagulation mechanism are reflected by abnormalities in all the routine laboratory tests. These include prolongation of the prothrombin time, the activated partial thromboplastin time, and the thrombin time. The concentration of "split products" in the serum is elevated, and tests of paracoagulation, as described earlier, may be positive. The test tube clot is small and easily broken up. Serial measurements of the routine coagulation tests, platelet count, fibrinogen concentration, and Factor VIII level may help to make the clinical decision about the presence of and the course of a suspected case of extensive intravascular clotting. Laboratory confirmation may be difficult in mild cases.

Treatment varies with the individual circumstances. In acute syndromes, the prompt and vigorous treatment of the primary underlying cause and the correction of shock are the most important measures. Heparin is sometimes used in order to arrest the deposition of fibrin, but not without fear of increasing the bleeding tendency. Repletion of coagulation factors and platelets may be indicated. Replacement therapy is best combined with heparin if the process has not been arrested and fibrin deposition is continuing. Inhibitors of fibrinolysis such as epsilon aminocaproic acid are contraindicated, since they will delay the physiologic resolution of the fibrin clots within the vasculature.

Primary fibrinolysis is an acute severe bleeding state which resembles intravascular clotting but must be distinguished from it because the treatments differ. The high levels of circulating plasmin which set up this state are sometimes secondary to metastatic carcinoma of the prostate, thoracic surgery, injury to the genitourinary tract with extravasation of urokinase-containing urine into tissues, or cirrhosis or shock with impaired ability to clear plasminogen activators from the circulation. Plasmin attacks circulating fibrinogen and causes a decrease in its concentration along with the appearance of fibrinogen degradation products in the circulation. These unfor-

tunately cannot be distinguished from the fibrin degradation products of disseminated intravascular coagulation. Other coagulation factor levels may also be depressed. However, in contrast to intravascular coagulation syndromes, the test-tube clot which initially forms completely dissolves within one or two hours, the platelet count is normal, the red cell morphology does not show fragmentation, and the bleeding improves with the therapeutic use of fibrinolytic inhibitors. Since the syndrome is primarily associated with the action of plasmin rather than thrombin, tests of paracoagulation on the plasma are negative. Under certain circumstances, such as metastatic prostatic carcinoma, primary fibrinolysis occurs together with disseminated intravascular coagulation and laboratory distinction of the two states is not possible.

Inherited disorders of fibrinogen are rare. Afibrinogenemia is a quantitative deficiency secondary to a profound lack of synthesis, while dysfibrinogenemia refers to a variation in the structure of the molecule, as discussed by Ratnoff and Forman. Only trace quantities of fibrinogen are detectable in *hereditary afibrinogenemia,* an autosomal recessive condition which is of clinical significance only in the homozygous form. Whole blood or recalcified plasma clotting times are indefinitely long and are not corrected with the addition of thrombin. Successful arrest of hemorrhage is achieved by replacement therapy sufficient to raise the fibrinogen level above 60 mg. per 100 ml. *Hereditary dysfibrinogenemia* is a mild or even asymptomatic disorder. Several different types have been described, presumably differing in the specific amino acid substitution in the molecule. The detailed abnormalities involved and the molecular mechanisms with respect to the altered function of the molecule remain for the most part to be worked out. Plasma coagulation tests may be broadly deranged. Fibrinogen concentration measured by immunochemical or physical methods is normal, but methods which depend on "clottable fibrinogen" give low values. The condition is autosomal, and affected heterozygotes therefore have normal fibrinogen along with the variant molecule. *Acquired dysfibrinogenemia* occurs in patients with severe liver disease (Martinez, Palascak, and Kwasniak, 1978). It has also been found in association with hepatoma.

Hereditary deficiency of Factor XIII is properly included among disorders of fibrinogen, since Factor XIII also affects clot structure. Deficiency is detectable in the laboratory by virtue of the fibrin clot solubility in 5 M urea. The defect, also autosomal recessive, is clinically severe and, as in hereditary afibrinogenemia, may first come to attention because of bleeding at the site of the sloughed umbilical cord. Wound healing is impaired because fibroblastic organization of the clot is not normal. Affected homozygotes have less than 1 per cent of the normal concentration and respond particularly well to replacement therapy because Factor XIII has a relatively long half-life and only small quantities are required. Factor XIII is among the factors consumed in disseminated intravascular coagulation, another explanation for a lowered level. Consumption or decreased hepatic synthesis account for low levels in patients with liver disease.

INTRINSIC AND EXTRINSIC SYSTEM DISORDERS

Hemophilia A and *hemophilia B* are hereditary deficiencies of Factor VIII and Factor IX, respectively. The two disorders are clinically indistinguishable except by laboratory test. Both are sex-linked and thus transmitted by asymptomatic carrier females to half their sons. Female homozygotes, offspring of affected fathers and carrier mothers, are exceedingly rare. Hemophilia A occurs with a frequency of 1 per 10,000, 5 to 10 times the frequency of hemophilia B. Severe hemophilia is characterized by repeated hemarthroses and ultimately by chronic arthritis and joint destruction. Ankles, knees, and elbows are most susceptible. The normal ineffectiveness of the extrinsic clotting system in the articular structures may explain the particular susceptibility of this tissue to hemorrhage in the face of severe deficiencies of the intrinsic system. Patients with hemophilia of moderate severity may have only occasional joint hemorrhages, whereas mild cases usually have normal joints. Deep hematomas may dissect along fascial planes and cause nerve compression or compromise the vascular supply of an extremity. Even with intensive treatment the surgical risk is great, and intracranial hemorrhage, often provoked by minor head trauma, may be untreatable and have a fatal outcome.

In severe hemophilia A Factor VIII_{AHF} is less than 1 per cent the normal level, in moderate cases 2 to 5 per cent, and in mild cases 6 to 30 per cent. The defect is limited to the procoagulant piece of Factor VIII molecule, VIII_{AHF}, which is either missing or is present but not functioning. Factors VIII_{Agn} and VIII_{VWF} are unaffected. It has been possible to classify patients with hemophilia A into two groups, based on reactions of their plasma with certain neutralizing antibodies to VIII_{AHF}. Plasma from about 10 per cent of patients with hemophilia A will neutralize these antibodies and is designated as cross-reacting material positive (CRM^+) or A^+. The remaining 90 per cent are CRM^- or A^-. The pathogenetic significance of this observation and its possible relationship to genetic polymorphism are still not clear. Similar immunochemical approaches suggest that analogous pathogenetic mechanisms also apply to hemophilia B.

The accurate diagnosis and classification as to degree of severity of hemophilia A and B ultimately rest upon the direct measurement of the levels of Factor VIII and Factor IX activity. The treatment of major hemorrhagic episodes or the preparation of patients for surgery also requires the ability to measure the specific factor level to ensure that it remains in excess of 30 per cent at all times. The partial thromboplastin time is sensitive to levels below 20 per cent and thus is almost always prolonged in untreated patients of any degree of severity. The prothrombin time and the bleeding time are normal. Female carriers cannot be identified with certainty because their functional levels, 25 to 75 per cent for hemophilia A heterozygotes and 9 to 90 per cent for hemophilia B heterozygotes, overlap considerably with the range of normal, 50 to 150 per cent. Ratnoff and Jones report 94 per cent accuracy in identifying female carriers of hemophilia A with the use of newer methods which compare the ratios between the levels of procoagulant (VIII_{AHF}) and antigenic activity (VIII_{Agn}). In hemophilia A heterozygotes the ratio is about half the expected value in normals.

Replacement therapy with plasma or plasma derivatives is effective in both hemophilia A and hemophilia B (Fig. 7–8). Treatment must be specific, however, an axiom which has become of crucial importance since plasma fractionation procedures have come into common use. Cryoprecipitate and other Factor VIII-rich preparations lack Factor IX activity, whereas fractions containing Factor IX and the other vitamin K-dependent factors lack Factor VIII. Factor IX is relatively stable and is present in stored plasma which is a poor source of Factor VIII. The longer biologic half-life of Factor IX (about 24 hours as compared to 12 for Factor VIII) is also of importance in that less frequent infusions of Factor IX are required to maintain its functional activity at the desired level.

Von Willebrand's disease is also a hereditary disorder of Factor VIII but, in contrast to hemophilia A, it is inherited as an autosomal dominant and in addition has an associated defect of platelet adhesion to injured blood vessels, causing a prolonged bleeding time. Platelet adhesion to glass beads is also impaired, but other platelet functions, such as the usual aggregation reactions and ADP release, are typically normal. Epistaxis, menorrhagia, and gastrointestinal hemorrhage are common, but joint hemorrhage is rare. The Factor VIII_{AHF} level is reduced below 50 per cent to as low as 1 to 5 per cent. The partial thromboplastin time is not adequate to detect those cases with less severely depressed levels. Factor VIII_{AHF} levels fluctuate in individual cases,

FACTOR VIII LEVEL
(%)

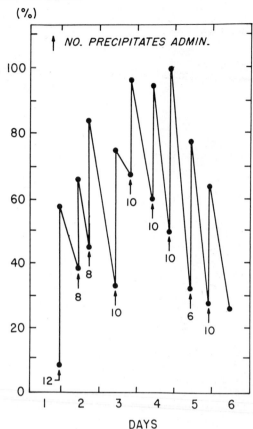

Figure 7–8 Plasma Factor VIII$_{AHF}$ levels measured during treatment of a patient with hemophilia A by repeated infusions of cryoprecipitate. (Redrawn from Pool, J. G., and Shannon, A. E.: N. Engl. J. Med., 273:1443, 1968. Reprinted by permission.)

in contrast to their constancy in hemophilia A. Pregnancy stimulates an increased Factor VIII$_{AHF}$ level, as in normal women, and thus may ameliorate hemorrhagic manifestations.

"Classic" von Willebrand's disease is associated with deficits in all three aspects of the Factor VIII molecule — procoagulant activity, antigenic level, and "ristocetin cofactor" concentration are reduced. However, Gralnick and his associates have summarized evidence that several variants can be characterized. The "classic" cases are considered to represent quantitative deficiency of the VIII$_{VWF}$ locus, which by the nature of the Factor VIII molecular structure described above requires an equal loss of VIII$_{Agn}$ and VIII$_{AHF}$. In one variant the levels of VIII$_{AHF}$ and VIII$_{Agn}$ are normal and only the bleeding time is long in association with a low level of "ristocetin cofactor." These cases are considered to represent a qualitative defect of the VIII$_{VWF}$ locus which is nonetheless structurally represented and thus unassociated with abnormalities of the other two aspects of the Factor VIII molecule. Another variant appears to be a combination of quantitative and qualitative defects in which the degree of reduction of VIII$_{Agn}$ and VIII$_{AHF}$ is not as profound as that of VIII$_{VWF}$.

One of the most intriguing differences between hemophilia A and von Willebrand's disease lies in their response to plasma infusions. The increase in VIII$_{AHF}$ level in hemophilia A is entirely accounted for by the amount of infused material; the maximum occurs immediately after infusion and the declining level thereafter follows the known biologic half-life of VIII$_{AHF}$, about 12 hours. Plasma infusions given to patients with von Willebrand's disease actually stimulate the production of VIII$_{AHF}$. Levels, reaching a peak at 4 to 24 hours, are higher than those which could be explained on the basis of the amount of infused material. The subsequent decline to original pretreatment levels occurs slowly over several days (Blatt and associates, 1976) (Fig. 7–9). Donor plasma taken from patients with hemophilia A indeed has more potent VIII$_{AHF}$ stimulating activity than normal plasma. The correction of the prolonged bleeding time, if it is corrected at all, is much more transient and may last only a few

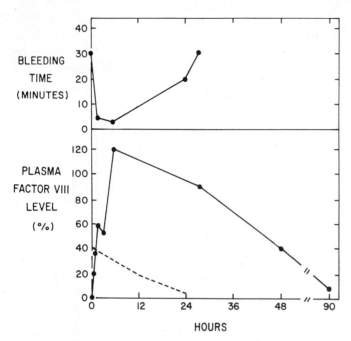

Figure 7–9 Response of Factor VIII$_{AHF}$ level and of bleeding time in a patient with von Willebrand's disease after, given at time zero, a single infusion of a fraction prepared from normal plasma. The interrupted line represents the response in Factor VIII$_{AHF}$ level to be expected in a patient with hemophilia A. (Modified from Williams, W. J.: *In* Williams et al. (Ed.): Hematology, McGraw-Hill Book Co., New York, 1972, p. 1340.)

hours. The persistence in the circulation of VIII$_{Agn}$ and "ristocetin cofactor" activity tends to be intermediate, less prolonged than the VIII$_{AHF}$ elevation but more prolonged than the period of bleeding time correction. The only sure conclusion that can be drawn from these observations is that the metabolic behavior of Factor VIII is complex. The explanation for the relative inefficacy of infusions in favorably influencing the bleeding time may point to the significance of intraplatelet and/or endothelial cell depots of VIII$_{VWF}$ which cannot be easily repleted by simple infusion of exogenous material. Platelet transfusion does not correct the bleeding time defect as it does in hereditary or acquired defects of platelet aggregation, further evidence that the poor platelet adherence in von Willebrand's disease is related to a plasma deficiency.

Ristocetin induced platelet aggregation is also deficient in the *Bernard-Soulier syndrome,* a hemorrhagic condition in which the intrinsically defective platelets are large, heavy, and decreased in number. In this disorder there is a deficiency in the platelet receptor for VII$_{VWF}$. There is no plasma deficiency of Factor VIII constituents.

Acquired defects in Factor VIII, other than those found in the intravascular coagulation syndromes, result from the pathologic production of autoantibodies directed against Factor VIII (Shapiro and Hultin). Somewhat paradoxically, about 5 to 20 per cent of patients with hemophilia A develop antibodies against Factor VIII after re-

peated replacement therapy. These greatly complicate successful therapy when they are present in high titer. Fortunately, the titer falls with time, and if the intervals between hemorrhagic episodes are sufficiently spaced, intensive replacement therapy may successfully arrest the bleeding before the anamnestic response to the infused Factor VIII raises the antibody titer to levels which would preclude successful treatment. Acquired antibodies to Factor VIII are also seen in association with such autoimmune disorders as lupus erythematosus, rheumatoid arthritis, ulcerative colitis, and regional enteritis. A third variant occurs days to weeks postpartum. A fourth type is found without obvious relationship to other coexisting factors, especially in older people. The antibody behaves as a natural circulating anticoagulant and its addition to normal plasma will delay its clotting time. Specific confirmation is made by measuring the neutralization of the Factor VIII activity of normal plasma by plasma containing the natural antibody. Therapy may be difficult if spontaneous disappearance does not alleviate the problem. Immunosuppressive therapy has been successfully used in a few instances. Concentrates of vitamin K dependent factors have been reported to be effective in the control of bleeding because of their content of Factor Xa, an artifact of the method of preparation, which bypasses Factor VIII. They are not without adverse effects, including thrombosis and hepatitis. Autoantibodies to other plasma coagulation factors have also been discovered, but the great majority have been directed against Factor VIII.

Hereditary deficiencies of the remaining plasma coagulation factors are uncommon. Of the surface-active factors, Factor XII deficiency is not associated with any bleeding abnormality, and the hemorrhagic diathesis of Factor XI deficiency is mild. Deficiency of Factor X, V, or II will prolong prothrombin and partial thromboplastin times. In Factor VII, only the prothrombin time is long. All are associated with mild to moderate bleeding manifestations.

Inadequate supplies of vitamin K cause depletion of the vitamin K-dependent factors: II, VII, IX, and X. Absorptive impairment secondary to gastrointestinal disease or to obstruction of the biliary tract causes clotting factor depletion which is correctable by parenterally administered vitamin K. The coumarin and indandione derivatives antagonize the hepatic synthesis of the vitamin K-dependent factors by competitive inhibition. A large number of medications interact with these anticoagulants by either increasing or decreasing their effects, as reviewed by Koch-Weser and Sellers. The Factor VII level is the first to fall because of its short biologic half-life. Factors II, IX, and X reach their nadir at about 5 to 10 days after anticoagulant therapy is begun. Vitamin K, occasionally required to arrest hemorrhage in patients treated with anticoagulant, will significantly increase the levels of the dependent factors within 6 hours. If more rapid correction is necessary, replacement therapy with plasma or with concentrates of the vitamin K-dependent factors can be given. Vitamin K therapy is ineffective if the low factor levels are the result of severe liver disease, which in addition to the vitamin K-dependent factors is associated with failure of synthesis of other factors, such as Factor V, fibrinogen, and Factor XIII along with a host of other defects (Walls and Losowsky, 1971).

The normal newborn infant has lower concentrations of the vitamin K-dependent factors than the adult, partially because of the immaturity of the fetal liver and partially because of low vitamin K stores. Prematurity exaggerates the phenomenon. Breast milk is a poor source of vitamin K, but cow's milk contains significant quantities. A hemorrhagic disease occurring two to three days after birth owing to low levels of the vitamin K-dependent factors has been associated with a sufficiently high mortality rate that prophylactic administration of a small quantity of vitamin K is considered warranted, even though only a partial correction of the coagulation abnormalities is achieved. The syndrome must be distinguished from other neonatal hemorrhagic syndromes, such as the thrombocytopenias, disseminated intravascular coagulation disorders, and hemophilia. The coumarin drugs cross the placental barrier and therefore are not given to pregnant women.

Hemorrhagic complications following heparin therapy are relatively infrequent, considering how extensively this drug is used. The duration of action of heparin is limited to 4 to 6 hours and thus the use of protamine, which neutralizes heparin, is rarely necessary in the management of hemorrhagic complications. Hemorrhagic complications may also occur following therapy with plasminogen activators, such as streptokinase or urokinase, but these agents are also rapidly removed if phagocytic clearing mechanisms are functioning normally.

Reviews on anticoagulant therapy have been written by Gurevich, by Rogers and Sherry, and by Wessler and Gitel. Bell has compared streptokinase and urokinase in a review of the status of fibrinolytic agents in therapy.

HYPERCOAGULABLE STATES

Pathologic thrombosis in the coronary or cerebral circulation, in the deep veins of the legs, in the heart interior, or in other vascular sites is among the most important of public health problems. Yet, with some exceptions to be discussed below, it has been impossible to predict which individuals will suffer this often devastating aberration of blood coagulation.

Table 7–5 lists a few selected conditions which are known to be associated with a thrombotic tendency, some to a striking degree. These are classified as diseases of the vascular integrity, of stasis of blood flow, cellular abnormalities of the blood, and plasma abnormalities, but overlap between categories frequently occurs. In several of these conditions the thrombotic tendency occurs concomitantly with a bleeding tendency.

Hereditary deficiency of antithrombin III is an autosomal dominant condition in which multiple members of affected families develop thrombotic tendencies in early or middle life. Since this is another one of the "consumable" plasma factors, low levels occur in disseminated intravascular coagulation. Antithrombin III lack is one of several possible explanations for heparin resistance.

HEMOSTASIS: VASCULAR FACTORS

The vascular wall stands closely juxtaposed to the normal process of hemostasis. Platelets adhere at cut surfaces and aggregate where collagen is bared. Serotonin is released by platelets, causing vasoconstriction which may assist the task of vessel plugging. Collagen also activates

TABLE 7–5   HYPERCOAGULABLE STATES

Altered Intravascular Surfaces
Atherosclerosis (and predisposing conditions such as
    diabetes mellitus, hypertension, the hyper-
    lipidemias, etc.)
Prosthetic heart valves
Vasculitis
*Thrombotic thrombocytopenic purpura
Homocystinuria
*Pseudoxanthoma elasticum

Stasis of Blood Flow
Deep venous thrombosis (and predisposing causes,
    such as immobilization, venous compression, valve
    incompetence, etc.)
Valvular heart disease
Congestive heart failure
Cardiac arrhythmia

Cellular Abnormalities of the Blood
*Polycythemia vera
*Thrombocythemia
Sickle cell disease
Paroxysmal nocturnal hemoglobinuria
*Leukemia

Plasma Abnormalities
*Disseminated intravascular coagulation
    (see Table 7–4)
Postoperative state
Pregnancy
Oral contraceptive use
Malignancy
Antithrombin III deficiency
*Dysfibrinogenemia
Plasminogen deficiency

*Also often associated with pathologic bleeding.

the intrinsic coagulation system. The vascular
endothelium then finally initiates the process of
clot lysis by releasing plasminogen activator.
However, intrinsic defects of the vascular wall
itself may be of pathogenetic importance in the
etiology of hemorrhage. The supporting structures around the vessels may lose elasticity and
turgor, an important factor in the *superficial purpura* commonly seen in the inelastic skin of normally aging individuals. This syndrome, somewhat injudiciously named "senile purpura," is
clinically benign and is not associated with clinical bleeding, its most serious consequence being
cosmetic. Hereditary disorders of connective tissues, such as *Ehlers-Danlos syndrome,* also decrease the compliance of perivascular tissues sufficiently to cause significant hemorrhage. *Scurvy,*
usually seen in combination with alcoholic liver
disease and other nutritional deficiencies, affects
the integrity of connective tissue of the vascular
wall. Perifollicular hemorrhages resembling pe-

techiae suggest vitamin C lack. Excessive
amounts of adrenal glucocorticoids weaken the
structure of the vascular wall. Purpura and ecchymoses of *Cushing's syndrome* are explained on
this basis. Amyloid deposition within vascular
walls is another example of an acquired intrinsic
disorder of the vessel wall. The abnormality in
hereditary hemorrhagic telangiectasia, an autosomal dominant condition, is still not understood
in terms of primary etiology but leads to localized
dilatations of small vessels which appear as tiny
punctate vascular spots which blanch on pressure. These non-pulsatile spots are found commonly on the lips and mucous membranes of the
mouth and nose as well as on the fingertips. However, internal involvement commonly occurs in
the gastrointestinal tract as well as in other
organs, including the lungs and the central nervous system. The telangiectasias usually do not
develop until the fifth or sixth decade of life,
when the weakened vascular wall finally becomes apparent. Epistaxis and gastrointestinal
hemorrhage are the most common symptoms.

Damage to the vascular wall as a consequence
of various infections has already been mentioned.
Immunologic vascular damage leads to the syndrome of *allergic purpura,* which resembles
thrombocytopenic purpura in the sense that a
petechial eruption forms with predilection for the
dependent portions of the body. The eruption appears more violaceous and more confluent than
thrombocytopenic purpura, and also has a tendency to involve the buttocks and flexor surfaces
of the legs. When the purpuric signs are combined in a triad together with gastrointestinal
hemorrhage and arthritis, the term "Henoch-
Schönlein purpura" is appropriate. The condition
may affect the pediatric age group, in which a
postinfectious cause appears to be most common,
or adults, in which case drug reactions may be
more likely trigger mechanisms (Cream, et al.,
1970). In either group, nephritis is the most
serious complication, as discussed by Meadow
and associates.

The diagnosis of the primary vascular purpuric
syndromes rests primarily on clinical recognition. Laboratory confirmation is at present unsatisfactory. The bleeding time and the tourniquet
test (in which the appearance of petechiae is observed after inflation of a blood pressure cuff to
the level sufficient to occlude venous return but
not arterial filling) are primarily tests of adequacy of platelet numbers and function, and although abnormalities may be detected in the primary vascular disorders, the information is not of
great assistance in establishing their presence.
The fact that almost 10 per cent of normal people
have a positive tourniquet test also diminishes
the diagnostic value of this procedure.

REFERENCES

Bell, W. R.: Thrombolytic therapy. A comparison between urokinase and streptokinase. Seminars in Thrombosis and Hemostasis, 2:1, 1975.

Blatt, P. M., Brinkhous, K. M., Culp, H. R., Kraus, J. S., and Roberts, H. R.: Antihemophilic factor concentrate therapy in von Willebrand disease. J.A.M.A., 236:2770, 1976.

Colman, R. W., Robboy, S. F., and Minna, J. D.: Disseminated intravascular coagulation (DIC): an approach. Am. J. Med., 52:679, 1972.

Cream, J. J., Gumpel, J. M., and Peachey, R. D.: Schönlein-Henoch purpura in the adult. A study of 77 adults with anaphylactoid or Schönlein-Henoch purpura. Q. J. Med., 39:461, 1970.

Davie, E. W. and Fujikawa, K.: Basic mechanisms in blood coagulation. Ann. Rev. Biochem., 44:799, 1975.

Donaldson, V. H., Glueck, H. I., Miller, M. A., Movat, H. Z., and Habal, F.: Kininogen deficiency in Fitzgerald trait: Role of high molecular weight kininogen in clotting and fibrinolysis. J. Lab. Clin. Med., 87:327, 1976.

Gralnick, H. R., Coller, B. S., Shulman, N. R., Andersen, J. C., and Hilgartner, M.: Factor VIII. Ann. Int. Med., 86:598, 1977.

Gralnick, H. R., Sultan, Y., and Coller, B. S.: von Willebrand's disease. Combined qualitative and quantitative abnormalities. N. Engl. J. Med., 296:1024, 1977.

Gurevich, V.: Guidelines for the management of anticoagulant therapy. Seminars in Thrombosis and Hemostasis, 2:176, 1976.

Hillenbrand, P., Parbhoo, S. P., Jedrychowski, A., and Sherlock, S.: Significance of intravascular coagulation and fibrinolysis in acute hepatic failure. Gut, 15:83, 1974.

Jaffe, E. A.: Endothelial cells and the biology of Factor VIII. N. Engl. J. Med., 296:377, 1977.

Koch-Weser, J. and Sellers, E. M.: Drug interactions with coumarin anticoagulants. N. Engl. J. Med., 285:487, 1971.

Marder, V. J., and Budzynski, A. Z.: Fibrinogen and its derivatives, hereditary and acquired abnormalities. Schweiz. Med. Wschr., 104:1338, 1974.

Martinez, J., Palascak, J. E., and Kwasniak, D.: Abnormal sialic acid content of the dysfibrinogenemia associated with liver disease. J. Clin. Invest., 61:535, 1978.

Meadow, S. R., Glasgow, E. F., White, R. H. R., Moncrieff, M. W., Cameron, J. S., and Ogg, C. S.: Schönlein-Henoch nephritis. Q. J. Med., 41:241, 1972.

Nossell, H. L.: Radioimmunoassay of fibrinopeptides in relation to intravascular coagulation and thrombosis. N. Engl. J. Med., 295:428, 1976.

Pool, J. G., and Shannon, A. E.: Production of high-potency concentrates of antihemophilic globulin in a closed bag system. N. Engl. J. Med., 273:1443, 1965.

Ratnoff, O.D., and Forman, W. B.: Criteria for the differentiation of dysfibrinogenemic states. Seminars Hematol., 13:141, 1976.

Ratnoff, O. D., and Jones, P. K.: The laboratory diagnosis of the carrier state for classic hemophilia. Ann. Int. Med., 86:521, 1977.

Rogers, P. H., and Sherry, S.: Current status of antithrombotic therapy in cardiovascular disease. Progr. Cardiovasc. Dis., 19:233, 1976.

Rosenberg, R. D.: Actions and interactions of antithrombin and heparin. N. Engl. J. Med., 292:146, 1975.

Shapiro, S. S., and Hultin, M.: Acquired inhibitors to the blood coagulation factors. Seminars in Thrombosis and Hemostasis, 1:336, 1975.

Spicer, T. E., and Rau, J. M.: Purpura fulminans. Am. J. Med., 61:566, 1976.

Walls, W. D., and Losowsky, M. S.: The hemostatic defect of liver disease. Gastroenterology, 60:108, 1971.

Wessler, S., and Gitel, S.: Control of heparin therapy. Progress in Thrombosis and Hemostasis, 3, 311, 1976.

8

Identity of Blood Cells

One of the earliest and most fundamental events in the emergence of life must have been the packaging of complex molecules into cells separated from the environment by membranes. These membranes provided the cell with both physical protection and metabolic discrimination, and during the further evolutionary development, the cell membranes have become the biologic expression of cellular identity.

Cell membranes are, in general, made up of a 45 Å.-thick lipid bi-layer containing free-floating protein globules (Fig. 8–1). The lipid component consists primarily of tightly packed phospholipid molecules with their hydrophobic fatty acid tails intertwined in the center of the membrane and their hydrophilic phosphoglycerol heads providing the intrinsic and extrinsic boundaries (Danielli and Dawson, 1935). At body temperature,

the lipid bi-layers exist in a semi-liquid form permitting considerable lateral movements within the membrane but owing to the layers of polar forces, little opportunity for movements across the membranes.

In nucleated cells, the lipid membrane can be renewed to compensate for loss from injury or from interiorization during processes of phagocytosis or pinocytosis (Fig. 4–3). In non-nucleated cells, such as in erythrocytes, considerable re-modeling may take place through a dynamic exchange with extracellular neutral lipids, especially cholesterol. However, structural membrane lipids cannot be replaced and the senescence of the red cells is associated with or caused by a loss in surface area.

The physiologic role of the lipids in the transport of molecules across the membrane is not

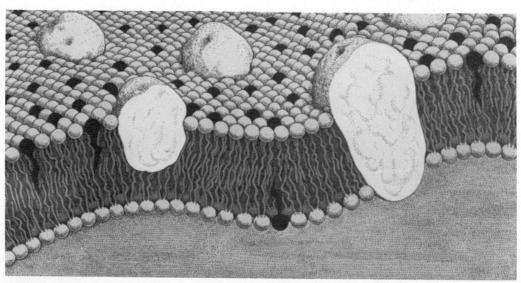

Figure 8–1 Floating iceberg model of cell membranes with globular proteins embedded in a bi-layer of lipids (grey) and cholesterol (black). The proteins make up the membrane's "active sites." Some pass entirely through and may contain transport pores. (From Singer, S. J.: Hosp. Practice, *81*, May 1973.)

clear. The lipid bi-layer appears best suited to serve as an impenetrable insulator. Actually, the membranes with the least transport function, such as the myelin coating of the nerves, are the ones with the highest content of lipid, and the membranes with the most transport obligations, such as the mitochondrial membranes, contain very little lipid. Recent studies have suggested that most if not all membrane transport is mediated by protein globules floating like icebergs in the semi-fluid lipid matrix (Singer, 1974). These protein globules can be visualized directly by electron microscopy of freeze-cleaved red cell membranes (Fig. 8–2). It is assumed that these globules have a hydrophobic half deeply embedded in the hydrophobic lipid center and a hydrophilic half emerging from the surface. Some proteins may even be banded like woolly bears with their hydrophobic center band embedded in the hydrophobic lipid center and their hydrophilic ends emerging from both interior and exterior surfaces (Fig. 8–1). Such protein bridges would alone or in groups be well suited to mediate molecular transport across the membranes. In mature red cells the transmembranous proteins are attached on the inner side of the membrane to rodlike proteins, spectrins (Fig. 8–3). These abundant proteins have so far not been identified with an enzymatic function and they may merely serve as a reinforcing scaffold for the lipid bilayer. On the outer side of the membrane, the proteins serve as metabolic receptors and as anchors for sialic acid groups and for branching antigenic oligosaccharides.

The floating iceberg concept of membrane structure has been strongly supported by the observation that cross-linking antibodies to membranous proteins will move the proteins together into one spot, so-called capping. Because of the above-mentioned attachment of red cell transmembranous proteins to spectrin, this capping phenomenon is not observed in red cells (Singer 1974). In summary, it appears likely that all membranes consist of a lipid bi-layer that acts as a non-specific insulating component, and protein globules that act as receptors or transport enzymes, providing the cells with their functional identity.

In addition to functional identity, cells also have individual identity achieved by the presence and configuration of specific systems of sugar and protein molecules on the membranes. This fingerprint individuality of the membrane surface apparently is needed for the phagocytes to distinguish between self and non-self and probably plays a major role in the recognition and destruction of altered or foreign cells. It is also of importance for blood transfusions and organ transplantations, and the unravelling of blood and tissue types has had both theoretic and practical rewards (Fudenberg and co-workers, 1978).

The ABO system was the first recognized sys-

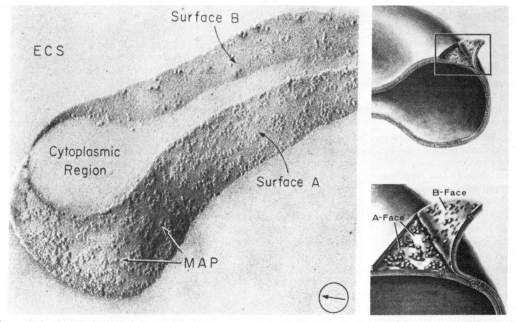

Figure 8–2 Artist's conception and actual electron microscopic view of a freeze-cleaved human red cell ghost membrane. Its A surface is oriented toward the extracellular space (ECS), and is partly covered with clusters of 100 Å membrane-associated particles (MAP). Surface B has fewer particles and faces the cell's interior. (From Weinstein, R. S., and McNutt, N. S.: Seminars Hematol., 7:259, 1970.)

POLYPEPTIDE   COMPONENT   APPARENT   DESIGNATIONS
BANDS   MOLECULAR
                            WEIGHT

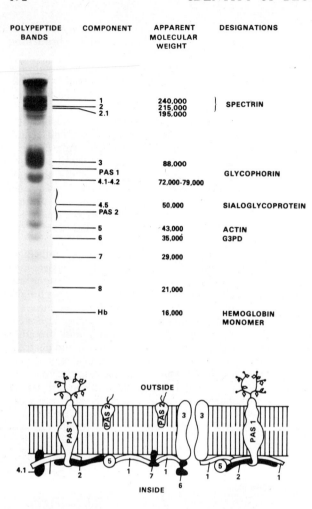

Figure 8–3 Characterization of the protein components of the red cell membrane and diagrammatic representation of its macromolecular architecture. Polyacrylamide gel electrophoresis after solubilization with sodium dodecyl sulfate shows a series of membrane components represented as numbers 1 to 8 with the addition of hemoglobin monomer at the lower portion of electrophoretic gel. Molecular weights of these components range from 240,000 down to 16,000 daltons. Several of the membrane protein components have been isolated and identified as indicated at right. Below is a diagram of a macromolecular model of the red cell membrane, showing the approximate locations of known red cell membrane protein components relative to the lipid bilayer. PAS-1, or glycophorin, is the transmembrane protein which bears the oligosaccharides and charged sialic acid groups at the external membrane surface. At the internal surface it presumably makes contact with spectrin components 1 and 2. These spectrin components form a continuous meshwork on the internal aspect of the membrane and interact with component 5, actin. Component 3 is a large-molecular-weight transmembrane protein which may contain a central aqueous core and serve in transmembrane transport of cations and other substances. Component 6 represents glyceraldehyde-3-phosphate dehydrogenase, an enzyme component localized to the internal membrane surface. (Courtesy of Lessin, L. S., and Bessis, M.: Hematology, 2nd Ed. McGraw-Hill, New York, 1977, p. 103.)

tem of specific, individual surface markers. This system is expressed on all cells in the body, but owing to its practical importance for blood transfusions, it has been identified with red blood cells (Marcus, 1969). The prime members of the system, the A, B, and H antigens, are branching carbohydrate chains that extend above the membrane and are attached to specific sphingolipid protein sites in the membrane. These sites begin to appear during the early maturation of nucleated red cells (Minio, et al., 1972) and, at the time of release from the bone marrow, each red cell has about 1 million ABH sites. The ABH antigens (Watkins, 1966) are derived from a common precursor substance consisting of a chain of four sugars terminating in a galactose (Fig. 8–4). A genetic locus with the allelic genes H and h determines the first step of differentiation (Fig. 8–5). The H gene codes for an enzyme that transfers fucose to the terminal galactose of the precursor substance producing the antigen H. Since this antigen is needed as substrate for the production of A and B antigens, individuals without the H

gene, or in other words, homozygous for h, will not make any of the ABH antigens. People with this rare phenotype called "Bombay" will have all three isoantibodies, Anti A, Anti B, and Anti H, and the only compatible donors will be other individuals of the Bombay type.

After the production of H antigens, the final determination of the specific blood type is controlled by three allelic genes in the ABO chromosomal locus. The A gene codes for an enzyme that transfers acetylgalactosamine to the terminal galactose and changes the H antigen to an A antigen. The B gene codes for an enzyme that transfers galactose to the terminal galactose and changes the H antigen to a B antigen. The O gene does not code for any recognized transferase and the H antigen remains unchanged. (See reviews by Mollison and by Giblett.)

About 20 per cent of individuals with A antigens belong to the clinically important subgroup A_2 (Table 8–1). The difference between this antigen and the common A antigen, so-called A_1, is, in part, quantitative rather than qualitative.

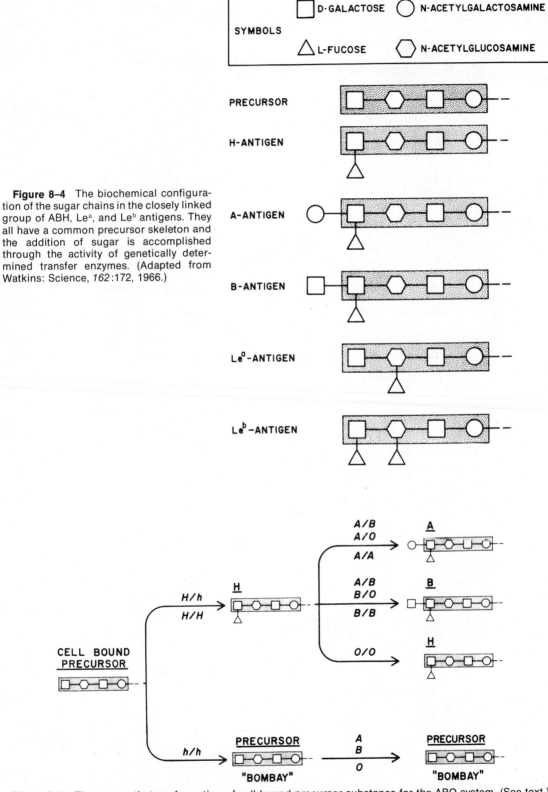

Figure 8–4 The biochemical configuration of the sugar chains in the closely linked group of ABH, Le^a, and Le^b antigens. They all have a common precursor skeleton and the addition of sugar is accomplished through the activity of genetically determined transfer enzymes. (Adapted from Watkins: Science, *162*:172, 1966.)

Figure 8–5 The enzymatic transformation of cell bound precursor substance for the ABO system. (See text.)

TABLE 8–1 ABO SYSTEM

Subgroups	Antigens	Antibodies
0	H	Anti A + Anti A₁ + Anti B
A₁	A₁	Anti B
A₂	A₁ + H	(Anti A₁ in 1% of subjects)
B	B	Anti A + Anti A₁
A₁B	A₁ + B	None
A₂B	A₁ + B	(Anti A₁ in 25% of subjects)

The transferase, coded by the A_1 gene, transforms almost all the H-substrate to A_1 antigen while the transferase coded by A_2 is less active and leaves considerable amounts of unchanged H on the surface. This explains why A_2 red cell agglutinates in vitro—both with Anti-A_1 and with Anti-H. The occasional but potentially dangerous presence of Anti-A_1 antibodies in the plasma of the A_2 individuals, however, cannot be explained merely by the low density of A_1 antigen on the cell surface; and it seems likely that there are additional subtle differences in transferases or substrates.

The same precursor substance attached to cell surfaces is also present in body fluids. In its solu-

ble form, it is attached to a circulating lipoprotein and serves as a substrate for the ABO determined transferases. The elaboration of soluble antigens, however, is more complex, since it involves the interaction of two closely related genetic loci—the "secretor" and the "Lewis" loci (Fig. 8–6).

About 20 per cent of all individuals lack the secretor gene (Se) and are homozygous se/se. In these individuals, the soluble precursor substance cannot be altered by the transferase produced by the H, A, and B genes. They are so-called non-secretors and have no ABH antigens in their saliva, regardless of their capacity to produce ABH antigens on cell surfaces. If they are also Lewis negative (le/le), they do not secrete Lewis blood groups either. However, if they are Lewis positive (Le/le or Le/Le), as is 90 per cent of the population, the Lewis gene will code for a fucosyl transferase that transfers a fucose to the next to the last sugar molecule of the soluble precursor substance and changes it into a Lewis antigen — so-called Le^a substance. This substance in turn will be passively absorbed to the membrane of circulating red cells providing the cells with the phenotype Le$^{(a+b-)}$ (Table 8–2).

About 80 per cent of all individuals possess the secretor gene (Se/Se or Se/se), and in these indiv-

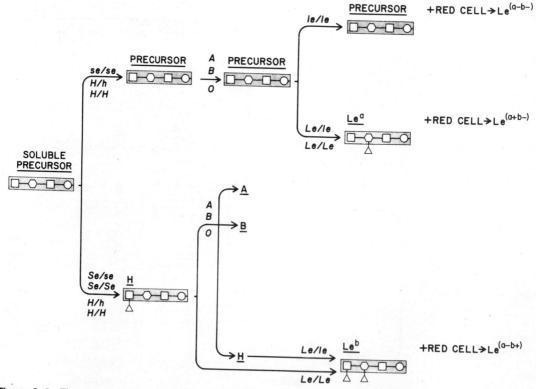

Figure 8–6 The enzymatic transformation of soluble precursor substance for the ABO Le system. (See text.)

TABLE 8–2   H-ABO-Se-Le SYSTEM

Genotype				Phenotype	
H (99.9%)*	ABO (100%)*	Se (80%)*	Le (90%)*	Soluble	Red Cells
+	+	−	−	− −	ABO $Le^{(a-b-)}$
+	+	−	+	− Le^a	ABO $Le^{(a+b-)}$
+	+	+	−	ABO −	ABO $Le^{(a-b-)}$
+	+	+	+	ABO Le^b	ABO $Le^{(a-b+)}$

*Incidence of genes in population.

iduals, the transferases coded by the H and the A and B genes can act on the soluble precursor substance and make specific soluble antigens parallel to their action on the precursor substance on the red cells. Ten per cent of these individuals are Lewis negative, and no soluble Lewis substance will be produced or passed on to the red cells. In the 90 per cent who have the Lewis gene, however, the precursor substance will be exposed to two fucosyl transferases, one coded by the Lewis gene and capable of transferring a fucose to the next to the last sugar molecule, and the other coded by the H gene and capable of transferring a fucose to the last sugar molecule. The result is the production of an Le^b substance that in turn will be absorbed to red cells, and render them $Le^{(a-b+)}$ (Table 8–2).

Of the other blood group systems, the Ii system is the most closely related to the ABO and Lewis systems. The antigens are carbohydrates; they are present in secretions as well as on cell membranes; they are present in close proximity to the ABH antigens on the red cell surface, and they are associated with naturally occurring isoantibodies. The phenotypic expression of the Ii system bears a remarkable resemblance to that of the fetal-adult hemoglobins. Antigen i is present during fetal development and is gradually replaced by antigen I at time of birth (Giblett and Crookston, 1964). In some individuals and in certain hematologic disorders, however, the antigen i reappears in a fashion analogous to that of fetal hemoglobin. Anti I is a cold reactive antibody present in small amounts in all adults and in large amounts in patients with atypical (mycoplasma) pneumonia, and in some patients with cold-reactive, acquired hemolytic anemia.

Naturally occurring isoantibodies may also be directed against antigens of the MN and P systems. The antigens in all systems with isoantibodies appear slowly during fetal maturation and are still not fully expressed at time of birth. The isoantibodies are usually not found until three to six months after birth, and if present

earlier, are acquired passively from the mother. The isoantibodies of the ABO system are primarily of the complement-binding IgM type. Even isoantibodies of the IgG type, however, will bind complement and cause hemolysis, presumably due to the great density of the ABH sites on the red cell surface. Antibodies of the IgM type cause visible agglutination in vitro because their pentameric structure provides enough length to bridge the gap between cells. The IgG antibodies, on the other hand, usually cannot do so unless the negative repelling charge of red cells is decreased by trypsin or papain treatment or by coating with albumin. Albumin may also cause clustering of antigenic sites, thereby facilitating IgG-induced agglutination of cells sparsely covered by antigens (Victoria, et al., 1975). The addition of antibodies against IgG molecules or complement (Coombs serum) leads to visible agglutination of IgG-coated red cells. The immunologic origin of the naturally occurring isoantibodies is still unknown. They may be genetically determined, but it seems more likely that they are acquired during early infancy in response to AB-like exogenous antigens absorbed through the immature gastrointestinal mucosa.

In a number of blood group systems, such as Rh, Kell, and Duffy, naturally occurring antibodies are absent, and sensitization occurs first after repeated parental exposures to their antigens. Of these systems, the Rh system is of most importance, since the strong antigenicity and early fetal emergence of the D antigen make it a frequent offender in transfusion reactions and in the development of erythroblastosis fetalis.

The Rh antigens are lipoproteins rather than glycolipoproteins, and they are present in a much smaller number on the red cell surface than the antigens of the ABO system. This low antigenic density, about 10–20,000 sites per cell, may explain the fact that IgG immune Rh antibodies rarely fix complement or cause intravascular hemolysis. The biochemical structure of the antigenic sites is poorly understood. They appear,

TABLE 8–3 NOMENCLATURE AND FREQUENCY OF Rh-Hr SYSTEM

Separate Gene Hypothesis (Fisher-Race) Gene and Agglutinogen	Single Gene Hypothesis (Wiener)		Frequency in Caucasians (Race and Sanger, 1962)
	Gene	Agglutinogen	
DCe	R'	Rh_1	41%
DcE	R^2	Rh_2	14%
Dce	R^0	Rh_0	3%
DCE	R^z	Rh_z	<1%
ce	r	rh	39%
Ce	r'	rh′	1%
cE	r''	rh″	1%
CE	r^y	rh_z	<1%

however, to be integral parts of the lipid surface layer, rather than elevated above it as in the case of the branching polysaccharide chain of the ABH sites. This conclusion is supported by the fact that in the absence of all Rh sites, as found in the rare genetic condition, Rh null, the red cells are defective and short-lived, while in the absence of all ABH sites, as found in the Bombay type, the red cell surface is presumably normal, since the red cells survive normally in the circulation (Levine, et al., 1973).

It has been proposed that the Rh sites in the surface layer of the membrane consist of three connected loci; the first containing either C (rh′) or c (hr′), the second containing either E (rh″) or e (hr″), and the third containing either D (Rh$_0$) or no known antigen. Only the D is a strong antigen and the antigenic behavior of the eight possible combinations (Table 8–3) is mostly determined by the presence or absence of D. Although the concept of three separate but connected loci (Fisher and Race) is attractive and easy to understand and remember, family studies indicate that each of the eight possible combinations behaves as the product of a single gene (Wiener), a finding justifying the use of the Rh-Hr terminology, at least by blood bankers. Since the blood type of each individual is determined by a pair of genes, 36 genotypes are possible resulting in the production of 18 different phenotypes. This multitude of

types are of great importance for genetic mapping, but for transfusion reaction and erythroblastosis, the presence or absence of the D (Rh$_0$) antigen is still the prime concern.

Although the ABO and possibly also the Rh genes express themselves on all cell surfaces, the major antigens of the leukocytes and platelets do not belong to these systems. These antigens, also ubiquitous in distribution, are the histocompatibility antigens of the HL-A system (for Human Leukocyte Antigens) as well as a few antigens presumably specific for each cell type. During the last decade, histocompatibility antigens have become of prime importance for skin and organ transplantation and for platelet and leukocyte transfusions (reviewed by Bach and van Rood, 1976). They are glycoproteins and so numerous that about 1 per cent of all proteins found on the lymphocyte membrane are HL-A antigens. They undergo continuous production and turnover, and it seems likely that soluble HL-A antigens in tissue fluids originate from cell membranes. The genetic locus controlling the production of the HL-A antigens consists of a complex of subloci which in man are located in close proximity on chromosome No. 6 (Fig. 8–7).

The two major subloci HLA-A and HLA-B (new nomenclature) are serologically defined or, in other words, their numerous allelic antigens can be detected by specific antibodies. The antigens of

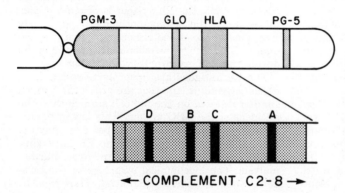

Figure 8–7 Chromosome #6 with the HLA D, B, C, and A regions and some established loci for other gene complexes (PGM-3 = Phosphoglucomutase-3, GLO = Glyoxylase, PG-5 = Urinary pepsinogen-5). Complement C2 is situated in a specific locus close to HLA-D while other complement loci are less defined although situated in the HLA region. (Adapted from McKusick, V. A. and Ruddle, F. H., 1977.)

TABLE 8–4 THE HLA SYSTEM

Sublocus A	Sublocus B	Sublocus C	Sublocus D
	Recognized Antigens, 1977		
HLA–A1	HLA–B5		
HLA–A2	HLA–B7		
HLA–A3	HLA–B8		
HLA–A9	HLA–B12		
HLA–A10	HLA–B13		
HLA–A11	HLA–B14		
HLA–A28	HLA–B18		
HLA–A29	HLA–B27		
	Provisionally Identified Antigens, 1977		
HLA–Aw23	HLA–Bw15	HLA–Cw1	HLA–Dw1
↓	↓	↓	↓
HLA–Aw43	HLA–Bw42	HLA–Cw5	HLA–Dw6

sublocus HLA-C also produce circulating antibodies, but only a few alleles have been detected. The antigens of the important HLA-D locus are presently identified only by the mixed lymphocyte culture test (Table 8–4).

The serologic test, i.e., HLA microcytotoxicity test, depends on complement fixation to lymphocytes in the presence of a specific antibody. Complement fixation will damage the cell membrane and permit a dye to enter the cell or a ^{51}Cr-labeled cytoplasmic component to be released. Using a battery of antibodies obtained from multiparous women, patients with skin grafts or patients having received multiple transfusions of leukocytes, it has been possible to identify eight antigens determined by sublocus HLA-A and eight antigens by sublocus HLA-B (Table 8–4). A great number of additional antigens have been described and have received the designation w for workshop. In the inheritance of these HLA genes, the loci are so close together that there is rarely any crossover and the genes are passed on in fixed groups (Fig. 8–8).

The mixed lymphocyte culture or response test, so called MLC or MLR, is an in-vitro representation of the in vivo lymphocyte response to foreign antigens. It consists of culturing lymphocyte suspensions from two individuals together for several days. The lymphocyte suspension from the unknown is "the responder," while the lymphocytes from an individual with a known HLA type serve as "the stimulator." The stimulating cells are prevented from responding by previous exposure to mitomycin C. The degree of DNA synthesis induced in the responding cells and measured by ^{3}H-thymidine incorporation is a measure of the genetic difference between individuals.

The antigens in the two serologically identifiable subloci of the HLA system underlie the matching grades in use for kidney transplantation (Table 8–5) and in case of cadaver transplant there is usually too little time for mixed lymphocyte culture matching. However, serologic matching alone is inadequate and immunosuppression is needed even for excellent A- and B-matches. In case of transplantation from live donors, more thorough tissue typing and cross-matching by means of a MLC test can be carried out. This is especially needed for bone marrow transplantation in which both host versus graft and graft versus host reactions play a role. Cross-matching or cross-culturing of lymphocytes from HLA-in-

INHERITANCE OF HISTOCOMPATIBILITY ANTIGENS

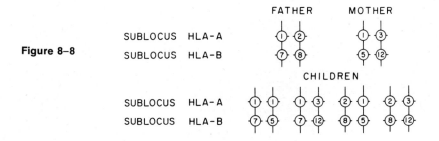

Figure 8–8

TABLE 8–5   MATCHING GRADES FOR HL-A
SYSTEM

Grade

A	Identical siblings
B	Identical unrelated or no antigen in donor not present in recipient
C	1 Incompatibility
D	2 Incompatibilities
E	3 Incompatibilities
F	Positive crossmatch or ABO incompatibility

compatible individuals will, of course, result in DNA synthesis and blast transformation, but it may also be positive in perfectly matched individuals, suggesting the existence of additional genes not yet recognized by our serologic and MLC techniques for tissue typing. The enormous complexity of these systems has limited the therapeutic use of bone marrow transplantation and of platelet and leukocyte transfusions between unrelated individuals. Owing to the close genetic linkage of tissue types, however, such procedures carried out between matched siblings are often successful and, as summarized by Storb and co-workers, can provide dramatic therapeutic benefits.

REFERENCES

Bach, F. H., and van Rood, J. J.: The major histocompatibility complex — genetics and biology. N. Engl. J. Med., *295*:806, 872, 927, 1976.

Danielli, J. F., and Dawson, H.: A contribution to the theory of permeability of thin films. J. Cell. Comp. Physiol., *5*:495, 1935.

Fudenberg, H. H., Pink, J. R. L., Wang, A. C., and Douglas, S. D.: Basic immunogenetics, 2nd ed. Oxford University Press, New York, 1978.

Giblett, E. R.: Erythrocyte antigens and antibodies. *In* Williams, W. J., et al. (eds.): Hematology, 2nd ed. McGraw-Hill Book Co., New York, 1977, p. 1497.

Giblett, E. R., and Crookston, M. C.: Agglutinability of red cells by anti-i in patients with thalassemia major and other hematologic disorders. Nature, *201*:1138, 1964.

Lessin, L. S., and Bessis, M.: Morphology of the erythron. *In* Williams, W. J., et al. (eds.): Hematology, 2nd ed. McGraw-Hill Book Co., New York, 1977, p. 103.

Levine, P., Tripodi, D., Struck, J., Jr., Zmijewski, C. M., and Pollack, W.: Hemolytic anemia associated with Rh null but not with Bombay blood. Vox Sang., *24*:417–424, 1973.

McKusick, V. A., and Ruddle, F. H.: The status of the gene map of the human chromosomes. Science, *196*:390, 1977.

Marcus, D. M.: The ABO and Lewis blood-group system: immunochemistry, genetics and relation to human disease. N. Engl. J. Med., *280*:994, 1969.

Minio, F., Howe, C., Hsu, K. C., and Rifkind, R. A.: Antigen density on differentiating erythroid cells. Nature (New Biology), *237*:187, 1972.

Mollison, P. L.: Blood Transfusion in Clinical Medicine, 5th ed. Blackwell, Oxford, 1972.

Race, R. R., and Sanger, R.: Blood Groups in Man, 4th ed. Blackwell, Oxford, 1962.

Singer, S. J.: Architecture and topography of biologic membranes. Hosp. Pract., *8*:5, 81, 1973.

Singer, S. J.: Molecular biology of cellular membranes with applications to immunology. Adv. Immunol., *19*:1, 1974.

Storb, R., Prentice, R. L., and Thomas, E. D.: Treatment of aplastic anemia by marrow transplantation from HLA identical siblings. J. Clin. Invest., *59*:625, 1977.

Victoria, E. J., Muchmore, E. A., Sudora, E. J., and Masouredis, S. P.: The role of antigen mobility in anti-$Rh_0(D)$-induced agglutination. J. Clin. Invest., *56*:292, 1975.

Watkins, W. M.: Blood group substances. Science, *162*:172, 1966.

Weinstein, R. S., and McNutt, N. S.: Ultrastructure of red cell membranes. Seminars Hematol., *7*:259, 1970.

APPENDIX

NORMAL ADULT LABORATORY VALUES*

		Old System	New System
Red cell count	Men:	4.6–6.0 (5.1) $\times 10^6$/mm.^{3}	$\times 10^{12}$/l.
	Women:	4.1–4.8 (4.5) $\times 10^6$/mm.^{3}	$\times 10^{12}$/l.
Hemoglobin	Men:	14.5–16.7 g./100 ml.	g./dl.
	Women:	12.2–15.0 g./100 ml.	g./dl.
Packed cell volume	Men:	42–49%	.42–.49 l./l.
	Women:	38–45%	.38–.45 l./l.
Erythrocyte indices:			
Mean corpuscular volume		82–92$\mu.^3$	fl.
Mean corpuscular hemoglobin		27–32$\mu\mu$g.	pg.
Mean corpuscular hemoglobin conc.		32–36 g./100 ml.	g./dl.
White cell count		5,000–10,000/mm.^{3}	5–10 $\times 10^9$/l.
Differential:			
Neutrophils (segs)		54–62%	%
Neutrophils (bands)		5–10%	%
Absolute neutrophil count		3,000–7,000 mm.^{3}	3–7 $\times 10^9$/l.
Eosinophils		0–3%	%
Basophils		0–1%	%
Lymphocytes		18–35%	%
Monocytes		3–7%	%
Platelet count	Men:	210,000–340,000/mm.^{3}	210–340 $\times 10^9$/l.
	Women:	208,000–380,000/mm.^{3}	208–380 $\times 10^9$/l.
Reticulocyte count		0.5–2.6%	%
Absolute reticulocyte count		25,000–125,000/mm.^{3}	25–125 $\times 10^9$/l.
†Prothrombin time		12–15 sec.	sec.
†Partial thromboplastin time		50–90 sec.	sec.
†Partial thromboplastin time, activated		25–46 sec.	sec.
†Thrombin time		20–26 sec.	sec.
Fibrinogen		198–434 mg./100 ml.	1.98–4.34 g./l.
Bleeding time (Ivy method)		2–7 min.	min.
Euglobulin lysis time		more than 2 hrs.	hrs.
Fibrin degradation products		0 1μg./ml.	mg./l.
Factor VIII and other coagulation Factors		50–150% of normal	0.5–1.5 U./ml.
†Serum iron		80–180μg./100 ml.	14–32μmol./l.
†Total iron binding capacity		250–425μg./100 ml.	45–76μmol./l.
% saturation		20–50 (35) %	%
†Serum ferritin	Men:	20–200 ng./ml.	μg./l.
	Women:	10–200 ng./ml.	μg./l.
†Serum B_{12}		200–1100 pg./ml.	ng./l.
†Serum folate		1.9–14 ng./ml.	μg./l.
†Schilling test	Stage I	10–40 (18)% of dose	%
	Stage II	10–42 (18)% of dose	%
Haptoglobin (hemoglobin binding capacity)		50–150 mg./100 ml.	.5–1.5 g./l.
Bilirubin (total)		0.1–1.2 mg./100 ml.	1–12 mg./l.
Bilirubin (direct)		0–0.3 ng./100 ml.	0–3 mg./l.
Serum lactic dehydrogenase		100–225 mU./ml.	0–90 I.U./l. 30° C.
Hemoglobin A_2		1.8–3.3%	%
Hemoglobin F		<2.0%	%
Erythropoietin (plasma)		3–20 mU./ml.	mU./ml.
Erythropoietin (urinary excretion)		2–5 U./24 hr.	U./24 hr.

*Ranges given in terms of ±2 standard deviations. Mean values in parentheses.
†Normal values vary with technique used.

INDEX

Page numbers in *italics* denote illustrations; (t) refers to tables.